The Archaeology of Disease

The Archaeology of Disease

SECOND EDITION

CHARLOTTE ROBERTS AND
KEITH MANCHESTER

CORNELL UNIVERSITY PRESS
ITHACA, NEW YORK

First published in 1983 by the University of Bradford

First published in this second edition in the United States of America in 1995
Cornell University Press

First printing Cornell Paperbacks, 1997

Reprinted 1999

Library of Congress Cataloging-in-Publication Data

Roberts, Charlotte A.
    The archaeology of disease / Charlotte Roberts and Keith Manchester. —
2nd ed.
      p. cm.
      Includes bibliographical references and index.
      ISBN 0–8014–3220–0 (cloth : alk. paper)
      ISBN 0–8014–8448–0 (paperback: alk. paper)
      1. Paleopathology. I. Manchester, Keith. II. Title.
      [DNLM. 1. Paleopathology. QZ 11.5 R643a 1995]
  R134.8.R62 1995
  616'.009'01—dc20
  DNLM/DLC
  for Library of Congress
                                         95–15961
                                         CIP

Cover illustration: healed head injury from medieval York (University of Bradford).

Typeset in 11/12 Ehrhardt.
Typesetting and origination by
Sutton Publishing Limited.
Printed in Great Britain by
Butler & Tanner, Frome, Somerset.

Contents

Dedicated to
Ann Manchester and
Ann Hunter

Acknowledgements

The authors would like to thank the following people for all the help they have given us to complete this book: Ann Manchester and Simon Fowler for their patience and tolerance; everybody working in the Calvin Wells Laboratory of the Department of Archaeological Sciences for understanding; the University of Bradford, Mark Pollard and Chris Knusel for creating the time for one of the authors (CR) to work on this book; Dave Lucy for helping with the bibliography and Richander Birkinshaw, secretary in the Department of Archaeological Sciences, for helping in times of need. Jean Brown, photographer in the Department of Archaeological Sciences, produced the majority of the illustrations and her dedication to the project is much appreciated. The University of Bradford Photography Department (David Berryman) also aided in the final production of some of the figures. For their help, guidance and encouragement over the years the authors would also like to thank Johs Andersen, Arnold Aspinall, Cecil Hackett, William Jopling, Don Ortner and Freddie Wells.

The illustrations were enhanced by the kind cooperation of colleagues both in the UK and elsewhere, who provided original photographs and gave us permission to use them. Particular thanks go to Pia Bennike (on behalf of the Museum of Medical History, Copenhagen), Patricia Bridges (Queens College, City University of New York), Diane France (France Castings, Colorado), Anne Grauer (Loyola University, Chicago), Robert Jurmain (San Jose State University, California), Charles Merbs (Arizona State University), Don Ortner (Smithsonian Institution), Juliet Rogers (Rheumatology Unit, Bristol), Tony Waldron (Institute of Archaeology, London), and the late Calvin Wells for his tremendous slide collection held at Bradford. Other institutions that allowed reproduction of photographs of their material include the Manchester Museum, Royal College of Surgeons, London, Wellcome Institute for the History of Medicine, London, and Reading Museum.

The authors are also grateful to a number of archaeological organizations for the provision of skeletal material now curated at Bradford for teaching and research. This material has provided invaluable data and illustrations for this book. Particular thanks are due to Malcolm Watkins (Gloucester City Museum) and Malcolm Atkin (formerly of Gloucester Archaeology Unit, now Hereford and Worcester Archaeology Unit) for all the cemetery sites in Gloucester, to Northamptonshire Heritage for the Raunds cemetery, to Alec Detsicas for the Eccles cemetery, to John Magilton (Southern Archaeology and Chichester

District Council) for the Chichester site, to Gil Burleigh (Letchworth Museum) for the Baldock material and to Susanne Atkin for the index.

Finally, Charlotte Roberts would like to thank the Calder Valley Fell Running Club who probably learnt a lot of what is in this book during our cold, wet, winter training sessions on the hills of Mytholmroyd; I am grateful to you all for taking an interest and keeping me running. May your joints remain free of osteoarthritis!

Any mistakes in this volume are the responsibility of the authors alone.

The Archaeology of
Disease

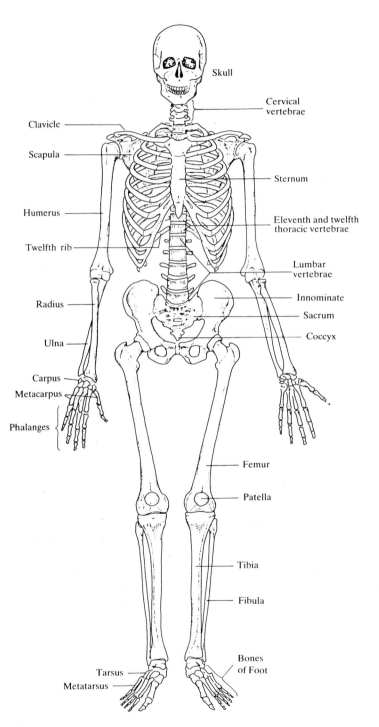

Skull

Cervical
vertebrae

Clavicle

Scapula

Sternum

Humerus

Eleventh and twelfth
thoracic vertebrae

Twelfth rib

Lumbar
vertebrae

Radius

Innominate

Sacrum

Ulna

Coccyx

Carpus
Metacarpus

Phalanges

Femur

Patella

Tibia

Fibula

Bones
of Foot

Tarsus
Metatarsus

The human skeleton

CHAPTER 1

The Study of Palaeopathology

I desire you would use all your skill to paint my picture truly like me, and not to flatter me at all; but remark all these roughnesses, pimples, warts, and everything as you see me . . .

(Oliver Cromwell 1599–1658)

DEFINITIONS

The study of palaeopathology examines the evolution and progress of disease through long periods of time and examines how humans adapted to changes in their environment. It provides primary evidence for the state of health of our ancestors and, combining biological and cultural data (the biocultural approach), palaeopathology has become a wide-ranging holistic discipline. The future of palaeopathology is exciting and is discussed further in the final chapter of this book.

Pathology is the study (*logos*) of suffering (*pathos*). In practice, pathology is defined as the scientific study of disease processes. Palaeopathology was defined in 1910 by Sir Marc Armand Ruffer as the science of diseases whose existence can be demonstrated on the basis of human and animal remains from ancient times. Palaeopathology can be considered a subdiscipline of biological anthropology. The study of palaeopathology is multidisciplinary in approach and concentrates on primary and secondary sources of evidence. Primary evidence derives from skeletons or mummified remains. Secondary (and more subjective) forms of evidence include contemporary documentary and iconographic data. Unfortunately, artists and authors in the past have illustrated and described the more visual dramatic diseases and ignored those which were more commonplace; the mundane, common illnesses and injuries are lost to the palaeopathologist. For example, the mutilating deformities of the infection leprosy and the curiosity factor in dwarfism have led to abundant representations of these conditions in art. In antiquity, those diseases with the greatest impact in terms of mortality, personal disfigurement or social and economic disruption, probably evoked the greatest response from society (and its authors and artists). In the past, attitudes towards illness have been due to the failure in understanding the nature of the disease itself. However, when interpreting disease in the past from secondary sources care must be taken – opinions and preferences about what should be described and drawn will affect what is read and seen. Imprecise and incomplete representation may transmit incorrect information. All literary works must be studied carefully within the traditional framework in which their facts are presented (Roberts, 1971). Those aspects of an illness which we consider to be of vital importance in the understanding of a disease may have been considered of no consequence to the observer in the past and may not therefore have been given due prominence in the record. There are circumstances where disease descriptions do not correspond with any known disease in the modern world. This may be because it actually does not exist or the disease is just not recognized because of the inaccuracy of representation. However, the diseases which are not displayed in the skeletal record, i.e. those only affecting the soft tissue, may only be recorded in art and documentary records and therefore, in these cases, this type of evidence is especially invaluable.

The correlative study of human remains within their cultural context, i.e. their period, geographic area and material culture, aids in the interpretation of the history of disease. For example, precise dating of skeletons with bone changes consistent with syphilis is important for the discussion of the pre- or post-Columbian nature and origin for this disease (Baker and Armelagos, 1988). Some researchers also study populations in geographic areas which sustain contemporary traditional societies. In these cases it is useful to interpret the archaeological (dead) population in the context of the living group if it is accepted that the latter bear close resemblances, in terms of culture, to the dead population. Of course, there are many limitations to this type of study, not least the vast differences in time and space between the living and dead populations in many cases. However, these societies are often unaffected by change (in the modern western sense) and their health and the effect of disease on their bodies is 'natural' and not influenced or changed by drug therapy. They are, thus, useful analogues.

WORKING FROM A CLINICAL BASE

The study of palaeopathology naturally starts with understanding how disease affects the body in the modern clinical sense and, more specifically, the skeleton, since most of the human-derived material palaeopathologists work with is skeletonized. It is only at this stage that this knowledge can be applied to an archaeological context. But why should palaeopathology be studied? The discipline illustrates how people interacted with their environment and adapted to it over many thousands of years. In modern studies of disease, a doctor may only be considering a patient's progress over a few weeks, months or years. It is sometimes more instructive to consider the disease over a longer timespan when significant changes in environment, climate or economy, for example, may have affected a population's predisposition to disease. The disease processes studied reflect the condition as seen on the skeleton or soft tissues without any influence from drug therapy, the chronic form of the disease. It is also possible that some disease processes today may not have been present in the past and, likewise, some pathological processes may have been present in the past but not seen today. For example, rheumatoid arthritis is a common condition today but in the archaeological record there are few convincing examples (Kilgore, 1989; Waldron and Rogers, 1994). There may be several reasons for its absence – non-diagnosis due to non-recognition, confusion with another joint disease or•that it really was rare in the past. It is a disease whose aetiology (cause) is ill understood. Climate, diet and environment may all have their part to play and may not, because they were different in the past, have predisposed populations to the disease.

Palaeopathology can contribute to knowledge in modern medicine. For example, Møller-Christensen's work in the 1950s and 1960s on the skeletons buried in medieval Danish leprosy hospital cemeteries (Møller-Christensen, 1953) highlighted a number of bone lesions characteristic of leprosy which had not been recognized by clinical leprologists at that time; this work helped diagnosis of modern leprosy sufferers. A second example can be illustrated in a study by Rogers *et al.* (1990) where a palaeopathologist's and a radiologist's observations were compared. The bone changes of joint disease were recorded for 24 knee joints macroscopically by the palaeopathologist and radiographically by a radiologist. The results showed that subtle bone changes were not observed by the radiologist but the palaeopathologist could, on the basis of her findings, diagnose the early stages of osteoarthritis.

HISTORY OF STUDY

Palaeopathology has been studied since the eighteenth century when non-human disease was considered in case studies of 'interesting' finds by scholars such as Esper and Cuvier. This was followed by a concentration on human palaeopathology, again as individual case studies or, more exceptionally, concerning aspects of human skeletal variation such as cranial deformation. Jarcho (1966: 5), in fact, noted the 'cranial fixation which has not been fully overcome in our own time . . . [and] abstraction-bound student(s) who, having mainly crania at his disposal, slipped into the comfortable assumption that some diseases ended at the foramen magnum'. The case studies produced in these early years were useful sources of information for, for example, illustrating when and where diseases appeared in the archaeological record but ' . . . we learn[t] little about population dynamics or disease evolution' (Buikstra and Cook, 1980: 435). Wood *et al.* (1992: 344) also note in recent years the move away from, '. . . a particularistic concern with individual lesions or skeletons to a population-based perspective on disease processes . . .'.

Buikstra and Cook (ibid.) note that palaeopathology has had four stages in its development: the nineteenth-century 'descriptive' phase, the early twentieth-century 'analytical' period, a period between 1930 and 1970 characterized by specialisms, and the final phase from 1970 to date where studies have become much more interdisciplinary. However, it was not until the early twentieth century when scholars such as Ruffer, and Elliot-Smith and Wood Jones (1910), writing on Egyptian human material, began to take a closer look at disease at the population level. Hrdlicka, and Hooton and Morse were prominent in these studies of human palaeopathology in South and North America, respectively, again at the population level. From this time scholars world-wide began to utilize larger populations for the study of particular disease processes and their evolution through time (e.g. Møller-Christensen (ibid.) on leprosy and Hackett (1963) on the treponematoses). The emphasis was on the integration of data on skeletal or mummified remains with archaeological data: the biocultural approach. Calvin Wells, Andrew Sandison and Don Brothwell were prime movers in the field in the UK in the 1960s and the latter still retains a prominent position in the field. The creation of the Paleopathology Association in 1973 in the United States has brought together researchers in the field of palaeopathology with the common purpose of studying health in the past using the biocultural approach. Since the 1960s the discipline has become more probing and multidisciplinary with increasing use made of scientific methods of analysis resulting in, more recently, the study of microbial deoxyribonucleic acid (DNA) in bone and soft tissue to diagnose disease in past humans (e.g. Salo et al., 1994); palaeopathology goes from strength to strength, but new methods should not be assumed to answer 'all our prayers' as Sandison (1968: 206) pointed out!

METHODS OF STUDY AND TISSUE CHANGE

The methods of study in palaeopathology are many but usually, primarily, rely on macroscopic observation and description of abnormal changes seen in the human remains. A description of these changes and their distribution in the skeleton or soft tissues is a prerequisite to attempting a diagnosis of the disease process being observed although, as Waldron (1994: Table 3.2) points out, diagnosis in modern contexts is difficult even with the array of diagnostic tests available. In this description it is important to use unambiguous terminology so that readers and future workers who may wish to use these data understand its meaning.

The bone changes seen in palaeopathology represent chronicity, i.e. the individual adapted to the problem and the body reacted to it by forming and/or destroying bone. An individual with skeletal abnormalities may therefore represent a healthier constitution than one without, although lack of bone abnormality could either mean a healthy individual who died as a result of an accident, for example, or somebody who was unhealthy but died before bone change occurred; absence of evidence does not mean evidence of absence in all cases! Wood et al. (1992: 357) suggest that 'different disease processes interact with each other and also with an individual's constitutional susceptibility to stress in determining frailty', and hence what is observed on the skeleton. However, the degree of frailty in a population is not known for the past, nor is its association with the development of abnormal lesions. In addition, knowledge of the amount and length of exposure a person had to a disease-causing organism is not known.

The bone changes of disease may be proliferative, i.e. bone forming and initiated by osteoblasts (bone forming cells), or destructive, i.e. bone destroying and initiated by osteoclasts (bone destroying cells). There may also be a mixture of the two activities. In the normal physiological state there is a balance between osteoblast and osteoclast activity which allows continuous remodelling and turnover of bone. Pathological stimuli may induce an imbalance in this activity, producing changes of atrophy, hypertrophy, hyperplasia or metaplasia. The cellular changes in bone are stimulated by a change in oxygen supply to the tissues – high blood oxygen tension stimulates osteoclasts and low blood oxygen tension stimulates osteoblasts. Hypertrophy involves increase in cellular size and may be induced physiologically, e.g. the person has a heavy manual occupation and the muscles used become increased in size. Atrophy means that there is a decrease in cell size, e.g. when a limb is not being used in, say, paralysis of whatever cause. Hyperplasia indicates cellular division and an increase in cellular content of the tissue, and metaplasia involves the change in differentiation of cell type, i.e. a cell assumes the morphological and functional characteristics of another cell (under pathological stimulus), e.g. in a tumour.

The bone formed in a disease process may be woven, immature or primary bone (porous, disorganized; Fig. 1.1), or more mature, older, organized, lamellar

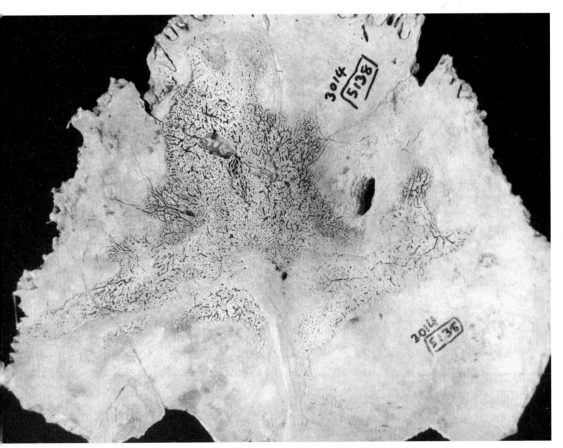

1.1 Woven bone formation on endocranial surface of occipital bone

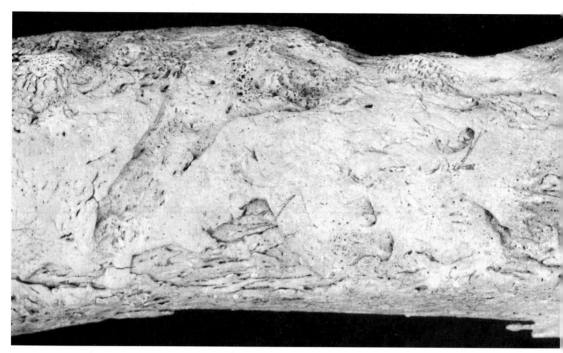

1.2 Lamellar bone formation on long bone

bone (Fig. 1.2). The former indicates that the disease process was active at the time of death, and the latter may indicate that the process was quiescent or had been overcome. However, the presence of active lesions may not indicate the process was the cause of death but that, with other factors, it contributed. It is also of importance to study whether an abnormal lesion appears healed (smooth bone with rounded edges) or unhealed (sharp unremodelled edges) because this gives an indication of the disease state at the time of death and perhaps whether this abnormality had contributed to the demise of the individual. However, determining the ante- or post-mortem nature of unhealed lesions often proves problematic. It is essential to have a complete skeleton to study since observation of distribution patterns of abnormalities is necessary to attempt a diagnosis based on modern clinical criteria. Unfortunately, in archaeological contexts complete skeletons are not always the normal occurrence and the palaeopathologist is often working with incomplete data; it should also be remembered that several diseases may induce similar lesions of bone and occur on the skeleton at the same time, because bone can only react to a pathological stimulus in a limited number of ways. Consideration of a differential diagnosis for the abnormalities described is essential because of the potential for several disease processes to cause the same bony changes. This means recording the bone abnormalities and their distribution and considering all potential disease processes which could have caused the patterning; by a process of gradual elimination on the basis of known patterning in modern clinical circumstances a most likely diagnosis may be made.

Many workers in the field also like to attach some degree of severity to lesions observed; their appearance may not necessarily reflect a gradation in the disease, but if grades are to be included a definition of the grades (including photographs) should be given so that future researchers understand the meaning of the definitions. Recording detailed descriptions of abnormal changes, although accepted as essential, does take up space in a report. It is therefore advocated that an archive is kept for all reports. Recently, advances in the storage of both visual and textual data (Roberts and Rudgewick-Brown, 1991) may help this problem to be solved in the future. Of especial interest to the palaeopathologist is the study of disease prevalence through time but basic data needs to be collected before true prevalence rates can be obtained (see Waldron, 1994 for a discussion of prevalence and incidence and past human skeletal populations). For example, if the prevalence of left hip joint disease is to be studied then the observers need to know how many left hips they have observed in order to determine what the prevalence of hip joint disease may be – this is essential data which should be included in all reports. The nature of the (often) fragmentary state of human skeletal material means that one cannot assume all bones are represented in all skeletons and, if prevalence rates for disease are presented according to individuals, i.e. five out of ten people had leprosy, the assumption has to be that all bones were present for observation.

In addition to macroscopic examination of the skeleton, radiography plays a large part in the diagnosis of disease and trauma (Roberts, 1989a) especially in the

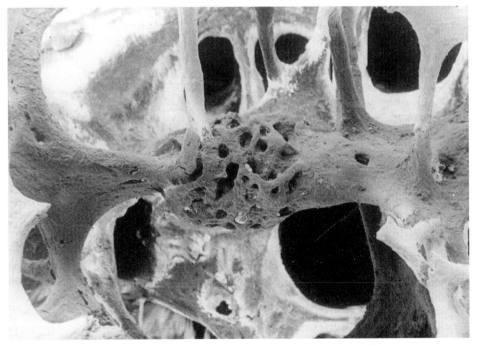

1.3 Scanning electron microscopy of vertebral section showing healed microfracture. Lumbar vertebra, 8th century AD, Britain

case of unwrapped mummies (Notman, 1986). In addition, light, transmission and scanning electron microscopy (Wenham, 1987; Bell, 1990; Martin, 1991; Roberts and Wakely, 1992) add an extra dimension and increase accuracy for diagnosing disease (Fig. 1.3) and also pseudopathological changes, i.e. those post-mortem changes which appear to be pathological but are not. Physical and chemical techniques of analysis have been used increasingly over time to diagnose disease (e.g. lead poisoning, Corruccini *et al.*, 1987) and also to examine dietary status (Price, 1989; Schwarz and Schoeninger, 1991; Katzenberg, 1992) and, of course, the latter has a bearing on a person's likelihood of acquiring a disease. More recently, work has focused on identifying disease at the molecular level and advances in this area are anticipated over the next few years (Cattaneo, 1991).

Recently, attempts have been made to suggest how abnormalities should be recorded and a minimum set of data which should be generated for skeletal population studies (Rose *et al.*, 1991; Buikstra and Ubelaker, 1994). To be able to compare data between different cemetery groups, methods of recording and data generated must be comparable if palaeopathology is to be recognized as a scientific discipline.

TERMINOLOGY

There are several terms to become familiar with which will appear in later chapters. Aetiology refers to the cause of the disease, pathogen is the foreign life-form which is capable of stimulating disease (e.g. *Mycobacterium tuberculosis* causes tuberculosis), and pathogenesis refers to the mechanism and development of tissue change in a disease. An affected individual's physical signs and symptoms are clinical features (e.g. the swelling and pain of joint disease), and a lesion refers to the individual tissue manifestations in a specific disease. Epidemiology studies the incidence (or prevalence), distribution and determinants of diseases in populations. For example, pollution in an environment may determine the prevalence of upper respiratory tract infections. Mortality refers to death and morbidity describes the occurrence of illness. Clearly, there may be many factors contributing to the occurrence of disease – genetic predisposition, age, sex, ethnic group, physiological state, prior exposure to the micro-organism, intercurrent or pre-existing disease and human behaviour, e.g. occupation, diet, hygiene (see Polednak, 1989 on racial and ethnic differences in disease). A person may have natural (i.e. inherited) immunity to a disease independent of any previous exposure to specific pathogenic micro-organisms. In addition, an acquired adaptive immunity may be stimulated by exposure to foreign proteins of invading pathogenic micro-organisms and the immune system will be dependent upon the properties of specific circulating white blood cells called lymphocytes. Adaptive immunity is characterized by the retention of a specific memory for the invading pathogen so that a 'tailor-made' defence mechanism for future invasion by the specific pathogen is in place. The problem with immunity in past human groups is that the level of natural and acquired immunity cannot be ascertained.

LIMITATIONS OF PALAEOPATHOLOGICAL STUDY

There are several limitations to the study of palaeopathology, as Wood *et al.* (1992) stated. In any discipline there are limitations to study but some can be overcome. The hazards of selective mortality, individual variation in a person's risk of disease and death (i.e. there is an unknown mix of individuals who varied in susceptibility to death and disease, depending on biocultural factors), and the non-stationary nature of populations were highlighted by Wood *et al.* as major problems which may not be possible to solve in palaeopathology.

The populations being studied in palaeopathology are dead and therefore may not be representative of the living group; biological anthropologists are dealing with a sample of a sample of a sample . . . of the original living population, and total excavation of a cemetery is unusual. Partial excavation of a cemetery is the most common occurrence in archaeology and therefore only a portion of the original buried population will be examined; the differential disposal of males, females and subadults and their subsequent excavation means biases in the produced data are inevitable. In addition, skeletal material is often fragmentary and poorly preserved, with non-adult skeletons commonly suffering, and therefore observation of the distribution pattern of abnormal changes is not possible; hence an attempt at a diagnosis cannot be made. Researchers in biological anthropology often deal with small numbers of individuals and therefore cannot say much about disease prevalence at the population level because the group of skeletons being examined can only be a small sample of the original living population; sample representivity is often difficult to assess.

Acute infective disease is likely to have killed people very quickly in antiquity, especially if the individual had had no previous exposure or experience of the invading organism. Therefore, no evidence of abnormal bone change would be visible (or expected) because the person died before the bone change developed. Many diseases also only affect the soft tissues and therefore would not be visible on the skeleton. It is therefore quite possible that skeletons from the younger (subadult) members of a cemetery population were victims of an acute or soft tissue disease because frequently they do not have any signs of abnormal bone change. Pathological bones are inherently fragile structures and may, in some circumstances, become damaged while buried and not survive to be excavated, which precludes examination and recording; thus their prevalence may be under-represented.

A further factor to consider is the inability, in most circumstances, to ascribe a cause of death to an individual. Without, for example, a weapon embedded in the skeleton in the grave, or an unhealed injury, it is often guesswork determining a cause of death. The observation of the posture of a skeleton within its grave may be an indication of cause of death. The live burials recorded from Kingsworthy, Dalton Parlours and elsewhere in Britain (Hawkes and Wells, 1975; Manchester, 1978a) were dependent for interpretation upon the observed posture. However, complete bodies such as those from north-west European bogs (Brothwell, 1986) may indicate a more obvious cause of death because of the survival of soft tissue. What can be indicated are the disease processes an individual may have been suffering from in life and whether the disease was active or not at the time of

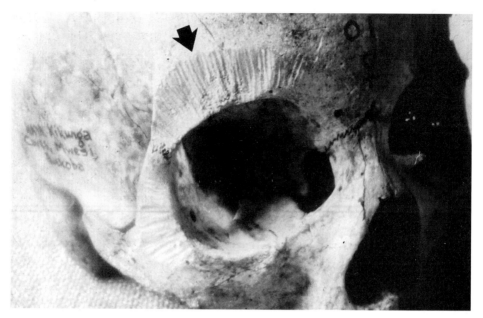

1.4 Pseudopathological lesions on skull (gnawing of orbit)

death. There is, finally, the problem of deciding whether an abnormal bone change is the result of a disease or due to the post-mortem effects of deposition, burial and excavation of the body, or pseudopathology (Fig. 1.4 and Wells, 1967; Hackett, 1976; Bell, 1990).

THE BIOCULTURAL NATURE OF DISEASE FREQUENCY

Despite these limitations, a striking feature in the study of the history of disease is the constant nature and the different distribution of disease with the passage of time. Many diseases which have been recognized in skeletons from distant antiquity present the same physical characteristics as those diseases today. Diagnoses in palaeopathology are made with reference to the knowledge of modern pathology. The agents of disease stimulate bone reactions which were the same for the palaeolithic hunter as they are for the twentieth-century office worker. It is the overall world frequency of disease and the differing geographical patterns of disease which have changed during the history of human populations.

Travel, trade and contact by people have spread disease, sometimes with devastating effect. The environmental changes brought about by people have eliminated some diseases and made others rife at local level. Techno-scientific developments of the twentieth century have given rise to the radiation-induced diseases and, with the potential of bacterial warfare, diseases of unprecedented horror have been unleashed on human populations. When one population moves from the region to which it has become adjusted to another, it shows increased susceptibility to the diseases of the area into which it moves (Banks, 1959). This fact was noted with cynical effect in Kent in the nineteenth century. At that time, and for many years before, the north coast of Kent was an important focus of endemic malaria. The area was marshy and the frequent hot, dry summers resulted in outbreaks of the disease (Smith, 1956). Indigenous males appeared to be immune to a strain of the malaria parasite and so did not readily succumb to the disease.

Of perhaps greater interest and significance to palaeopathologists are those diseases which were transported to new ground by moving populations. The human infectious diseases have achieved world-wide status through the migrations of humans and the animals associated with them. Within this population spread the temporary movements of people and their diseases should not be forgotten. For several thousands of years armies have crossed frontiers and seas and travelled on campaign to distant lands. Crowded together, poorly nourished and usually exhausted by the stress of battle, soldiers on active service are notorious for their spread of infectious disease, often of the enteric types.

Unlike the immunity of indigenous populations as, for example, in the tropical diseases, people transporting infectious disease from one region to another were probably overtly infected themselves. With the notable exception of typhoid fever, there are very few asymptomatic carriers of human infectious disease. The population into which the disease was introduced was no more and no less susceptible than the people actually transporting the disease. Climate *per se* has a profound effect upon the incidence of certain diseases (Brimblecombe, 1982). The constant relationship of respiratory disease to the winter climate is well known to all living in northern Europe. What may not be quite so well known is the seasonal and climatic variance of such diseases as meningitis, poliomyelitis, glaucoma and mental disease. It is possible that a knowledge of the geographical prevalence of specific diseases will provide clues to their causes (Learmonth, 1988). The ability of people to adapt to a totally new environment and associated diseases is perhaps one of our most valuable characteristics.

Until the advent of agriculture in all parts of the world, many people lived in reasonable harmony with their environment. The equilibrium was destroyed with deforestation and agricultural development. Ploughing, crop-rearing and tending flocks increase exposure to tetanus. Cultivated soil with organic refuse, particularly animal dung, is a good medium for survival of the spores of the tetanus bacillus. People cultivating land were liable to develop this disease, which in antiquity was almost invariably fatal. In common with most of the acute infectious diseases, tetanus is not recognizable in the human skeletal record. Environmental change has been a feature of all periods of time. In association with the change in environment, be it deforestation, land cultivation or urbanization, people have come to live in closer relationship with a variety of animals. Cattle, horses, sheep and pigs were accumulated and people lived a life of close proximity to them, often sharing their houses. Only later were the dog, cat and a multitude of animals seen as companions and pets. These animals are all subject to their own parasites which may or may not cause disease within them. Cattle are subject to tuberculosis, the pig to *Taenia solium* and the dog and sheep to hydatid disease, to name but a few. In fact, many of our human diseases may have originated from animals (Waldron, 1989: Table 3). Increasing domestication of animals brings people not only closer to animals but also closer to their parasites, be they worms, bacteria or viruses, and it may have been during this time of increasing contact with animals that people first became infected with the parasites of animal origin (zoonoses – see Brothwell, 1991). Close contact with dogs and canine distemper may have been responsible for the introduction of measles to humans. The measles virus, which, at present, appears to have no primate ancestral parallel, is similar to the virus causing canine distemper. This transfer may have been the stepping-stone for the recurrent endemic and, at times, life-threatening disease of measles with which modern populations are so familiar. As noted earlier, however, the community size at the introduction of the measles virus must have been large enough to sustain it as an endemic infection. The rise of urban communities, which perhaps gathered momentum towards the later medieval period in Europe certainly, pushed people into closer contact, often in poorly ventilated, unhygienic houses, creating a situation that allowed transmission of infectious diseases more readily (Keene, 1983; Woods and Woodward, 1984; Cohen, 1989; Dyer, 1989).

In the early and somewhat haphazard stages of village and town development, little thought was given to waste disposal (Keene, ibid.). The health hazard of the open sewer and its attendant flies was not realized. The inadequacy of communal water supply was unrecognized. It is within this framework of public health ignorance that the largely water-borne infections of cholera, typhoid and infantile gastroenteritis flourished. These are the debilitating, sometimes fatal, illnesses of adulthood and the almost invariably fatal illnesses of infancy and childhood. The almost careless, at least unwitting, proximity of water supply and effluent discharge in the narrow medieval town streets of Europe allowed the easy transference of bacteria and viruses from one public service to the other. Later in time, a specific example in London reveals the problem of having a water supply which may not be beneficial to health. In 1854 the Soho area of London was subject to an epidemic of cholera and its source was centred on a pump in Broad Street (now Broadwick Street); this suggested that the water supply had been infected, a common method of transmitting the disease (Learmonth, 1988).

In more recent times the health hazards of the large conurbations of industrial development have become apparent, albeit poorly understood. Lung cancer and chronic bronchitis show a high incidence in the large centres of population in Britain (Howe, 1970). The coal-miner's pneumoconiosis and anthracosis, also seen in past humans (Munizaga et al., 1975; Walker et al., 1987), the business executive's coronary thrombosis and the ubiquitous mental illness are but a few of the many penalties of human adaptation to changing circumstances. The phenomenon is not new but may be better documented.

Not all environmental change has favoured the parasite. Sometimes, quite unintentionally, people have altered the environment and destroyed the natural habitat of the vectors of some diseases and so effectively eliminated the particular disease. Drainage of marshlands and maintenance of adequate dykes were responsible for the eradication of malaria in the late nineteenth century in some parts of Britain. This environmental improvement, carried out by the farming community for reasons of economy, led unwittingly to the elimination of the mosquito by destroying the habitat favourable to it.

The commonplace infections which killed or debilitated humans in antiquity are rapidly treated with antibiotics in modern Western societies. Unfortunately, the use and, perhaps, misuse of the earlier antibiotics has led to the development of resistant strains of bacteria, for example in tuberculosis today (Brown, 1992) and in some instances the parasite has regained its former upper hand. The manufacture of more and varied antibiotics has, however, once more mastered some diseases.

The infectious diseases due to viruses are in a different class since at present no universal totally effective antiviral agent exists. The diseases of the common cold, influenza, measles and smallpox, for example, are incurable once established. Success against them depends upon preventing their establishment. With very few exceptions, however, these viral diseases are not manifest in palaeo-pathological material and for this reason will not be discussed further.

More important for Western populations is the increasing significance that circulatory, degenerative and neoplastic disease has in modern society. By their adaptability and knowledge, humans have exchanged one group of diseases for another. The conquest of cancer, AIDS and circulatory disease is a goal of the present. The increase in incidence of these diseases may be more apparent than real and due in part to the increased longevity of modern Western populations. They are also due to environmental change and industrialization of the past 200 years.

It is not only the change in landscape which results in disease variance. Occupation of unchanged land itself may encourage the development of certain diseases. It has been suggested, for example, that people living in districts with a high soil content of copper, zinc and lead have a higher than average incidence of multiple sclerosis (Warren et al., 1967). Such problems of relationship between disease and environment are ill-understood today. Their significance for the diseases of antiquity may remain unknown. An association between disease incidence and geographical characteristics can be assessed and checked in contemporary societies.

The causal relationship between the development of goitre and a nutritional deficiency of iodine is well known. This deficiency, due to a low iodine content of water, is most common in inland mountainous areas of the world, especially in parts of America and Switzerland (Bloom, 1975: 402). In Britain the deficiency gave rise to the now classic Derbyshire neck. The significance of fluorine as a nutritional trace element is a recent concept, although as early as 1892 it was suggested that a dietary deficiency of fluorine was related to the high prevalence of dental caries in Great Britain. The properties of fluorine at the correct levels in the prevention of dental caries are now well known. It is also known, however, that excessive levels of fluorine in water can cause fluorosis (Singh et al., 1962). However, to differentiate between a disease caused by a deficiency or lack of a dietary element noted in skeletal and dental remains and the infiltration of soil elements into the bone or teeth is probably only a theoretical proposition and needs great care in interpretation (Price et al., 1992).

There is a factor in the causation of disease which is beyond the influence of the environment and which may have a bearing upon the differing geographical prevalence of certain diseases of antiquity. In 1953 it was reported that there was a significant association between cancer of the stomach and individuals of blood group A (Aird and Bentall, 1953). Since that time investigation has extended to many diseases and blood group associations (Polednak, 1989), including the relationship of disease to certain proteins of the blood (Cattaneo, 1991). The results of these investigations are not without their critics (Weiner, 1970), but, as is observed, blood group frequencies do separate geographically, even in the present days of widespread travel.

The problems of disease today in relation to environmental change, to advances in medical treatment and the very nature of humans themselves are complex and the subject of continuous change. The understanding of disease in antiquity and the analysis of the changing patterns of disease throughout history are equally complex, but may be of paramount importance in the interpretation of medical problems of today.

In the following chapters diseases that potentially affect bones and teeth are discussed. Both congenital and acquired diseases will be considered. Congenital disease is present at birth, and acquired disease is developed during life. This latter classification encompasses:

1. Infectious disease: caused by invading living organisms (viruses, bacteria, parasites or fungi).
2. Traumatic lesions: due to injury or malformation of the skeleton and associated soft tissues.
3. Joint disease: diseases that affect the joints of the body and their associated soft tissues.
4. Neoplastic disease: 'new growths' which may be benign (localized to the site of growth) or malignant (progressive growth which invades and destroys surrounding tissues and spreads to more distant sites in the body).
5. Metabolic disease: caused by a disturbance in the normal processes of cell metabolism.
6. Autoimmune disease: diseases that result from an abnormal function of the immune mechanism, where the immune system fails to recognize 'self'. The immune tissue response is unleashed on the body's own cells and not the invading organism.
7. Endocrine disease: caused by over- or underactivity of the endocrine glands which secrete hormones.
8. Dental disease. Although dental diseases encompass many of the above classifications they will be treated as a separate entity for the purposes of this book.

In a book such as this it is not feasible to consider all the possible skeletal and dental diseases that occur in past human remains; it is the intention to deal with those disease processes that are more commonly seen, with the aim of providing guidelines for scholars in the discipline and other interested readers about the commonly occurring palaeopathological lesions and their interpretation within a cultural (archaeological) context.

CHAPTER 2

Back to Basics

If the world was repeopled from 8 persons after the Flood and that England was peopled originally by 2 persons, or by a number not exceeding 20 persons, such first peopling was about the year of the World 2200 or 2300, that is 600 years after the flood.

(Gregory King 1648–1712)

INTRODUCTION: POPULATION SIZE AND FLUCTUATION

These words of Gregory King written in the seventeenth century with the confidence of Old Testament authority seem to us strangely anachronistic. Yet the earliest date for which the population of the world can be estimated even to within 20 per cent accuracy was the mid-eighteenth century (Coale, 1974). For populations before that time the error is even greater and we find that the global population at the time of Augustus, using the Roman and Chinese Imperial records, cannot be estimated with any more accuracy than a factor of two. It is within this broad framework of inaccuracy that the estimation of population growth since the emergence of humans has to be made. Before complacency sets in about our contemporary accuracy, however, it is well to remember that recent censuses in the USA have undercounted the population by 2 or 3 per cent.

The Malthusian theory proposes, in essence, that population increases faster than its means of subsistence and is subject to the checks of war, famine and pestilence. To what extent the doctrine operated in earlier communities and by what means it was overcome is central to the study of palaeodemography; it is also an essential aspect of archaeology and may be vital to the future survival of human populations. And yet population statistics for earlier communities, so germane to all aspects of archaeological research, are often so limited by inaccuracy.

For the major part of the human past, no records of population size exist. The earliest census in world history was made in China around 2000 BC, with a further and perhaps more reliable one in AD 2 during the Han Dynasty. In the Western world, a Roman census was conducted in the sixth century BC (Hollingsworth, 1969). However, it is not known what sections of society were included in these censuses and therefore their value is limited. In England the Domesday Survey was carried out in the eleventh century, largely for taxation purposes and therefore is probably inaccurate for the country as a whole. For the remainder of the Middle Ages population counts were made by the clergy, and it was not until AD 1848 in England that regular censuses were taken, although regular census taking had been introduced in Sweden by AD 1749 (Eversley *et al.*, 1966). Therefore, it is for only about 0.5 per cent of the time since the emergence of *Homo sapiens* that population statistics based on reliable census data exist. The evidence for population size and growth for the remainder of the human past is circumstantial and the result of retrospective calculation.

For all the inherent inaccuracies of method, asessments of world population size have been made and patterns of growth projected. Such figures and patterns are of immense value to archaeologists and to palaeopathologists; a circular feedback of data operates to calculate population size and growth and then to explain it in terms of technological evolution. The figures and trends are of value to the palaeopathologist and to the modern clinical researcher in determining disease prevalence in antiquity. Its changing pattern may have a bearing on modern disease and its possible causation.

Important factors are the rate and pattern of growth of the population, the relation of these to epidemic disease, famine and technological innovations of antiquity, and the whole complex interrelationship of these to changing birth and death rates. Of course, not all areas of the world have contributed uniformly to the growth of the population. Probably the initial upsurge, which may have been coincident with the development of tool making, occurred on the African continent. The growth in the Fertile Crescent with the advent of agriculture may have contributed disproportionately to population increase, as did the European population expansion of the post-medieval industrial revolution.

In general terms, however, the traditional view that population growth has been a steady, continuous and uniform process is no longer regarded as valid (Nag, 1977). It is probable that human populations have been subject to three major increases in population size followed by long periods of relative stability (Deevey, 1960). These periods of stability have been characterized by minor and usually localized fluctuations only, due to such factors as epidemic disease, famine and war. The significance of epidemic disease was probably of no more than temporary influence in population decrease and had not the general and prolonged effect on people as was sometimes thought (Bean, 1962). The three principal periods of population upsurge have corresponded with the advent of tool making, with the change from hunter-gatherer subsistence to settled agricultural communities, and with the post-eighteenth-century techno-scientific revolution. The period of stability following this last upsurge has not yet made its appearance and for this reason predictions of impending Malthusian doom seem to be unanswerable.

POPULATION NUMBERS AND AGRICULTURE

The first two periods of upsurge of human numbers are associated with increased food and material prosperity, consequent upon mastery of the environment by new-found technologies. The advantage of the tool-user compared to the non-tool-user in the killing and the preparation of food, and some of the advantages of settled, controlled farming with its regular year-round food supply, are the most obvious factors accounting for population increase. But these factors are not the entire explanation. The increased likelihood of infectious disease in larger and more closely huddled settlements may have operated to decrease numbers. This may have been offset by a more regular food supply and an ability to withstand disease, although studies of hunter-gatherer and agricultural populations suggest that in the past food supply of the latter may have been difficult to maintain (Cohen, 1989) and quality of diet may have suffered. The increase in population may, however, be a consequence of more food being available, together with the more settled life that it heralded.

An improvement in the quality and quantity of protein consumption leads to a reduction in the age of female sexual maturity and increase in female fecundity, thus increasing the reproductive life of females (Hassan, 1973). The more settled and stable life of the Neolithic village could have resulted in a narrowing of the spacing of births (Sussman, 1973), so that not only was the female reproductive life lengthened but, because of both factors, the number of children born and reared was increased. However, it should not be forgotten that frequent childbirth does create maternal health stress, and childbirth was likely to have been hazardous in the past (Fig. 2.1 and Gelis, 1991); these factors may act adversely on population growth by increasing female mortality in the reproductive phase of life. However, it has been shown that settled communities may have been eating less protein (Cohen, 1989). The practice of birth space narrowing, if it existed, was probably for economic subsistence reasons, which were, in some measure, eliminated by the agricultural revolution. An additional and, in some respects, related reason for this practice was the difficulty of rearing a further child when there was already a child of breast-feeding age within the family (Nag, 1977).

It is possible, but unproven, that induced abortion and infanticide were practised in hunter-gatherer populations. Even today some societies do practise these population control methods, whether because of the traditional requirement for the numbers of females to be controlled, or for general population control. For similar reasons, birth control in the form of sexual taboo and prolonged postpartum

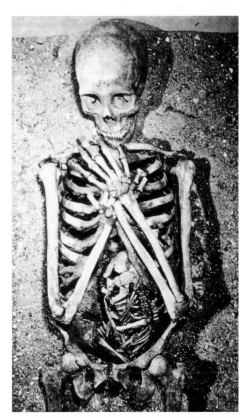

MUSEUM OF MEDICAL HISTORY, COPENHAGEN/PIA BENNIKE

2.1 Pregnant female (Æbelholt cemetery, Denmark)

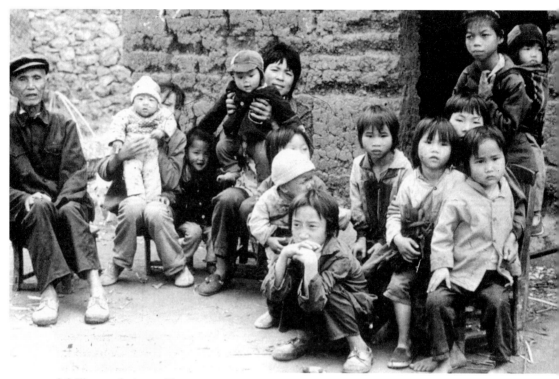

2.2 The population problem

sexual abstinence may have been practised; in addition, prolonged lactation would have induced a contraceptive effect.

During the palaeolithic period the population increase was at an estimated rate of about 0.02 per 1,000 per year, and the rate of increase probably did not exceed 1 per 1,000 per year until the seventeenth century. Since then the rate has risen progressively to 20 per 1,000 per year (Hauser, 1964). It is perhaps this rate of increase rather than the increase *per se* which is the present cause for concern (Fig. 2.2). Important in this discussion of population size is disease load in a population, and size of population will determine health status. For example, settled communities living in close proximity facilitate the transmission of infectious disease more readily.

The association between community size and infectious disease permanence has been proved by the study of modern isolated societies. Using measles as an infection that is acute, easily diagnosed, of frequent occurrence and purely human, study has been carried out in the Faroe Islands in the North Atlantic. This and similar acute infections which are of short duration are only spread by human to human contact and will not smoulder and cause periodic major outbreaks unless the community size is of the order of a quarter of a million. In communities below that size, the acute diseases such as measles and German measles either kill the individual, or infect and consequently immunize him or her. The virus, having no intermediate animal host and not being carried dormant by humans, dies out. Further outbreaks within the community will only occur on reintroduction of the virus from outside the community. The implication is that at the same time as one isolated group of people is free from and immune to such a disease, a neighbouring group is in the throes of an epidemic. It is only by inter-group contact in succeeding generations that the acute, infectious and totally human diseases will continue to thrive.

A further implication is that these diseases could not have made a lasting appearance in human populations until the size of these groups was large enough. The point in history at which population size reached the critical level for various infections is of course not known. These acute infections do not leave evidence on the skeleton, except possibly in the rare case of smallpox (Jackes, 1983). What is likely, however, is that our distant hunting ancestor was free from the common acute virus infections with which we today are so familiar.

Although an increase in the birth rate, consequent upon the adoption of a stable, settled agricultural way of life, contributed to the expansion of the population, this cannot be the sole cause. It is said that a decrease in the mortality rate was perhaps the main cause of population expansion (Durand, 1972). The decrease in mortality may in itself be related to settled community life and a more predictable food supply. By destroying the equilibrium between birth and death rates, humans have opened the door to infectious disease. It has been realized for some time that acute infections, particularly those due to viruses, will not gain a permanent foothold in communities that are below certain critical levels of size, and the implications for the antiquity of infections have only recently been stated (Cockburn, 1977). A decrease in death rates will allow population numbers to increase and provide just the conditions necessary for infectious disease to develop.

Interpreting the circumstantial and material evidence for population size requires the combined work of archaeologists, environmental specialists, biological, social and cultural anthropologists. Population can, of course, be considered at two levels: on the one hand there is the number of people living in a single, perhaps isolated, community; on the other hand there is the total world population.

PALAEOPATHOLOGY AND THE QUESTION OF NUMBERS

The valid consideration of palaeopathology is not possible without knowing basic facts about the population being studied. Many factors determine a population's susceptibility to developing disease in modern contexts, already discussed in Chapter 1; some of these factors may or may not be known. In the context of an archaeological group of individuals those predisposing factors may not be fully understood. The use of a multidisciplinary approach to palaeopathology is a prerequisite; studying skeletal or mummified remains in isolation from their cultural context, although being the primary evidence for disease, cannot produce the most convincing interpretations about the history of disease.

It is important to know how many people were at risk of becoming ill as a first step to understanding why some diseases were more prevalent than others. There

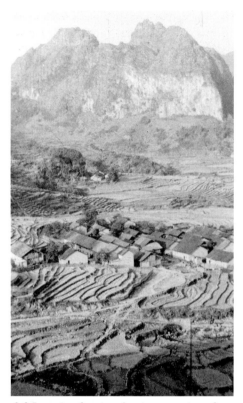

2.3 Intensive farming showing terracing of land: China

are several lines of enquiry to be considered when looking at population numbers. A population can only increase and be successful if the carrying capacity of the area in which that population lives is large enough. Current thinking on population size in the world today suggests that there are major problems with maintaining a steady food supply for the increase in population. Intensification of food production (Fig. 2.3) is one solution to the problem, yet this may exhaust soil fertility. Contraceptive education may be another, but access to this education could be the limiting factor. The shift from hunter-gathering to agriculture around the world has been seen as a response to population increase, but is also due to an expansion into poor game environments and the disappearance of large game animals (Cohen, 1989: 56). However, even though this move may have created enough food to support the population, it also brought with it new problems (Cohen and Armelagos, 1984; Larsen, 1982: Fig. 3; Cohen, ibid.). Furthermore, natural checks may decrease a population if it is increasing faster than its means of subsistence (the Malthusian Theory). In general terms, health appears to deteriorate, with infections of increasing significance appearing with the transition to agriculture; in many studies there also seems to be a reduction in longevity (Cohen and Armelagos, ibid.: 586). Dietary status and susceptibility to infection are closely linked, as many studies show, and increasing population density is an accepted factor in precipitating infectious disease transmission.

CALCULATING POPULATION SIZE

The direct evidence for the population size from which the sample being studied derived is the people themselves (or their remains). There are also secondary sources of evidence, e.g. material remains from the archaeological record and historical sources, which could be utilized provided they are contemporary with the skeletal evidence; this will vary by era and geographic area. Historical records such as tombstones, parish records, wills and taxes, and associated settlement evidence such as the number of artefacts, ecofacts, grain storage pits and refuse, plus the size of habitation structures, may all be used to indicate population numbers (Hassan, 1981), but there are considerable problems in using these secondary sources of evidence. Ethnographic analogy (i.e. studying modern developing societies as a comparison) and environmental carrying capacity and climate of an area today are additional sources of evidence which should be considered.

Certain assumptions, such as the size of a family occupying a single house and the minimum area of land required to maintain each individual, are necessary. Validity of these assumptions may be increased by drawing upon information obtained by ethnographic analogy. The number of occupants per house may decrease with increasing affluence and does therefore vary, not only with time, but even within a single community. Also, the area of land per individual changes with increased intensity of farming and increased farming mechanization. Such factors complicate the assumptions drawn from comparative anthropological studies.

The sample of skeletons at a biological anthropologist's disposal will be biased in a number of ways which will inevitably affect any conclusions about the population numbers being studied. Waldron (1994: 1 and Fig. 2.1) summarizes the losses in skeleton numbers through various processes and emphasizes that what is studied may be a small proportion of the original contributing population. The same can be said for numbers of individuals indicated in documentary records and in modern population censuses. However, censuses at all periods of our history are difficult to interpret.

Determining population numbers using skeletal evidence must start with the mere counting of numbers of left and right elements of the skeleton, to determine the minimum number of individuals present. This is particularly appropriate for mixed and/or disarticulated burials where individual burials cannot be isolated. For example, the presence of six left femurs and seven right femurs in an assemblage means that there was a minimum number of seven individuals. Skeletons are often fragmentary and therefore counts of bones from a total assemblage is the most reliable method of determining numbers. This bone count is also a prerequisite for determining the prevalence of disease in a population, e.g. if three left femurs of a total of six show evidence of tumours then the prevalence of tumours for left femurs is 50 per cent. This is a simple example but illustrates the point that describing prevalence of disease as a percentage of total bones examined is more accurate than describing the percentage of the total individuals affected when some of the bones of some of those skeletons may have been absent due to post-mortem factors. When calculating the number of individuals present through a period of time in a cemetery or geographic area, the calculation becomes increasingly difficult. Some cemeteries span several hundreds of years, and dividing burials into subperiods within the cemetery is usually not possible, although there are exceptions (Stroud and Kemp, 1993). In reality, a palaeopathologist may be dealing with 500 skeletons over 500 years but archaeological evidence may not allow subdivisions into smaller units of time. Therefore, examining the prevalence of disease through time, for example, may only be possible in a general sense.

DEMOGRAPHIC STRUCTURE: AGE AND SEX

Not only are population numbers studied but also their age and sex structure, because these factors are instrumental in determining the contraction and transmission of disease (Reichs, 1986a, b). The age and sex distribution within a population may also be biased and this could be determined by many factors. When, where and by which method was the body buried? Were leprous individuals, or infants, buried elsewhere from the main cemetery? What happened to the body while it was in the ground, e.g. disturbance and decay processes? How was the body excavated and how much of the cemetery site was retrieved? These factors can all 'erode' the final numbers, and affect their preservation (Boddington *et al.*, 1987; McKinley and Roberts, 1993). The possible sex bias in skeletal populations may be highlighted in the following example. It may be expected that cemeteries associated with monasteries and battleground cemeteries would contain more males than females. This situation was found in the cemetery of over 400 skeletons at St Andrew, Fishergate, York, England (Stroud and Kemp, 1993); it contained, in the monastic phase, 228 adult individuals and of those 173 (76 per cent) were male. There is also the problem of under-representation of juvenile individuals from many archaeological sites; the factors responsible for this situation could be, for example, burial away from the main cemetery or non-survival due to fragility of the bone. There are, however, some suggestions that the latter factor may not be always the case (see Saunders, 1992 for a comparison of documentary records and skeletal numbers in an historic population).

METHODS OF ANALYSIS FOR AGE AND SEX

Determining the age and sex distribution of a cemetery population is the first step towards establishing a palaeodemographic profile for a group of skeletons, and provides numbers for the group under study. Methods for age and sex determination have been developed over many years using skeletal populations with known age and sex (Bass, 1987). For example, the Terry Collection is a group of over 1,700 skeletons collected in the 1920s and curated in the Smithsonian Institution, Washington DC and the Hamann–Todd Collection is a group of over 3,000 skeletons curated at the Cleveland Museum of Natural History, Ohio, both in the United States; work on both groups has generated methods of analysis used on archaeological skeletal material. However, it should be remembered that in archaeological contexts the biological anthropologist may or may not be dealing with large numbers, and this could determine how accurate sex attribution is. The sexually dimorphic traits observed may vary in their expression in different population groups. In addition, the application of methods of age assessment derived from specific 'modern' skeletal populations may not be applicable to archaeological material. For example, quality of diet very much determines the rate at which people grow and age.

Three areas of the skeleton may indicate the sex of the individual: the pelvic girdle, skull and measurements of certain dimensions of the skeletal elements, particularly the femur (see Krogman and Iscan, 1986 for a summary of methods).

The pelvic girdle is accepted to be the most sexually dimorphic area of the body, with the skull and long bones being less reliable. It should be noted that some skeletons show mixtures of male and female traits, and occasionally it may not be possible to assign a definite sex to the individual. The expression of many of the cranial traits and metrical data used relate to the robusticity of the person in life, so that, in theory, males will be more robust than females; this does not always apply, because some females may have very strenuous occupations leading to the development of a robust skeleton. The determination of the sex of an individual who had not attained adulthood at death is not possible with any degree of accuracy at the present time (see Saunders, 1992 for a summary of methods). In addition to the skeleton itself, other associated features may help sex the individual, e.g. grave goods, fetal bones in the pelvic area, clothing, circumstances of burial (e.g. war cemetery), presence of disease (some diseases affect the sexes differentially), and associated documentary evidence (e.g. Molleson and Cox, 1993). Obviously, the sex of complete bodies rather than skeletons (e.g. the 'Iceman'; Spindler, 1994) may be easier to identify due to the survival of soft tissue.

The age at death of a population helps us to understand and interpret its health status; for example if a group of people have all died very young then an epidemic disease process must be considered as a possible cause of death. The attribution of age at death in the subadult and young adult skeleton (up to about 25 years of age) is relatively straightforward; ageing an older adult is much more difficult because people age at different rates. Dental development, calcification and eruption of teeth, and the development of the skeleton, including fusion of the epiphyses, are considered reliable methods for age attribution of subadult individuals (Ubelaker, 1987). In the adult, as Maples (1989: 323) says, 'age determination is ultimately an art, not a precise science'. Following development and eruption of all the dentition, and full development of the skeleton to its adult state, the body degenerates. Many methods of ageing skeletons have been developed and a multimethod approach is encouraged, i.e. applying methods to different parts of the skeleton, as some parts of the body may degenerate faster than others (Bedford et al., 1993). Wear (attrition) on the teeth (Brothwell, 1989), closure of the cranial sutures (Masset, 1989), degeneration of the joint surfaces at the pubic symphysis (Meindl and Lovejoy, 1989) and auricular (sacral) surfaces of the pelvis (Lovejoy et al., 1985), and at the sternal rib ends (Loth and Iscan, 1989), radiography and histology of the bones (Ascádi and Neméskeri, 1970; Stout, 1992) and teeth (Hillson, 1986) comprise the main methods used in biological anthropology for adult age attribution. Some of the methods require knowledge of the sex of the skeleton before they can be used. There has been some debate as to the accuracy of adult ageing methods in use (Molleson and Cox, 1993). Sex, race and socio–economic status may all affect how fast a person ages, and there are problems with implementing all the methods described.

The determination of the age and sex of individuals from a cemetery population should always consider the representivity of the population; if there are more males, is this representative of the whole site, or only the part of it that was excavated? If all the individuals are subadults (meaning aged less than about

20 years), does this represent a major acute disease killing people very young or does it mean that only that part of the cemetery containing juveniles was excavated? It is possible to consider life-span estimates once age at death and sex have been determined, i.e. how long did people live? For juveniles it is easier to provide an answer because of the accuracy of ageing methods relative to adults; for adults it is more problematic. Data from the eighteenth/nineteenth-century crypt excavation at Spitalfields, London (Molleson and Cox, ibid.), where known ages at death and historical data were compared, suggest that some of the methods of ageing used could underestimate the age of an adult by up to 20–30 years. It seems that people under the age of 40 years were being overaged and those over 70 years at death were being underaged (Molleson and Cox, ibid.: 169). There is no reason to doubt that, once a person survived the hazardous years of infancy and childhood, they would live to a reasonable age. A typical mortality profile for an archaeological group may be expected to look like Fig. 2.4 but in reality this may be invalid, considering the previous discussion; in reality very young individuals where high mortality would be expected are usually under-represented in the actual skeletal record. However, most authorities accept that in the past the mortality curve often reflected high mortality in infancy and childhood (Fig. 2.5) from, for example, acute infections, and a lower mortality than for modern populations for older individuals; death rates from congenital abnormality *per se* have probably remained fairly constant throughout history. The conquest of infection has brought about the dramatic change in mortality seen today. Respiratory infections and gastroenteritis were probably the chief causes of infant death in antiquity. Notwithstanding the fact that the latter disease is less common in breast-fed infants (and that this method of feeding was probably the norm), improved medical management and the advent of antibiotics have reduced respiratory and gastrointestinal mortality. However, it may well be that people in the past actually did live longer than estimated.

Today, in developing countries, the mortality profile is often similar to past populations, with high numbers of children dying young. In Westernized societies, medical advances and improvements in socio-economic status have enabled infants to survive into adulthood (which has a profound effect on population growth), and adults to survive into old age. Interestingly, females now appear to live longer than males, and one of the explanations may be that childbearing and childbirth are safer, and women, having had to bear children, develop better innate immunity (Stini, 1985; Stinson, 1985).

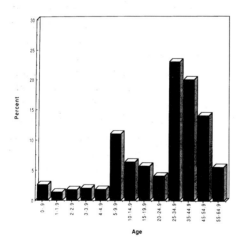

2.4 Age at death distribution St Helen-on-the-Walls, York. (Reproduced with permission of Anne Grauer 1991: Fig. 7.1.)

MORTALITY

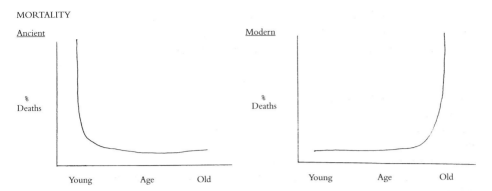

2.5 Graph showing basic differences between modern and ancient mortality

The age group 20–25 years is part of the female reproductive period of life during which time pregnancy and childbirth were fairly frequent. Before the twentieth century and the advent of modern obstetric care, childbirth was a hazardous process indeed. Reproductive death is not merely a problem of parturition but is a potential hazard throughout pregnancy. In respect of certain complications, particularly the haemorrhagic complications of birth, the greater the number of pregnancies, the greater is the likelihood of such complications; and the number of pregnancies in antiquity may have been high by modern Western standards. This increased female mortality in the reproductive period of life may be due to the deaths associated with childbirth, either during pregnancy or during or following parturition.

This unilateral and totally explicit view may not be the true answer, however. Undoubtedly it was a major contributory factor, and examples of female skeletons with fetal bones *in situ* have been recorded (Wells, 1978) as have female skeletons with the remains of young, possibly new-born, infants. One other factor to bear in mind is the accuracy of sex attribution. Although in past populations more males seem to survive into old age, it has been shown (Weiss, 1972; Walker, 1994a) that older people develop skeletal structures which are more robust, and a skeleton may be attributed mistakenly for a male rather than a female. Various authors have proposed that men and women in the past were unequally treated in society and that females may have received less than an adequate diet, and were expected to work long and hard hours. This may have been the case for some, but not all, and the assumption is probably naïve; perhaps the question to ask is do young females in a death assemblage look more stressed than males in terms of pathological abnormalities? If there is a problem with 'finding' older females, i.e. beyond the childbearing years, then the hypothesis that females died young because of childbearing may not be supported.

STATURE AND HEALTH

Of relevance to the occurrence of disease is stature. A reduced stature may indicate less than adequate nutrition and poor health when the person was growing. Nutritional status, genetic make-up, environment and disease will all affect the attainment of final stature. Over time, but especially more recently, stature has increased marginally (Huber, 1968) and final stature is reached earlier in life. The reasons for an increasing stature earlier in life are many. The most obvious factors contributing to this in modern society are improved childhood nutrition, with early vitamin supplements and improved medical care in the treatment and prevention of childhood disease.

Examples of the association of diet and stature are seen in the archaeological record; Nickens (1976) observed smaller mean stature in central and southern Mesoamerican skeletal populations than in a group from northern Mexico, with the interpretation that in Mexico there was less reliance on intensive food production, with less likelihood of suffering periodic episodes of stress with its effect on stature. Furthermore, many of the studies in Cohen and Armelagos (1984) showed a decrease in stature with the transition to agriculture; not only may this suggest a general problem with diet but it may reflect a decrease in protein. Less obvious, however, are those factors that depend on the structure of society itself. It has been observed in rural France, for example, that the height of a community is inversely correlated with the degree of inbreeding within the community. Inbreeding may lead to smaller people. No doubt in some of the closed societies of the past, which were more restrictive with increasing antiquity, inbreeding during generations took place. Failure of contact with neighbouring groups, either because of geographic, cultural or tribal restrictions, would predispose to inbreeding. Any benefit from reduction of inbreeding and increase in stature may have been offset by the more rapid spread of infectious disease that results from travel, trade and contact.

Of all the myths surrounding human populations in antiquity, perhaps the most widely believed and the most easily disproved is that concerning stature. The popular picture of a world inhabited by small people is manifestly untrue. The figures calculated from the measurements of human skeletal remains demonstrate that the man and woman of antiquity were more or less of the same stature as modern groups, at least until the mid-twentieth century in Western society. There has been a move, albeit less dramatic than at present, during the past 100 years for a steady increase in body size. It has been noted, for instance, that the mean maximum height of Norwegian males has increased by 3 cm between the medieval period and the twentieth century. Observations in the United States indicate that stature is still increasing. Height is the most easily obtained measure of stature, but with increasing height the other parameters of stature such as girth, weight, skin surface area and so on, must also increase. Humans have also been attaining their maximum stature at a progressively earlier age (Huber, 1968; Tanner, 1968).

If we accept that people below 160 cm in height are short and that those above 170 cm are tall, it is seen from Table 2.1 that most men in antiquity were in the tall class. Just as we are familiar with a range of height in the population of today, so it was in the past. The calculation of stature is undertaken using either the anatomical or mathematical methods (Krogman and Iscan, 1986: 302–51 for summary). The latter method is that most preferred by the majority of biological anthropologists. It involves the measurement of the maximum length of specific long bones. Regression formulae, developed on populations of known height are applied to the measurement and a stature obtained; the most commonly used formulae are those of Trotter (1970).

Table 2.1 Average British adult male height through time (cm)

Neolithic	171.8
Danish Neolithic	177.6
Bronze Age	176.4
Iron Age	167.8
Anglo–Saxon	173.2
British medieval	171.8
Swedish medieval	173.1
British 1979	175.0

MORBIDITY AND MORTALITY

Once age and sex have been attributed to a group of individuals it is possible to determine a mortality profile. Mortality, for the purposes of this book, is considered with respect to the occurrence of disease in a population. People may be intrinsically more susceptible to a specific disease in view of their age, sex or genetic inheritance (Stini, 1985; Stinson, 1985; Reichs, 1986a, b; Polednak, 1989). Likewise, extrinsic factors such as diet, living conditions, climate and occupation may also affect health (Learmonth, 1988).

Mortality is the relative frequency of deaths to population numbers. It affects all age groups but in differing frequencies depending on time period, geographic location and the intrinsic and extrinsic factors already referred to. The pattern of mortality has changed through time and there appears to be a distinct difference between mortality curves in earlier and more recent populations. High infant mortality in earlier and modern developing societies (see Malhorta, 1990), with fewer people dying in old age, contrasts with lower infant mortality and a more extended length of life in modern Westernized societies. The prehistoric curve with high infant mortality may be seen as reflecting the tenuous existence very young individuals may have had to experience in the past in terms of deficient diets and high disease loads. The same can be said for the fewer older people reflected in the curve, i.e. the presence of the necessary prerequisites for the development of disease and the absence of preventative medicine. However, already noted is the problem of accurate attribution of age to adult individuals and the notion that people may be underaged by up to 30 years. In modern Westernized contexts people do live longer because of improvements in living conditions, diet and medication. An increase in infant survival clearly has a profound effect on population growth, especially if birth rate remains constant. Palaeodemography aims to reconstruct the age and sex composition of a population, their mortality rates for different ages, length of life, fecundity, family and population size, and to consider the effects of nutrition and disease on demography.

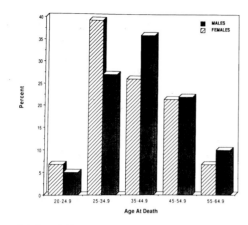

2.6 Sex differences in mortality at St Helen-on-the-Walls, York. (Reproduced with permission of Anne Grauer 1991: Fig. 7.2.)

There are several problems with assessing these factors. One is the common lack of a progression through time in a cemetery's development. A biological anthropologist may be examining several hundred skeletons over many hundreds of years, with no further information available about the phasing of the cemetery, i.e. how many burials were from a particular period within that span. This means that mortality rates are determined for the whole group and a pattern of mortality over time cannot be assessed. In addition to the construction of a mortality curve (Ubelaker, 1989), where age at death for populations can be compared in specific age groups and by sex differences (Grauer, 1991a: 80 and Fig. 2.6), life tables are commonly constructed. Life tables compare and analyse the mortality of a biological population and summarize information on mortality and survivorship to a person's next birthday. The basic components are illustrated in Grauer (ibid.).

Using mortality curves and life tables, it is possible to compare these patterns with the evidence for disease load within the population. For example, if there is a high infant mortality rate then the question of whether there is any evidence of stress markers on the dentition or skeleton needs to be asked; their presence may suggest that the infants' diet was inadequate, which could, subsequently, have predisposed them to develop an acute infectious disease which led to their death. Unfortunately, children are under-represented in the archaeological record although as Roth (1992: 177) states, 'this material represents the most demographically variable and sensitive portion of the human life cycle . . .'. If a child survives into adulthood, this may reflect an inherent healthy immune system which overcomes acute disease or dietary deficiencies. However, it may also reflect a healthy living environment. Palaeodemography not only relies on age and sex data but historical, archaeological, ethnographic and environmental data, and each may vary in their availability for a particular cemetery population. However, they all may contribute to palaeodemographic reconstruction.

ETHNICITY AND DISEASE

Another factor to consider in the occurrence of disease is genetic predisposition, or ethnic origin. The concept of biological race has different meanings to many people and often becomes confused with religious and political issues. Phenotypic (appearance) and genotypic (units of inheritance) traits contribute to the different ethnic groups throughout the world, but, due to the admixture of these different groups today, populations tend to express traits that may be a mix of several distinct groups (Negroid, Caucasoid and Mongoloid are often portrayed as the main racial groups but these include many subdivisions). The skull is considered to be the main ethnic indicator by studying morphological and metrical data (Gill, 1986). What is important to note is that certain ethnic groups (Polednak, 1989) are more susceptible to developing some diseases (Reichs, 1986b). For example, sickle-cell anaemia occurs almost exclusively in Negroid populations or in populations from the southern Mediterranean (ibid.: 198), and blastomycosis (a fungal infection) is found most commonly in the United States today (ibid.).

Finally, the study of palaeopathology cannot be considered without examining the cultural context of the skeletal population samples. The time period, subsistence base and technology will all affect a population's predisposition to developing certain diseases. For example, tuberculosis developed as a human disease when cattle were domesticated in the Near East, but it was not until later periods when population density increased and people were urbanized that the disease became a major problem. Here, time and subsistence base become important areas to study.

The changing rates and patterns of mortality throughout history clearly reflect the changes in disease prevalence at different times of life. Quite possibly, the advent of new diseases brought about by modern complex industrial technologies and warfare will cause further change in mortality patterns of the future. Against this must be offset the improved health status of modern Western populations as indicated by their stature increase (albeit limited until very recently), an associated reduction in age of maturity and a longer life. The whole complex web of individual human development reflected in mortality rates, stature and maturity, is closely related to, and dependent upon, total population growth and the world-wide increase and spread of humans in antiquity, and their even more rapid world-wide travel today. What is more, basic underlying facts such as age, sex, stature and ethnicity are crucial to understanding disease occurrence both today and in the past.

CHAPTER 3

Congenital Disease

In every case disease is the fault of inheritance, and since they are visited upon the sons and daughters because of the sins of their fathers, they are true sins of inheritance.

(Von Walther 1781–1849)

INTRODUCTION

If one considers the skeletal characteristics of the males and females of all nations, it is noted that there is a marked similarity of form between them. The number and size of the bones are fairly constant. The marks of muscular attachment on bones are the same for all humanity. The internal soft tissue organs are likewise uniform. In terms of skin colour and hair form the ethnic groups exhibit wide differences. There are, however, quite marked differences in the shape of some bones, in particular the skull, in different ethnic groups. Berry and Berry (1967) have observed many morphological deviations from normal in the cranium and correlated some with a genetic origin, although later work (see Saunders, 1989 for a summary) suggests that these traits may have other causes, e.g. some may be occupationally related. These observations perhaps demonstrate that there is a remarkable degree of genetic constancy in the various ethnic groups. These facts are perhaps no more than evolutionary expectations.

And yet, at the individual level, problems of development do occur. Developmental abnormalities occur both in soft tissues and in the skeleton; these commence during fetal development and present themselves at birth or shortly thereafter. These developmental abnormalities constitute the range of congenital disease. This range of disease extends from the most minor anomaly of development which may never produce signs or symptoms in the individual, to the most severe abnormality which is incompatible with life itself. The full extent of abnormalities of fetal development are not, and may never be, known, since spontaneous abortion may, in some cases, be nature's way of eliminating the grossly abnormal. In contemporary societies the congenital diseases can, however, be documented, but in the less developed areas of the world even this may be an ideal not yet achieved. How much more difficult it is then to determine the range of congenital disease in antiquity.

Soft tissue abnormality is, of course, only recognizable in preserved bodies and these represent only a very small proportion of humanity of the past. In the context of biological anthropology, which covers the majority of extant remains, only the skeletal abnormalities can be catalogued and it is only in the fairly recent investigations that minor abnormalities of skeletal development have been recorded. Of the congenital malformations of live births in England and Wales between 1964 and 1977, approximately 40 per cent were skeletal, the remainder being divided between the nervous system, the alimentary system, and the heart and vascular system. Numerically, therefore, skeletal malformations are more significant than individual system soft-tissue malformations in live births. It must not be forgotten, of course, that in archaeological terms it is mainly the live births which are preserved and examined, and only rarely are still births recognized; even then they are usually too fragmented or poorly preserved to be of palaeopathological interest. The numerical significance of these skeletal malformations is clear, but their survival significance is not great; of still births, skeletal malformations represent only 15 per cent or so of the range of abnormality. Looking at the survival of malformed and of normal individuals, in a recent study (Table 3.1) it was noted that in the first year of life there is a great mortality difference between the two groups, and that this persists to the 5 year age group. Doubtless, the infant survival rate of antiquity was much less than today, so, bearing in mind the added disadvantage that malformation confers in terms of care, feeding and susceptibility to intercurrent infection, the discrepancy between the two groups in Table 3.1 would have been greater in antiquity than it is today. But, for the reasons of preservation just given, the recognition of such malformations in skeletal remains of these age groups is rarely possible.

In antiquity, the actual percentage of infant and childhood deaths attributable solely to congenital disease was probably low. Doubtless, many infantile deaths were due to the common infections of gastroenteritis and pneumonia, deaths which affected both normal and congenitally malformed infants. In the modern antibiotic era in which control of infantile infection is successful and commonplace, the percentage of deaths due directly to congenital disease has therefore increased. Numerically, though, the deaths attributable to the problem may have remained fairly stable; it is their significance relative to other infantile disease which has changed.

Table 3.1 Survival of malformed and of normal children to age 5 years (%) (after McKeown and Record, 1960)

Age	Malformed	Normal
28 weeks' gestation	100.0	100.0
Birth	83.5	98.2
1 day	76.5	97.5
1 week	69.6	96.9
1 month	63.0	96.8
1 year	53.8	96.0
5 years	51.3	95.7

In modern investigations it is noted that there is an association between different congenital malformations. An individual possessing one abnormality is likely also to possess a second and different abnormality. For example, an infant with a cleft palate or a club foot is more likely also to have an abnormality of the nervous system. Down's syndrome, for example, is commonly associated with a malformation of the heart (McKeown and Record, 1960). It is as if nature deals a double blow. The occurrence of such different and seemingly unrelated congenital abnormalities in a single individual is due, in fact, to a disruption of fetal development at a specific age. Any disturbing factor during the early life of the unborn child may affect several different areas of bodily development and so produce multiple abnormality. In many cases the association may be of skeletal and soft tissue malformation. In antiquity this latter is undetectable and such associations of malformation may be impossible to record, but they are likely to have the same pattern and, for reasons of causation, more or less the same prevalence in antiquity as today (Turkel, 1989).

Because they are abnormalities of development, the congenital malformations may be considered as the total failure of development, the partial development, the overdevelopment, or the abnormal development of part of the body, which in terms of the skeleton means one or more of the bones. Like most medical classifications, this is perhaps too simple, but is nevertheless practical and convenient.

Just as with other diseases, congenital abnormality can rarely be ascribed to a single cause. The abnormalities are caused partly by environmental influence upon the mother and partly by the hereditary constitution of the fetus. The environmental influences include such factors as virus infection of the mother, drug effects and radiation. Rubella (German measles) is perhaps the best-understood virus infection in this context of significance in palaeopathology. Maternal rubella is today known to be associated with cleft palate, spina bifida, Down's syndrome and microcephaly. This is not to say that rubella was the cause of these abnormalities in antiquity, but that it may, in some cases, have been a factor implicated in causation. Maternal measles, mumps, chicken pox and shingles are also virus infections known to cause congenital malformation today and perhaps in antiquity.

Although the connection between drug treatment and congenital abnormality is an emotive and well-known fact in modern practice, it should not be forgotten that drugs are not solely an invention of recent times. No doubt people in distant antiquity sought to remedy their physical ills with herbal remedies in many cases. By modern standards these crude, unrefined agents may not have been efficacious but they, too, may have had effects upon the development of the unborn. This is, of course, speculative, but these herbal remedies may have had a place in the aetiology of congenital disease in antiquity.

The interaction of the two main factors, genetic and environmental, predisposes to the development of the abnormality. In one case, the major influence may be hereditary factors; in another, environmental factors. Such differences account for the variation of congenital disease. Many congenital abnormalities can be attributed to single genes, and their transference through generations should follow the patterns of Mendelian inheritance. However, some individuals are so malformed that even if they survive to adulthood, they are unable to reproduce and hence their genetic abnormality will not be passed on directly to new generations. These individual malformations arise either by the mutation of a gene, or by the maternal and paternal combination of recessive genes for the abnormality. Evidence for a genetic influence in many congenital diseases rests upon the recording of the repetition of the abnormality in siblings and other close blood relatives. Such evidence can only be obtained from contemporary and closely documented families. Its relevance to the congenital abnormalities noted in skeletal material can only be inferred and must remain unproven. It is perhaps worthy of remark that the likelihood of congenital malformation is increased if parents are themselves close blood relatives. For example, marriage between first cousins is commonplace within certain religious groups today and it is found that there is an increase in the rate of congenital malformation in their offspring. Breeding between closely related males and females in the small isolated groups of antiquity, of necessity, may have been common and, if so, will have had a similar influence upon the malformation rate.

ACHONDROPLASIA

An example of genetically based congenital abnormality is the condition of achondroplasia, of theatrical dwarf fame. It is an abnormality of simple dominant inheritance but which, most commonly, develops as a result of a gene mutation, and today affects males and females equally. The problem arises in the process of ossification, or bone formation, in the skeletal precursors of the fetus. Simply stated, ossification takes place by two different methods: one by intramembranous ossification resulting in the bones of the skull vault, the face and the clavicle or collar bone; the remaining bones of the skeleton develop by the other method, i.e. intracartilaginous ossification. In achondroplasia the first method progresses normally whereas the second method is defective. Hence the skull vault, face and clavicle are normal and the remainder of the skeleton is manifestly retarded in development. Consequently, the dwarf stature and short-limbed appearance of the achondroplastic are quite characteristic (Fig. 3.1) and recognizable even from artistic work of antiquity. The modern incidence of the condition is 1 per 10,000 live births, and the incidence in antiquity was probably of the same order.

It is perhaps because of the distinctive appearance that the achondroplastic individual has drawn the attention of the artist in the past, and it is from pictorial sources that much of the evidence for the antiquity of achondroplasia comes (Enderle *et al.*, 1994). More than any other congenital abnormality of the past, achondroplasia is portrayed in statuettes, tomb illustrations and even in the Bayeux Tapestry. The role of the achondroplastic individual in society seems also to have achieved undue prominence. The Egyptian god Phtha (and probably Bes) was given dwarf status. Achondroplasia is the most common disorder of dwarfism; not only this form but several other dwarfism syndromes also achieved social and ritual significance in Egypt (Dasen, 1988). The Roman emperors Tiberius, Alexander Severus and Mark Antony retained achondroplastic dwarfs

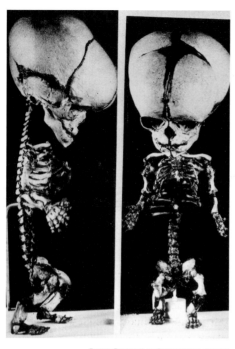

ROYAL COLLEGE OF SURGEONS, LONDON

3.1 Skeleton with achondroplasia

as counsellors (Johnston, 1963). The little figure of Turold in the Bayeux Tapestry clearly held a position of importance in the entourage of Duke William of Normandy (Denny and Filmer-Sankey, 1966). Their role as 'objects of interest' in the Middle Ages is shown by a record of a gift of nine dwarfs to Charles IX of France from the king of Poland. Precisely why such honours as Egyptian deification, Roman Imperial advisor, or medieval court entertainer should be bestowed upon the congenitally malformed, is impossible to say.

Although rare, and rather less emotive than the statuettes, there is the skeletal evidence of achondroplasia from both the Old World and the New World. The earliest recorded example of dwarfism is from Italy and of late Upper Palaeolithic date (Frayer *et al.*, 1987). What role (if any) in society such an individual played at this time can only be wondered at. Typical squat limb bones and characteristic skull shape have been described in remains from pre-Dynastic Egypt and from the Dynastic tombs of King Zer and King Mersekha (Brothwell and Powers, 1968). Several examples from North America have been described, and a single Neolithic example from Great Britain has been tentatively diagnosed. Two examples of achondroplastic adult skeletons have been described from Poland (Gladykowska-Rzeczycka, 1980). Fairly complete skeletons of an adult male and an adult female dwarf have been reported from a prehistoric Indian site at Moundville, Alabama. The height of the female was estimated to be 124 cm and the bones of the dwarfs were described as rugged and muscular (Snow, 1943).

Since the achondroplastic person is not mentally retarded and, as is evident, performed useful functions into adult life, it is expected that their skeletons will be preserved and not suffer the fate of the bones of the young, dying in infancy from their congenital malformations.

OSTEOGENESIS IMPERFECTA

A similarly generalized, genetically determined abnormality of bone formation is osteogenesis imperfecta. It is an abnormality of great rarity today and the evidence from the past consists of two skeletons only. As its name suggests, the disease is the result of the inadequate formation of bone tissue. The bones are, in consequence, brittle and distorted. Their fragility leads to frequent and multiple fractures. Although today the afflicted individual can be nurtured into adulthood, this may have been rare in the past. Death from fractures and their complications must have been the pattern in early childhood, as is indicated by the Egyptian infant of the XXI Dynasty (Gray, 1969). A single specimen from Britain, dated to the Anglo-Saxon period, has been described, but the evidence rests on the fractured and distorted femur (Wells, 1965).

ANENCEPHALY

Perhaps the most severe congenital abnormality known in palaeopathological contexts is anencephaly. The abnormality is incompatible with independent life after birth and has a modern incidence of 1 per 1,000 (Rendle-Short *et al.*, 1978). There seems to be a genetic factor in the causation of the abnormality, but this is clearly not all the picture, since a difference in geographical incidence is found in modern societies, Eastern and African populations producing anencephalic infants more rarely than Western groups (Penrose, 1959). Quite possibly the same multifactorial causes operated with the same frequency in antiquity, but the failure of postnatal survival of the afflicted infants accounts for the extreme rarity of evidence from the past. The thin, fragile bones of neonates do not readily survive to allow for the recognition of skull vault abnormality.

The basic defect is the lack of development of the skull vault and the associated failure of brain development (Fig. 3.2). A mummy from the Catacombs of Hermopolis demonstrates the abnormality and, although considered at one time to be the mummy of an ape, it is in fact that of an anencephalic human (Brothwell and Powers, 1968). The failure of postnatal survival of the anencephalic child is a problem of equal significance today as it must have been in antiquity. Because of the very nature of the defect, medical management is powerless. Yet the personal grief of the new mother in the Neolithic village was probably as great as the mother of the 1990s. Notwithstanding the resigned acceptance of infant death in antiquity, pregnancy, then as now, held an expectation of success. The delivery of an anencephalic baby must have been psychologically traumatic.

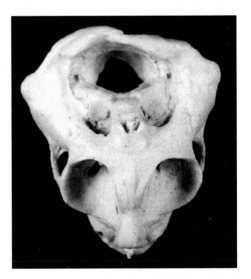

FRANCE CASTINGS, COLORADO, USA

3.2 Anencephaly of cranium. Original specimen: AFIP 1001019, Anatomical Collections, National Museum of Health, Washington, DC

A less severe congenital abnormality, but one which is of profound significance in social interpretation of antiquity, is microcephaly. This abnormality has genetic and environmental determinants and is characterized by a small cranial vault and generally severe mental impairment. It is a rarity in skeletal remains, but a review of recorded cases has been undertaken (Richards, 1985).

SPINA BIFIDA

Having some association with anencephaly, and also having a genetic basis, is the defect of the spine known as spina bifida. This spinal abnormality is associated in some cases with a severe defect of the central nervous system. The spinal cord may be exposed at the body surface and, in consequence, be subject to injury and overwhelming infection. The deficiencies of bladder control and lower-limb paralysis merely compound this life-threatening affliction. Unlike the affected neonate of today, given the benefit of sophisticated surgical techniques, the severely affected child of antiquity would have died shortly after birth.

As with anencephaly, the diagnosis of severe spina bifida (cystica) in human skeletal material is not likely, and its presence in the past must be inferred from its modern incidence of about 1 per 400. However, there is a lesser degree of the deformity, spina bifida occulta, which is readily detectable in skeletal material, being found on average in 2.7 per cent of some early British skeletons (Brothwell and Powers, 1968), but this prevalence is higher for some populations. There is merely a defect in the bony spinal canal which does not produce significant symptoms (Fig. 3.3). Examples from archaeological sites are clearly of this insignificant spina bifida occulta type because, as already stated, the more severe type is not compatible with survival. The defect is commonly of one or more pieces of the sacrum but may occur at other points of the spine. The posterior parts of the vertebrae enclosing the spinal cord are absent. The spinal canal is thus exposed, but it must be remembered that this bony defect was, in life, bridged by cartilage or membrane. These abnormalities, as seen in the adult remains of the past, were of no significance to their possessors, who would have been quite able to function satisfactorily.

The lower parts of the spine are also the site of another, but probably developmentally related, abnormality. This, too, is insignificant but may, as a complication, become symptomatically serious. The defect to some extent bridges the gap between the congenital and the acquired abnormalities. In the bony union of parts of a vertebra early in life, the bone development may be disorganized and, due to the continual stresses and strains of the upright bipedal posture, may fracture early in

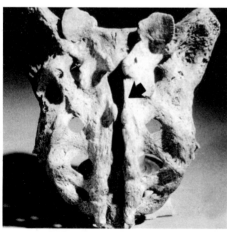

3.3 Spina bifida occulta showing open posterior sacrum

adult life. This defect is known as spondylolysis and is recognized in skeletal material as a separate and seemingly ununited posterior part of a vertebra. In most instances the defect does not create symptoms. Occasionally, however, the defect creates sufficient instability of the spine to allow one vertebra to move in alignment upon its neighbour and this may compress the spinal cord and the nerves issuing from it, and so create symptoms of pain in the legs and back. This dislocation, known as spondylolisthesis, is only rarely recognized in skeletal material. Spondylolysis is further discussed in Chapter 5.

CONGENITAL DISLOCATION OF THE HIP

In modern medical practice the congenital diseases of anencephaly and the gross spina bifida are readily apparent. In the former case the lesion is totally

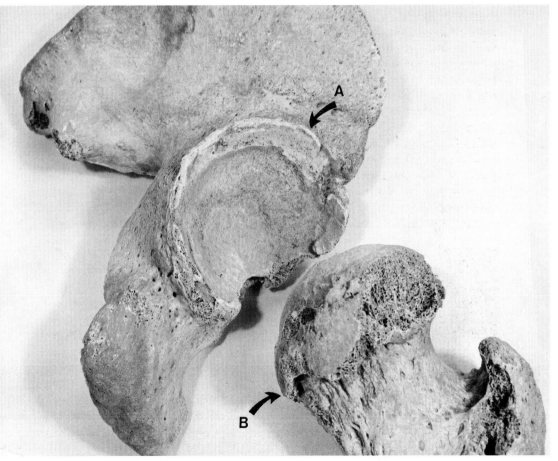

3.4 Congenital dislocation of hip joint: A: Eburnation of roof of shallow acetabulum; B: Osteophyte formation at edges of flattened femoral head (17th century adult male, Sandal Castle, Yorkshire, England)

untreatable and in the latter case the lesion is sometimes treatable, allowing survival of the affected infant. In past societies, both lesions were obvious and both were universally fatal. There is also a congenital defect with genetic factors of causation which, with modern knowledge, is both diagnosable and curable shortly after birth. The neonate of antiquity was not so fortunate. The problem is that of congenital dislocation of the hip joint, perhaps more correctly termed congenital acetabular dysplasia, indicating that the defect is in the development of the acetabulum of the hip joint. In past societies the abnormality became apparent only when the child started to walk, by which time treatment, had it been available, would have been ineffective. The swaying gait due to the recurrent dislocation of the joint on weight bearing is characteristic. The abnormality predisposes to the early development of degenerative arthritis in the hip joint. Figure 3.4 shows the abnormality and its sequelae in all stages. The socket is shallow and has a smooth area at its upper rim due to the tendency to dislocation of the joint. The upper end of the femur is flat and has a grossly irregular edge due to arthritis.

Clearly, with such an abnormal gait and with such severe arthritis the individual would have been unable to perform any activity efficiently which involved walking. The individual would also have had constant incapacitating pain. His or her role in society in the past, particularly those societies dependent for their existence upon hunting or agriculture, must have been restricted. The modern incidence of the condition in Great Britain is 1.5 per 1,000 live births and, in more than half the individuals affected, the condition is of both hip joints. There is marked geographical variation in incidence and perhaps both genetic and environmental factors are responsible for this. The abnormality has been recognized in skeletons from many periods from both the Old and New Worlds (e.g. Wakely, 1993). At present, the earliest skeletal evidence for the condition is from a French Neolithic context, but there is no reason to suppose that it did not exist in earlier times. An indulgence and tolerance towards the afflicted was obviously necessary in the past.

CLUB FOOT

A less common abnormality in palaeopathology is the individual with club foot. The most numerous and perhaps visually convincing evidence is in pictorial sources from Egypt, backed by evidence from mummies. The classically inverted feet of this abnormality of talipes equinovarus are admirably demonstrated in drawings. Recognition of the abnormality in skeletons is difficult and perhaps it was more common in the past than the reported evidence suggests. Because of the difficulties in skeletal diagnosis, palaeopathological examples of talipes equinovarus are rare. Perhaps the earliest recorded specimen is of Neolithic date from Nether Swell (Brothwell, 1967a). Later examples have been identified and their anatomy admirably described and analysed (Mann and Owsley, 1989; Owsley and Mann, 1990). Careful examination of skeletal material and reappraisal of all evidence is just as necessary for the recognition of club foot as for many other abnormalities in palaeopathology. Just as with congenital dislocation of the hip, the main problem of club foot is in walking, and no doubt the same restriction of activity would have applied.

CLEFT PALATE

Although encouraged to do otherwise, many mothers in modern Western society choose to feed their offspring artificially with bottle and teat. In the past, breast feeding must surely have been the norm (Stuart-Macadam and Dettwyler, 1995). A new-born baby needs to be able to suck in order to feed adequately at the breast. The normal infant does not find this a problem, but the infant with cleft palate, in which there is an open connection between the mouth cavity and the nasal cavity, is unable to perform this simple function. The bony defect of cleft palate, which is due to a failure of bone union of the two halves of the palate during fetal development (Fig. 3.5), may be associated with a defect of the upper lip and bone beneath, called the cleft or hare lip. The modern incidence of the two conditions is 1 per 600 live births, but of cleft palate alone, 1 per 1,000 live births (Ferguson, 1978).

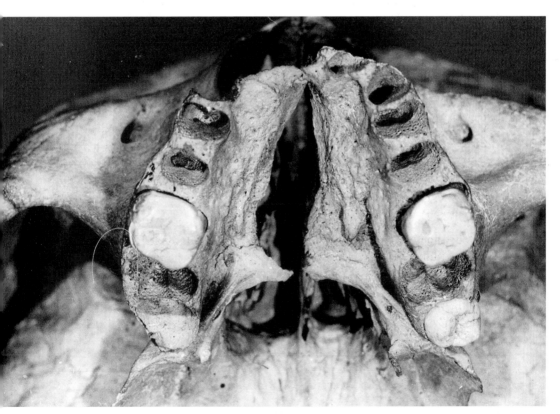

DON ORTNER

3.5 Cleft palate: NMNH 316482, adult female, date unknown, south-west Colorado, USA

The two problems of cleft palate and lip, and of cleft palate alone, are in fact two somewhat distinct entities with different causative factors. Approximately 80 per cent of cases of cleft palate and lip have a family history of such a condition and are therefore predominantly genetic in origin. The problem was probably as common in the past as it is today. The majority of cases of cleft palate alone demonstrate no previous family history. These are likely to be primarily of environmental origin and the prevalence in the past may not have been the same as today.

Neonates with cleft palate require very time-consuming and laborious spoon-feeding of maternally expressed milk, or specialized artificial teat adaptation. Such care is accepted and can be provided in modern Western societies, but may have been unacceptable or impossible in earlier people. Neonatal death of babies with cleft palate may therefore have been common in the distant past. In fact in many developing societies, both today and in the past, deformed neonates, including those with manifest cleft palate and hare lip, were probably killed or, at least, no effort was made to ensure their survival. Such actions may have been motivated by socio-economic attitudes. It is recorded, for instance, that North American Indians believed that a mother who gave birth to an infant with a hare lip had broken a food taboo of pregnancy and had eaten rabbit meat and, in consequence, produced the leporine abnormality. Such was the state of ignorance concerning congenital disease that to strive to rear an abnormal infant may have seemed contrary to the laws of the society. Such an action was not, however, universal in the past; in fact, in an early South American population the reverse was practised. Individuals with cleft palate were held in high esteem and positive efforts to ensure their survival were made after birth. Of even greater significance in the history of socio-medical care is the record of surgical correction of a hare-lip deformity in Anglo-Saxon Britain (Vrebos, 1986), but this depth of attention must surely have been unique in the annals of congenital abnormality. These examples reflect the differing cultural attitudes to disease and deformity, and even to life itself.

The preservation of fragile neonatal skulls is rarely good enough to allow diagnosis of cleft palate to be made. There are, however, examples in older individuals from archaeological contexts. An adult female with an extensive palatal defect has been described from the XXV Dynasty, Egypt, and, no doubt, this case posed a problem of feeding to the mother. A child from sixth to seventh-century AD Britain has been illustrated (Brothwell, 1981), but in this case the palatal defect is incomplete and may not have been associated with a deficiency of the soft tissue of the palate. Crania exhibiting both cleft palate and deformities of the maxilla indicative of hare lip have been excavated in California and dated to 2,000–4,000 years BP (Brooks and Hohenthal, 1963). These native American individuals were between the ages of 25 and 35 years at death. The child from Britain may have been able to breast feed but quite probably these other examples were not. Feeding by spoon, or some other modification lost to us through time, would have been employed. In addition to the difficulty of infant feeding, the person with cleft palate has a speech defect which does not, however, create any problem other than possible social embarrassment. These examples show that, maybe contrary to general practice in many communities, parental devotion to infant rearing is not just a phenomenon of our times but was also an ethic of distant antiquity, and the use of palaeopathology to show evidence for 'care in the community' has been discussed (Dettwyler, 1991).

DOWN'S SYNDROME

It should appear from the foregoing examples that care by the parents and community of the physically deficient child of the past was by no means lacking; the outcome may not have been as successful as in our present society, but the motivation was the same. Care of the mentally deficient child of the past is much more difficult to assess. Except in very few instances, mental defect is not associated with gross skeletal manifestation. It is mainly upon skeletal manifestations that palaeopathological evidence rests, and that is clearly lacking in mental deficiency states.

Down's syndrome is an abnormality resulting from a chromosome anomaly, and is characterized by mental defect and by certain typical physical features. The skeletal features are principally of the skull and consist of a relative shortening of skull length associated with some flattening at the back. These features, together with a retardation of growth of the base of the skull and the facial skeleton, give rise to an overall reduction in the capacity of the skull.

The condition has been described in at least two cases from archaeological contexts. The first case in archaeological literature is of late Saxon date (tenth to eleventh century AD) from Breedon-on-the-Hill in Leicestershire, England. This child was about 9 years of age at death. It is suggested that survival to this age was because of care given to it in the late Saxon monastery at the site (Brothwell, 1960). A second case is described from the late Hallstatt period (350 BC) at Taubischofsheim, Germany, showing characteristics similar to the example from Breedon-on-the-Hill (Czarnetski, 1980). Although a child with Down's syndrome may be born to any mother, it is much more common in women who are over the age of 40 years at childbirth. In early population groups, the number of women surviving and subsequently bearing children at that age may have been small. Down's syndrome may therefore have been an extremely uncommon abnormality in antiquity and, for this reason, the extant evidence may also be rare. Of course, as with many other congenital abnormalities, those affected children dying in infancy will go unrecognized in archaeological material; it is only the survivors to late childhood or to adulthood that present the preserved bone manifestations of their misfortune.

HYDROCEPHALUS

Of all the multitude of abnormalities of development affecting people, few are more dramatic in their presentation than hydrocephalus. Literally, hydrocephalus means water on the brain, but, in strict terms, it is applied to the condition in which there is an enlargement of the normal fluid-containing spaces within the brain substance, associated with increased pressure therein. The usual clinical presentation is of a rapidly enlarging head in infancy or childhood and, as such, will be recognized in skeletons from the past. The condition may arise as a congenital abnormality, in which case the unborn fetus itself has a large head. The condition may also arise due to acquired disease, and it is found that in modern populations most cases are due to the latter and arise in the first 6 months of life (Laurence, 1958).

Because of enlargement of the unborn child's head, congenital hydrocephalus was probably not compatible with fetal or maternal survival in antiquity. Such a case would result in obstructed labour which, notwithstanding the documentary classics of Caesarean section, was a fatal problem of childbirth of the past. Safe Caesarean section is a relatively modern concept; in fact as recently as the early nineteenth century, Osiander wrote of the operation, 'Before then undertaking this procedure one should allow the patient to draw up her will and grant her time to prepare herself for death'. What chance then had the woman of long ago in labour with a hydrocephalic fetus?

The diagnosis of hydrocephalus from archaeological contexts rests upon the recognition of skull enlargement and upon the anatomical configuration of the facial and cranial skeleton (Richards and Anton, 1991). Hydrocephalus developing in later childhood may not result in appreciable enlargement of the head (Vaughan and MacKay, 1975). Therefore the specimens of palaeopathological interest probably had their origin within the first 6 months of life. Survival of such children, many of whom must surely have physical disabilities, indicates a caring attitude in the society of antiquity. If, in addition, the child was mentally subnormal, the care and attention given must have been considerable and would have been a particular burden to a small, intensive social group. In these same specimens the progress of the disease may have become arrested and not ended in death. In modern groups Laurence (1958) noted that 46 per cent of cases arrested this progress between the ages of 9 months and 2 years, and a similar state may have existed in antiquity.

Hydrocephalus is a term that describes an abnormality, but which does not, *per se*, determine its cause. Infection of the brain substance by the viruses of mumps and measles is a known cause of hydrocephalus today. Notwithstanding the limitations of these infections imposed by the group population sizes of antiquity, these viruses may also have been a cause in the distant past. Bacterial infections, which today are cured by antibiotics but which, nevertheless, may still result in hydrocephalus, were probably fatal in antiquity before creating hydrocephalus. The parasitic infection of toxoplasmosis as a cause of hydrocephalus may have been of more importance in the past than today. The infection is known to be associated with eating undercooked meat and this may have been a common practice in earlier people. The possibility of a slowly growing tumour within the skull causing hydrocephalus must also be remembered, but this, too, is speculative. These causes of hydrocephalus are of changes in soft tissues and must therefore remain hypothetical in palaeopathology.

In palaeopathological records hydrocephalus is rare. It has been presented as a definite diagnosis in only eight or so cases (Gejvall, 1960; Brothwell, 1967a; Manchester, 1980a; Richards and Anton, 1991). The earliest case hitherto recorded in Britain is of Romano-British date. It is an adult with a cranial capacity of 2,600 cm^3 compared with the normal of about 1,500 cm^3 (Trevor, 1950). The condition in both a Saxon child of the sixth century AD, aged 14–16 years of age at death (Manchester, ibid.), and a medieval child of 16–18 years from Westerhus, Sweden (Gejvall, 1960) was probably caused by an intracranial tumour. A young adult Egyptian male of the Roman period has asymmetry of the limbs suggestive of paralysis associated with his hydrocephalus (Derry, 1913). In a modern study (Laurence, ibid.), most hydrocephalic individuals have been found to be of normal intelligence and the same considerations probably applied in the past. The cases recorded from archaeological contexts, albeit rarely, probably fulfilled a useful role in society if mental capability is the yardstick. However, today only 33 per cent of affected individuals are free from significant physical handicap and this, in an early work-centred society, may have been a limiting factor in determining the role of the individual.

In this outline of the palaeopathology of congenital disease, only the most dramatic and significant abnormalities have been discussed. The less significant abnormalities and the myriad of skeletal features, which may be counted as variations of normal, have been omitted. The diseases discussed were of grave significance to their possessors and to the community. They illustrate also the caring and the tolerance shown by communities of those less fortunate men, women and children of past society.

CHAPTER 4

Dental Disease

For there was never yet philosopher that could endure the toothache patiently.

(William Shakespeare 1564–1616)

INTRODUCTION

Teeth are often the only part of the body that survives to be excavated from a cemetery, due to their hard and robust structure, which is fortunate as they provide a wealth of information about, for example, diet, oral hygiene and dentistry, stress, occupation, cultural behaviour and subsistence economy. The mouth functions primarily as a food processor (Lukacs, 1989: 261); food type determines the micro-organisms present in the mouth, and the condition of a person's teeth reflects the composition of the food that has come into contact with those teeth. The oral cavity also produces sound, and is involved with respiration, and heat and fluid regulation, among other functions. As the teeth survive well (they are the hardest and most chemically stable tissues in the body), their analysis and interpretation contributes a considerable amount to the reconstruction of past human behaviour. Dental disease and anomalies are, with the joint diseases, the most commonly occurring abnormalities reported for ancient human populations and, when integrated with other forms of evidence from an archaeological site, are valuable sources of information about individuals and populations (Gilbert and Mielke, 1985). They provide evidence of diet, physiological adequacy of diet, method of procuring diet and oral hygiene. Their study may involve macroscopic and microscopic analysis, and the use of art, documentary, archaeological and ethnographic evidence to supplement the dental data.

Infectious disease is one of the more common dental diseases in archaeological populations, e.g. caries, whereas the degenerative diseases of the jaws include ante-mortem tooth loss following periodontal disease or recession of the bone of the jaw, usually as the person ages; developmental problems include enamel defects and genetic anomalies, which incorporate, for example, lack of or more than the expected number of teeth. It has to be emphasized here that the dental diseases do not develop in isolation from one another; there is a complex relationship between them. For example, a person could develop calculus deposits on their teeth which irritate the soft tissue (gingivitis) and underlying bone (periodontal disease) which, in turn, may lead to reduction of alveolar bone and ante-mortem tooth loss.

Today there is a great emphasis on caring for our teeth; use of toothpaste and dental floss, and visiting the dentist play a regular and consistent part of most people's lives. In the past, access to dental surgery and efficient dental cleaning implements and substances, although evidently available to some individuals in some populations (see below), was perhaps not seen consistently across all populations. In effect, it is likely that the dental problems observed in archaeological populations are not affected or influenced by significant oral hygiene or dentistry, and are more a pure reflection of particular dietary components eaten by the individuals being studied.

Although teeth survive well in archaeological contexts, care is needed in processing and cleaning them and the jaws that contain them, once out of the ground. The mandible, or lower jaw, is more robust than the maxilla, or upper jaw, and the latter does tend to suffer fragmentation during burial and/or excavation. Great care is needed with cleaning this area, where soil may become impacted in the nasal aperture and the integrity of this part of the facial skeleton may be affected. The reader is referred to Van Beek (1983: 5, 100) for the structure of a tooth and the numbers and type of teeth expected in the deciduous and permanent dentitions. Obviously, as the dentition develops there will be a mixture of the two types of teeth until all the deciduous teeth are lost to be replaced by the permanent teeth. The single-rooted teeth often become separated from the jaws during burial and/or excavation or during processing and care should be taken in their preservation; the multirooted teeth (e.g. the molars) are more stable in the jaws. Vigorous brushing of the teeth and jaws to clean them is inadvisable in an archaeological context; calculus deposits are easily dislodged and should be treated carefully, and the alveolar bone surrounding the teeth can be very fragile and become damaged. Loss of evidence is to be avoided. ·

There are several different dental diseases and anomalies which occur frequently in the archaeological record. These are now considered in terms of their aetiology, appearance on the dentition, methods of recording, where appropriate, and case studies. In some respects the use of modern clinical observations as a base for interpretation is more appropriate for the dental diseases than for bone disease. Dentists today can observe the tooth surface (as in an archaeological situation), although they cannot visualize the surrounding bone. However, for the doctor, the skeleton of an individual is usually viewed through radiography; but for the biological anthropologist the skeletal elements themselves can be observed directly.

DENTAL CARIES

Dental caries (Latin: *caries*, or rottenness) is perhaps the most common of the dental diseases (Fig. 4.1) and is reported for archaeological populations more frequently than other dental diseases; it may occur as opaque spots on the enamel surface or as large cavities (Hillson, 1986: 287). An infectious disease, it is the

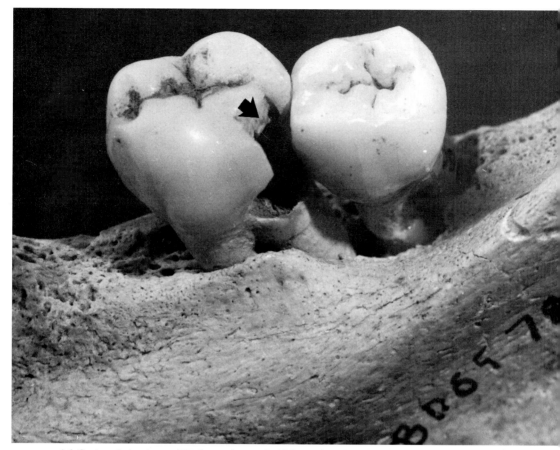

4.1 Carious lesion in mandibular molar tooth (4th century AD, Britain)

result of fermentation of food sugars, especially sucrose, in the diet by bacteria that occur on the teeth, e.g. *Lactobacillus acidophilus* and *Streptococcus mutans*. It is a transmissible disease in which progressive destruction of the tooth structure is initiated by microbial action on the tooth surface (Pindborg, 1970: 256). If the correct combination of plaque bacteria and sucrose occurs, then the acids produced demineralize the teeth and leave cavities. Any part of the tooth structure that allows the accumulation of food debris and plaque could predispose to development of caries. Powell (1985: 317) usefully divides the epidemiology of caries into several areas; environmental factors (e.g. trace elements in food and water), pathogenic agents (the bacteria causing the disease), exogenous factors (e.g. diet, oral hygiene) and endogenous factors (e.g. the shape and structure of the teeth).

These factors should all be considered in an archaeological population study. In fact, a recent study of caries in 12-year-old children in 90 countries found no strong relationship between the amount of sugar consumed and the occurrence of caries in Westernized countries (Woodward and Walker, 1994); this supports the multifactorial aetiology of caries. Some trace elements may prevent or predispose the person to develop caries (Powell, 1985: 315). For example, certain levels of fluoride may protect a person's teeth, and Sibbison's study (1990) suggests that children in fluoridated areas in the US suffer 18 per cent less caries, but elevated levels may lead to fluorosis which affects the integrity of the teeth. Other dental diseases may weaken the teeth and allow caries to occur. For example, deciduous teeth with developmental defects in the Libben (Late Woodland, Ohio) population of fifty-seven subadults were found by Duray (1990) to show a moderate increase in caries when compared to normal teeth. The theory was that the normal structure of the teeth was already weakened and therefore more susceptible to carious attack. Severe wear on the surfaces of the teeth may weaken the tooth structure, allow the entry of bacteria into the pulp cavity and abscess development at the root of the tooth, another infectious lesion.

Recording of caries should involve stating the tooth affected, the position of the caries on the tooth and the size of the lesion. Lukacs (1989: 267) describes a grading system incorporating four grades: no caries, less than half the tooth crown destroyed, more than half the tooth crown destroyed and all the crown destroyed. Care should be taken not to record caries when caries does not exist, i.e. discoloured, darkened areas of teeth and soil in the occlusal surface fissures may be mistaken for caries. Obvious cavities should be recorded, and recording any lesion which is not immediately obvious or convincing increases prevalence rates unnecessarily. To be able to indicate the prevalence of dental disease in a population the number of teeth observed needs to be known so that caries prevalence as a percentage of the numbers of teeth can be determined. These data should be available for all population studies. In addition, some authors present prevalence of caries per individual studied, but this assumes that all teeth were preserved or that the teeth lost post-mortem were not affected by caries. Of course, the determination of prevalence by sex has implications for differential access to diet for males and females, for example, and, while age prevalence for caries is always given for archaeological populations, the correlation of age with caries is not clear. A person with caries, aged 40–50 years at death, may have developed the lesion two, five or even ten years before death. Consideration of caries prevalence in the very young can obviously provide more information about epidemiology than for somebody in adulthood (the speed of development of caries, for example).

Many studies have been undertaken on the prevalence of caries in past human and non-human populations around the world, and interpreted in terms of factors operating within the living environment of individuals, particularly their subsistence base. Larsen (1984) studied pre-agricultural (1000 BC–AD 1150) and agricultural (AD 1150–AD 1550) dentitions from thirty-one cemetery sites from the Georgia Coast in the United States. Caries appeared to increase by around 10 per cent with the shift to agriculture for both sexes and all tooth types. The frequency increases were more pronounced in females than males. He attributed the increase to the adoption of maize agriculture, as maize has a high sucrose content. A number of other studies have also looked at specific population groups to determine caries prevalence with a change in subsistence. For example, Perzigian *et al.* (1984) found that caries prevalence increased through time in the Ohio River Valley in Late Archaic, Middle Woodland and Fort Ancient populations. Of 159 permanent teeth from the Late Archaic (hunter-gatherers) only four teeth (2.5 per cent) were carious. The Middle Woodland prevalence was five times that of the Late Archaic, and in the Fort Ancient population 24.8 per cent of the teeth were carious. Some studies have also concentrated on caries rate change with the intensification of agriculture (Hodges, 1989; Lukacs, 1992). Hodges (1989) examined skeletal material representing time periods from the Formative (1400 BC) through Classic to Postclassic (AD 950) periods in the Oaxaca Valley, Mexico. Here, a decline in caries rate from 17.9 per cent in the Formative to 16.9 per cent in the Classic to 11.1 per cent in the Postclassic was observed. The frequency of caries therefore did not increase with agricultural intensification except in male posterior teeth, which suggests a similar level of carbohydrate through all periods (Hodges, ibid.: 68).

Useful studies have also been made in Europe. Meiklejohn *et al.* (1984) reported for Mesolithic populations (8300–4200 BC) a caries frequency of 1.9 per cent (33 of 1,780 permanent teeth). For the Neolithic period (4200–1800 BC), when farming was being adopted, the caries rate was reported as 4.2 per cent (69 of 1,654 teeth), with the difference between the Mesolithic and Neolithic samples being highly significant. Eighty Mesolithic and 51 Neolithic sites were examined. Bennike (1985) also produced similar figures for Denmark; no Mesolithic teeth of 423 available for examination had caries, whereas 160 of 7,062 Neolithic teeth (2.3 per cent) were affected.

In British populations caries also appears to have increased through time, and this appears to have a marked correlation with the introduction of large amounts of sucrose into the diet. If one compares three periods of time for which useful data exist, the Romano-British period (first century BC to fifth century AD), the Anglo-Saxon or early medieval period (fifth to tenth centuries AD) and the later medieval period (eleventh to sixteenth centuries AD), interesting patterns emerge (Table 4.1). During all these periods agriculture was being practised to a greater or lesser extent. During the Roman period levels were relatively high compared to the preceding Iron Age, whereas for the Anglo-Saxon period levels declined, with an increase in the later medieval period. Moore and Corbett (1973) also noted this in their study. It was not until the twelfth century that cane sugar, containing high amounts of sucrose, was imported into Britain and it is, 'unlikely that sucrose formed a significant part of the diet in Europe or in American aboriginal tribes before this date' (Moore and Corbett, 1971: 166). Both in the Roman and Anglo-Saxon periods, honey was probably the main sweetening agent, with bread being the main source of carbohydrate. Cane and beet sugar were unknown, with small amounts of fructose being consumed in fruit. In the Roman period it is conceivable that some individuals had access to luxury imports such as figs and dates.

Until the early sixteenth century cane sugar was generally unavailable to the majority of the population, but a study of seventeenth-century British teeth

Table 4.1 Caries rates for archaeological populations in the UK

Site	Total teeth	Carious	%	Ref.
Roman*				
Cirencester, Glos	3251	166	5.1	1
Kingsholm, Gloucester	828	45	5.4	
Baldock, Herts	1270	102	8.0	
Gambier-Parry Lodge, Gloucester	451	50	11.1	
Poundbury, Dorset	?	?	15.8	2
Anglo-Saxon†				
Iona, Scotland	463	2	0.4	3
Jarrow, Co. Durham	609	6	1.0	
Monkwearmouth, Co. Durham	953	10	1.0	
Caister-on-Sea, Norfolk	1759	31	1.8	
Barton-upon-Humber	2149	111	5.1	
North Elmham Park, Norfolk	1577	102	6.5	4
School Street, Ipswich	680	68	10.0	
Norton, Cleveland a	906	31	3.4	5
b	1325	45	3.4	
Staunch Meadow, Suffolk a	2040	21	1.0	
b	225	8	3.5	
Later and post-medieval‡				
Jarrow, Co. Durham	957	42	4.4	
St Helen-on-the-Walls, York	7806	345	4.4	6
St Nicholas Shambles, London	?	?	5.5	7
Blackfriars, Ipswich	461	28	6.1	
Glasgow Cathedral	716	46	6.4	
Blackfriars, Gloucester	1112	81	7.3	
St Giles, North Yorkshire	665	57	8.6	
Ensay, Scotland (AD 1500–1600)	774	163	10.2	8
Spitalfields, London	2140	385	17.9	9
Fishergate, York				
10th–12th century a	1406	61	4.3	10
12th–16th century b	2945	356	12.1	

*   all sites in the southern half of England.
†   North-east England, Scotland, east and south-east England.
‡   London, north and south-west England and Scotland.
?   Data not given.
Note: those sites with two sets of figures indicate two phases of the cemetery.
References: 1. Wells (1982); 2. Farwell and Molleson (1993); 3. Wells (1981); 4. Wells (1980); 5. Marlow (1992); 6. Dawes and Magilton (1980); 7. White (1988); 8. Miles (1989); 9. Whittaker (1993); 10. Stroud and Kemp (1993). (These sites are also referred to in Tables 4.2 and 4.3). Other unpublished data is acknowledged from S. Mays (School Street), S. Anderson (Brandon, Staunch Meadow, Jarrow, Monkwearmouth and Caister-on-Sea), and S. King (Glasgow Cathedral).

revealed an increase in caries rate (Moore and Corbett, 1975). At this time cane sugar industries became established in the New World and exports came mostly to northern Europe. In 1641 the first sugar factory was set up in the West Indies and, as the price of sugar fell, consumption increased. By the end of the nineteenth century sugar consumption was rated at 20 pounds per person per year. By AD 1900 90 pounds of sugar per person per year were being consumed, including large amounts of chocolate, treacle and jam. A complex situation of increased availability of sugar and fine white flour, with relaxation of import duties, contributed to caries increase from about the sixteenth century AD.

For some geographic regions and cultures, however, caries rates (along with those of other dental diseases) may not have changed significantly through time. Molnar and Molnar (1985) found a change in dental disease in dental remains from seven Hungarian populations covering 1,800 years (late Neolithic to late Bronze Age). However, the major difference was the caries rate, which ranged from 0 to 14.7 per cent over the seven cultural groups, increasing to 14.7 per cent for populations of the late Bronze Age. Studies such as these in one geographic area over a long period of time start to make possible a correlation of dental disease and subsistence economy through time. Caries is termed a disease of stagnation, where food particles including sugar and plaque bacteria work together to demineralize the tooth structure. Its rapid increase associated with the introduction of large amounts of sucrose to the diet testifies to this correlation.

DENTAL ABSCESS

Dental caries can predispose to the development of a dental abscess through exposure of the pulp cavity from attrition or trauma and infiltration of the cavity by bacteria. Abscess formation can also occur if an individual develops periodontal disease and a peridontal pocket. This is initiated by the accumulation of plaque between the soft tissue of the gum and teeth (Hillson, 1986: 306). Once micro-organisms accumulate in the pulp cavity, inflammation begins and a body of pus (dead cells, bacteria) collects and is termed an abscess. This can track to the apex or base of the tooth root and into the surrounding tissues (Hillson, ibid.: 316). As the pus accumulates, pressure builds up and eventually a hole, or sinus, develops on the surface of the jaw bone to allow the pus to escape (Fig. 4.2). At this stage in the process the abscess can be identified archaeologically. Prior to this stage identification is not possible unless radiography, showing translucent destructive areas at the tooth's apex, is undertaken.

It is likely that the estimate of prevalence of dental abscess in the past is an underestimate of the true prevalence, especially when the high prevalence of caries, calculus deposits and periodontal disease in some populations is considered; these are all predisposing factors to dental abscess formation. Recording of a dental abscess is variable between authors, a sinus presence often being accepted as evidence of abscess. However, especially in the

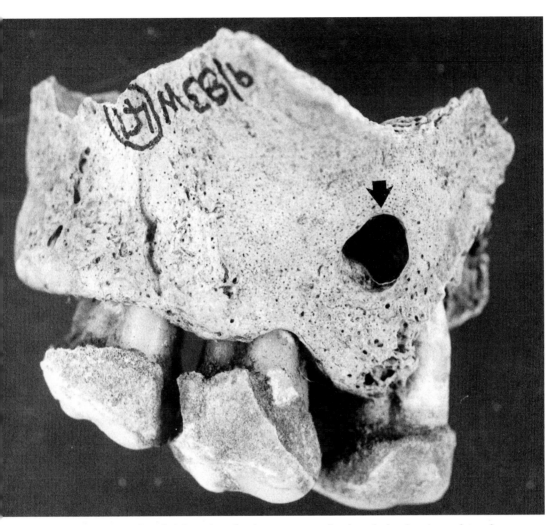

4.2 Dental abscess identified from sinus development; note also the calculus deposits on the teeth (4th century AD, Britain)

maxillary bone, pseudosinuses can be very convincing; identification of healed (rounded) edges to the sinus is indicative of ante-mortem disease. The teeth, especially in the anterior area of the jaws, are very close to the surface of the bone and post-mortem damage can occur, exposing the tooth root through a hole. Figures for dental abscess prevalence in Britain indicate that frequencies are indeed low, ranging from 1.2 per cent during the Romano–British period to 2.0 per cent for the medieval period (Table 4.2).

Table 4.2 Dental abscess prevalence rate from archaeological populations in the UK

		Tooth positions observed	Number	%
Romano-British				
Cirencester		4853	59	1.2
Baldock		2008	24	1.2
Anglo-Saxon				
Barton-upon-Humber		2735	22	0.1
Norton		1128	8	0.7
Addingham		911	8	0.9
Jarrow		843	9	1.1
North Elmham Park		2506	51	2.0
Monkwearmouth		1417	29	2.0
School Street		922	30	3.3
Caister-on-Sea		2441	131	5.4
Brandon	a	2366	59	2.5
	b	216	4	1.9
Later medieval				
Jarrow		1128	16	1.1
St Helen		9788	113	1.2
Blackfriars, Ipswich		1589	25	1.6
Glasgow		897	14	2.0
Blackfriars, Gloucester		644	14	2.3
St Giles		639	15	2.4
Fishergate, Period	4	?	?	1.9
	6	?	?	4.5

? Data not given.
Note: those sites with two sets of figures indicate two phases of the cemetery.

DENTAL ATTRITION

The predisposition of teeth to dental caries from dental attrition has already been discussed. Dental wear is the 'natural result of masticatory stress upon the dentition in the course of both alimentary and technological activities' (Powell, 1985: 308), and it usually occurs on the biting or occlusal surfaces of the teeth during grinding of the crowns of the teeth against each other. Another form of wear is erosion, where, for example, an acidic polluting environment or high acid-content foods may erode the tooth enamel. Abrasion usually occurs away from the occlusal surface and may be the result of cultural activities, e.g. brushing the teeth with an abrasive substance. Attrition is not a dental disease *per se* but can predispose to other dental pathological conditions, e.g. caries and abscesses. As the teeth wear, secondary dentine is produced under the worn enamel to protect the pulp cavity.

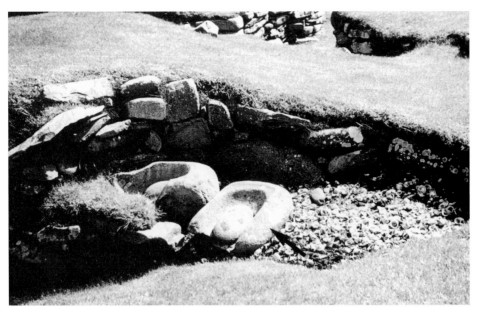

4.3 Stone mortars and pestles, Jarlshof, Shetland Islands, Britain

Today, modern Westernized diets tend to be much softer and easier to chew and digest than those in the past. One major factor affecting wear on the teeth is the processing of foods (Hillson, 1986: 183–4). For example, grinding grain on a stone mortar (Fig. 4.3) incorporates tiny particles of that stone into the grain and food produced from it; this will accelerate wear on the teeth. However, attrition may be somewhat beneficial to teeth in that it removes the fissures and pits on the biting surfaces of the molars which may trap food particles.

Methods of recording attrition have been developed, i.e. observation of the patterning and rate of dentine exposure for archaeological human groups as an age indicator (Murphy, 1959; Miles, 1963; Molnar, 1971; Scott, 1979; Brothwell, 1981; Santini *et al.*, 1990; Kambe *et al.*, 1991; Walker *et al.*, 1991), although attrition also reflects cultural factors within those groups. Clearly, attrition will vary between groups, time periods and geographic areas, and therefore one method developed on a particular group may not be applicable to another population. What is also clear is that the teeth compensate for wear by maintaining their height by 'continually erupting' (Levers and Darling, 1983; Whittaker *et al.*, 1985). Levers and Darling (ibid.) found that, by measuring the height of worn teeth from the inferior alveolar canal, worn occlusal surfaces maintained a more or less constant distance from the canal at all ages in the archaeological populations they studied.

The cause of severe attrition may be reflected in two other areas of the oral cavity. Degeneration of the temporomandibular joint may occur and has been observed in association with attrition in some archaeological populations. Richards (1990) considered two groups of Australian Aboriginal skulls and found significant differences in patterns of tooth wear and frequency of temporo-

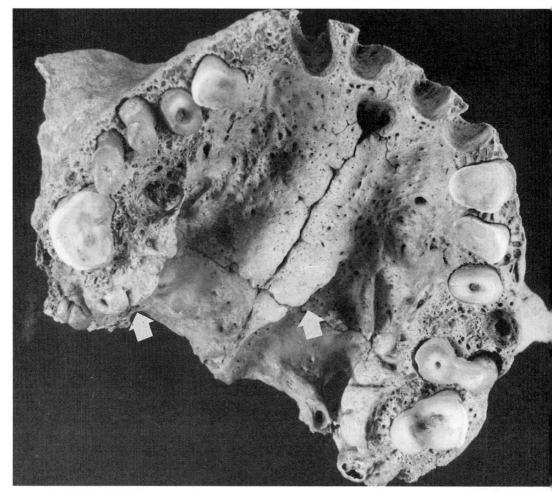

4.4 Maxillary and palatine tori, and severe attrition on maxillary teeth (8th–10th century AD, Britain)

mandibular joint changes between the two groups and sexes. Hodges (1991) also found an association of temporomandibular joint disease and attrition in 369 individuals from British populations and suggested that attrition predisposed to joint disease at this site.

Merbs' (1983) study of the Eskimo Inuit population also found a correlation between the two conditions, especially in females; this reflected the use of the jaws and teeth for cultural activities such as stretching and softening animal skins to make into clothing. Another condition seen in the oral cavity which may be present with heavy wear and temporomandibular joint disease are the mandibular, maxillary and palatine tori which, it is believed, reflect high levels of masticatory stress, producing a bony reaction (Fig. 4.4). Interestingly, they occur in high frequencies in Iceland and Greenland today (Halffman *et al.*, 1992).

CALCULUS

Other commonly observed dental diseases are calculus accumulation and periodontal disease. Dental plaque consists of micro-organisms which accumulate in the mouth, embedded in a matrix partly composed by the organisms themselves and partly derived from proteins in the saliva (Hillson, 1986: 284). It accumulates faster when there is sucrose in the diet. Plaque can become mineralized into dental calculus (Fig. 4.5) where crystallites of mineral are deposited in the plaque. Two types of calculus are seen: supragingival calculus (above the gum) is more common, is usually thicker and grey or brown in colour, and subgingival (below the gum), often seen on exposed tooth roots, is harder and green or black in colour. Calculus develops most commonly on the teeth nearest the salivary glands (tongue side of the lower incisors and cheek side of the upper molars) and appears to be a common finding on archaeological teeth, which perhaps reflects a lack of attention to removing plaque (and then calculus) from the teeth.

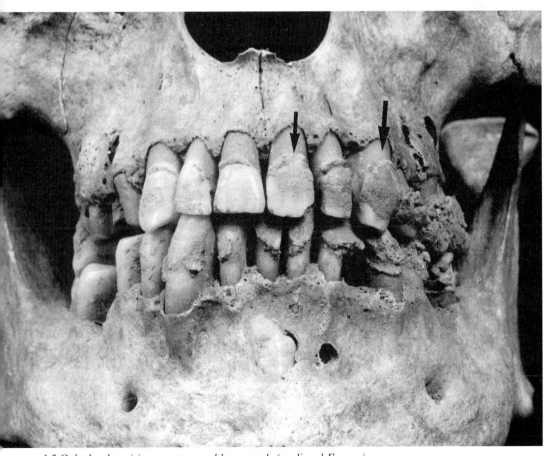

4.5 Calculus deposition on upper and lower teeth (medieval France)

Methods of recording calculus have developed and vary from the basic (Brothwell, 1981) to the more detailed (Dobney and Brothwell, 1987), where thickness and extent of deposit are considered. Calculus has also been analysed to assess its composition; this has provided valuable insights into more specific information about, for example, diet of an individual. Dobney and Brothwell (1988) used scanning electron microscopy to locate microscopic fragments of food debris in calculus on human and non-human teeth. Klepinger *et al.* (1977) also analysed calculus from skeletons from a population in Ecuador from 840 BC and later; the hypothesis in this study was that heavy calculus accumulation reflected habitual coca-chewing with lime. The site of calculus was different to its normal occurrence, i.e. the deposits were on the cheek side of all teeth. This was in accordance with the practice of holding the quid between the cheek and the teeth (ibid.: 506). Major and minor trace elements were analysed by X-ray diffraction. The magnesium concentration was higher than in modern calculus deposits, but magnesium is a consistuent of chlorophyll (present in plants) and a co-factor of some enzymes (ibid.: 507). It was suggested that the results did support the hypothesis posed.

Dental reports from archaeological human populations indicate that calculus was common in all periods, in the UK at least, although comparison between different groups suffers because most authors report calculus on the basis of individuals affected and not total teeth affected as a percentage of teeth observed.

PERIODONTAL DISEASE

Calculus accumulates in crevices between the tooth and soft tissue and bone of the jaw, forming periodontal pockets; it is a major predisposing factor in the development of periodontal disease. As the occurrence of calculus appears to have been so common in the past, it would be expected that the prevalence of periodontal disease would also have been high; this appears to be the case. Periodontal disease is also one of the most common dental diseases in modern populations and a major cause of tooth loss in those aged above 40 years. It commences with inflammation of the soft tissues (gingivitis) of the jaw and subsequent (but not always) transmission to the bone (periodontitis). Resorption of the bone and exposure of the tooth roots develop, and eventually loss of teeth occurs (Fig. 4.6). Details of the development of periodontal disease and its different types are described in Hillson (1986: 305–9).

Identification of this dental disease in archaeological material is problematic. Observation of the distance between the cemento–enamel junction and alveolar crest may increase, but this may not be due to periodontal disease (Clarke and Hirsch, 1991); it may merely be a reflection of continuing eruption from severe attrition (see above). Signs of inflammatory pitting or new bone formation on the jaw bones are more likely to secure a positive diagnosis for this dental disorder. Bone may be lost horizontally or irregularly, and age, oral hygiene and diets rich in sucrose are major predisposing factors, although this condition is multifactorial in cause. Even in an *Australopithecus africanus* dentition dated to 2.5–3 million years BP periodontitis has been recognized; this illustrates the antiquity of this disease (Ripamonti, 1988).

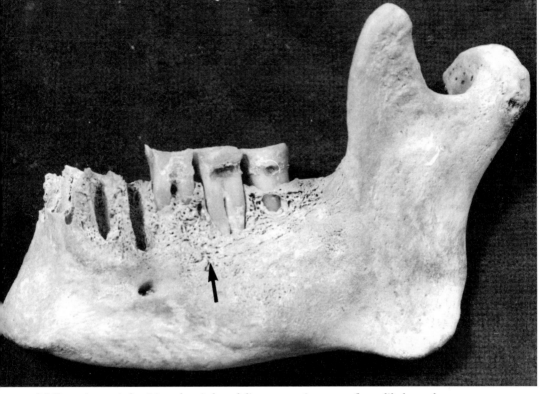

4.6 Extensive periodontitis and periodontal disease exposing roots of mandibular molars (8th–10th century AD, Britain)

The current suggestion is that periodontal disease is overdiagnosed in skeletal material and may only reflect the body's compensatory mechanism for extreme attrition. The problem with assessing the prevalence of this disease is a general lack of standardized recording and knowledge of what actually constitutes periodontal disease. Davies *et al.* (1969), Brothwell (1981), Levers and Darling (1983), Karn *et al.* (1984) and Lukacs (1989) all describe how to record and classify this dental disease. Apart from the problems already outlined, the post-mortem damage that occurs to the jaws often mimics loss of bone around the roots of the teeth; care in diagnosing this disease is required.

Whether periodontal disease leads ultimately to tooth loss cannot be suggested with confidence, but it is likely that it was a major factor in the past as it is today. Ante-mortem tooth loss can only be recognized if there has been some infilling of the affected sockets with new bone. Rates of tooth loss in some British populations are given in Table 4.3. The mean tooth loss for the three periods in UK populations is 13.9 per cent (Romano-British), 7.1 per cent (Anglo-Saxon) and 11.7 per cent (later medieval). These figures correlate with the figures for calculus and periodontal disease.

Table 4.3 Ante-mortem tooth loss prevalence in archaeological populations in the UK

		Total teeth	Teeth affected	%
Roman				
Cirencester		4710	399	8.5
Gambier-Parry Lodge		451	54	12.0
Kingsholm		873	132	15.1
Baldock		2008	403	20.1
Anglo-Saxon				
Jarrow		843	34	4.0
Iona		492	24	4.8
Barton-upon-Humber		3552	209	5.9
Addingham		992	58	6.4
Monkwearmouth		1417	104	7.3
School Street		?	?	10.5
North Elmham Park		2457	272	11.1
Later medieval				
St Nicholas Shambles		?	?	7.6
Jarrow		1399	128	9.1
Spitalfields		2140	341	12.5
St Giles		639	86	13.5
Glasgow		897	137	15.0
St Helen-on-the-Walls		9788	171	17.5
Blackfriars		1589	279	17.6
Fishergate	a	?	?	3.2
	b	?	?	11.4

Note: those sites with two sets of figures indicate two phases of the cemetery.

ENAMEL HYPOPLASIA

Teeth can also indicate other factors in a person's life, particularly during the growing years when bone and teeth are developing. In biological anthropology dental enamel defects (the most common being dental enamel hypoplasia) have attracted the attention of many researchers, in studies of both modern and ancient populations (Goodman and Capasso, 1992); they are often termed an 'indicator of stress' and are defined as 'deficiencies in enamel matrix composition' (Goodman, 1991: 281). Defects on teeth are, however, one of many stress indicators (see Chapter 8). Defects in teeth are observed as lines, pits or grooves on the enamel surface, usually more easily seen on the cheek surfaces of the incisors and canines (Fig. 4.7). These defects can occur only while the teeth are developing, and remain as a permanent record into adulthood. Many factors are relevant to enamel defect aetiology (see Table 2:1 in Hillson, 1986) but they can be categorized broadly into two groups: nutritional deficiency or childhood illness such as measles.

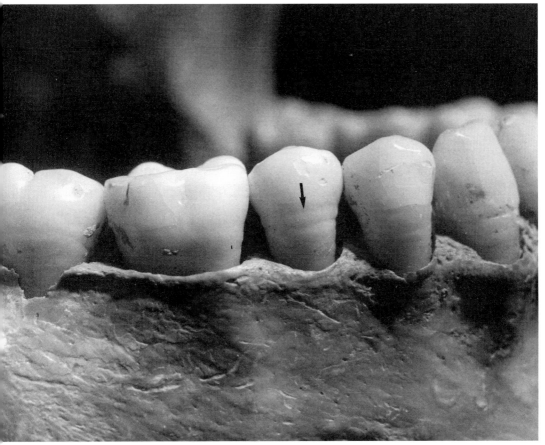

4.7 Enamel hypoplastic defects on buccal surfaces of mandibular teeth (8th–10th century AD, Britain)

Much of the work in palaeopathology in this area has concentrated on examining changes in defect prevalence with changes in subsistence economy and the influence diet might have. For example, Goodman *et al.* (1984) studied the Dickson Mound skeletal group from Illinois, dated AD 950–1300. Three groups of skeletons from different periods were considered: the Late Woodland (AD 950–1100), which consisted of a group practising hunting and gathering; the Acculturated Late Woodland (AD 1100–1200), representing a mixed hunter-gatherer/agricultural economy; and the Middle Mississippian (AD 1200–1300), representing an agricultural economy. Frequencies for enamel hypoplasia increased through time (ibid.: 285). Mean frequencies of defects per individual rose from 0.9 in the Late Woodland to 1.18 in the Acculturated Late Woodland and 1.61 in the Middle Mississippian. These findings were also supported by Larsen's work in prehistoric Georgia, looking at the change from hunting and gathering to agriculture (Larsen, 1984). In fact, many similiar studies have suggested that this change in economy led to increased stress. However, further agricultural intensification (as shown in an Oaxacan population; Hodges, 1989) may not affect the prevalence of enamel defects.

To explore the theme even further, not only have studies of ancient populations been undertaken, but populations from developing countries have been examined to determine a more specific cause for these defects; groups of children have been given supplemented and normal, unsupplemented diets and their defect rates have been compared. The results appear to support the hypothesis that diet may be one of the major causes of dental enamel hypoplasia (Dobney and Goodman, 1991; May et al. 1993). The identity of the dietary deficiency that contributes most to the development of enamel defects has been much researched, but more work is needed in this area. General socio-economic status may also affect the occurrence of hypoplasia, although many factors may be considered when assessing status, even for modern populations; diet may only be one factor contributing to the development of enamel defects but it is not known whether it is the overriding factor. Furthermore, when compared with other stress indicators (see Chapter 8), enamel defect frequency may be very similar or can be different, suggesting that many factors may be influencing stress indicator development. For example, Kolaridou (1991) found no correlation between Harris line formation and other stress indicators (including enamel defects) in a group of French medieval individuals, but Mittler et al. (1992) found a strong association between enamel hypoplasia and cribra orbitalia (see Chapter 8) in an ancient Nubian population.

As the chronology of tooth formation is well known, measuring where the defect occurs on the tooth helps to reconstruct when it occurred in the person's life, assuming that the rate at which the teeth develop was the same in the past (and this cannot be assumed). Recording of defects is usually undertaken macroscopically or using a binocular microscope with good lighting, but some researchers have developed more sophisticated methods (Hillson and Jones, 1989) or use comparative casts (Hillson, 1992). A recent study (Propst et al., 1994) showed that recording defects on casts rather than on the teeth themselves was easier, more productive and accurate. The Federation Dentale Internationale (FDI) developed a classification system for defects in enamel which Hillson (ibid.: 132) advocates as a standard. Number and type of teeth affected, number of defects, appearance and severity are all standard data which should be recorded.

A number of studies have also looked at the most common time for enamel defects to develop during a child's growth, and whether this is related to weaning and the stresses associated with that period of life. All these studies have to assume that standards for tooth crown formation (usually those of Massler et al., 1941; and Sarnat and Schour, 1941) were the same in the past as they are today and that there is no variation between and within populations of different time periods and geographic areas. Corruccini et al. (1985) examined children's teeth from a population of Barbados slaves dated to the seventeenth to nineteenth centuries AD and found that the majority of the defects occurred at the age of 3–4 years rather than between 2 and 3 years as found in non-industrialized populations. The suggestion was that slave children were weaned later than normal. Moggi-Cecchi *et al.* (1994) were able to correlate documentary records for nineteenth century Florence with data on enamel hypoplasia from eighty-three skulls of unclaimed indigents dated from 1870 to 1874. At this time weaning occurred between 12 and 18 months of age, and most defects occurred between 1.5 and 3.5 years, suggesting that these individuals were suffering stress following weaning.

DENTAL PROBLEMS AND ASSOCIATED DISEASES

Several other dental problems may be associated with specific disease processes. Of course, any person who has a health problem may develop dental enamel defects on his or her teeth, but there are specific patterns of dental affectation in certain diseases. For example, the more severe form of leprosy (lepromatous leprosy – see Chapter 7) can induce malformation of tooth root development, especially in the central incisors (Danielsen, 1970; Roberts, 1986b). Most of this work has been carried out on the medieval leprous skeletons from Naestved, Denmark, although no evidence has been reported from other leprous cemetery sites (e.g. at Chichester, Sussex, England, where a number of medieval skeletons were suffering from lepromatous leprosy). Likewise, the treponematoses (and more specifically congenital syphilis) can affect the normal development of the teeth, producing 'mulberry molars' and 'Hutchinson's incisors' (see treponemal disease in Chapter 7). A number of sites have reported the occurrence of these dental anomalies (e.g. Dutour *et al.*, 1994) but care should be exercised in diagnosis, especially in the case of molar malformations, when severe enamel hypoplasia could be considered a differential diagnosis.

CULTURALLY INDUCED DENTAL ALTERATION

As previously discussed, dental diseases have been strongly associated with cultural behaviour. To complement this account, the final area of study in this chapter focuses on evidence of direct cultural behaviour on the dentition, i.e. artificially produced abnormalities. A large literature exists both for modern and archaeological populations on how people and animals use their teeth for performing activities necessary, for example, in their subsistence economy. In addition, deliberate intervention (dentistry) for the treatment of dental disease is also occasionally seen.

Behaviourally induced dental modification may be evident macroscopically (Milnar and Larsen, 1991) or may be seen as microscopic striations (Teaford, 1991). Macroscopic alteration of teeth may be intentional, due to trauma (occupation, for example) or oral surgery (Milner and Larsen, ibid.: 357). Direct alteration of tooth shape, extraction of teeth and inlays of teeth with precious stones may be part of the behaviour of specific populations; these anomalies may represent a specific time or event in a person's life or may be used purely for decorative purposes.

Evidence for dental surgery in archaeological populations is rare but has been reported. Zias and Numeroff (1987) reported on an individual from Israel, dated to 200 BC, with a 2.5 mm bronze wire implanted in a tooth. Bennike and Fredebo (1986) also noted a skeleton dated to between 3200 and 1800 BC from a passage grave in Denmark (Middle Neolithic period). The individual had a drilled cavity between the roots of the upper second permanent molar and between the first and second molars; these teeth had evident carious cavities. One factor to consider is the problem of trying to differentiate between ante-mortem tooth loss and deliberate extraction. A more direct possible treatment for a carious tooth was described from Denmark by Møller-Christensen (1969a). A mature adult dated to the fifteenth century AD had dental caries in a mandibular tooth which was filled with a bone rosary bead (Fig. 4.8). Direct primary evidence for dental care is rarely observed, even though documentary and art evidence suggest that some populations in antiquity did practise dentistry. Primary evidence for dental hygiene is also rare, but evidence of grooves on adjacent teeth (Bahn, 1989) suggests that tooth picks may have been used as early as the French Middle Palaeolithic, 1.84 million years ago. There is further evidence of dental care, particularly from Etruscan populations living in Italy over 2,500 years ago (Becker, 1994). Whittaker (1993: 53–9) also found evidence in the Spitalfields post-medieval crypt population in London for gold-foil fillings and dentures in nine individuals; the dentures were composed of porcelain, ivory or bone and fitted using metal base plates and other stabilizing features such as gold pins. These are very recent examples of dentistry but provide a useful set of data for the history of dentistry.

Probably the most common alteration to teeth is that caused by activity. Patterns of tooth wear and alteration from normal shape may be induced by

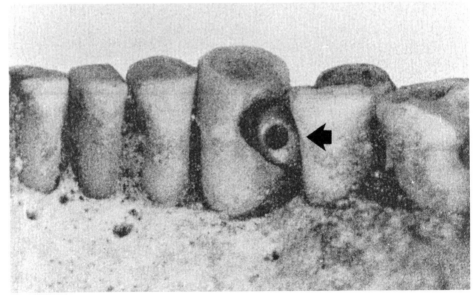

MUSEUM OF MEDICAL HISTORY, COPENHAGEN/PIA BENNIKE

4.8 Rosary bead in carious lesion

activities such as pulling materials through the teeth, e.g. plant fibres (Larsen, 1985; Lukacs and Pastor, 1988) or holding materials static in the teeth to allow manipulation. Differences in tooth wear between groups with different subsistence economies may be striking, allowing differentiation of hunter-gathering from agricultural groups. Hinton (1981) showed this in his study of aboriginal human groups where hunter-gatherers had labially rounded wear and agricultural individuals had little or no rounding but high frequencies of heavy cupped wear, the latter indicating heavy mastication. Some studies (both archaeological and ethnographic) have suggested that a considerable amount of pressure may be exerted on the teeth and associated structures when using them as tools which may lead to alterations in these structures and eventual loss (Molnar, 1972). In addition, not only will activities essential for survival induce dental changes but also activity related to leisure, particularly in modern populations, such as habitual pipe smoking or bagpipe playing. All surfaces of the tooth may be affected, but it is only by comparing patterns of tooth alteration from modern populations with past populations that suggestions for their modification by cultural behaviour may be made and, often, there are no available comparative data.

METHODS IN DENTAL DISEASE

Dental disease and modification of the dentition, through whatever means, provide the palaeopathologist with a wealth of information on diet, oral hygiene, dental care and occupation. However, use and comparison of these data is only possible when researchers utilize the same methods of analysis. Therefore, standardized methods of recording are developing and, once accepted, allow these comparisons to be made. Dental data are often presented in a variety of forms:

1. Teeth/tooth sockets affected as a percentage of the total teeth/sockets available for examination.
2. Individuals affected as a percentage of the total individuals examined; this assumes all teeth and sockets are preserved.
3. Number of pathological lesions per individual (again, assuming all teeth and sockets are preserved).

It is essential to present these data with reference to the age and sex of the populations being studied. If a person lives longer, dental disease will naturally be more likely to occur, and therefore a population composed mainly of older people with high rates of dental disease would be more readily accepted than a younger group. However, it has to be emphasized that, especially in the older age classes, the age at which the person developed the dental disease cannot be surmised. Differentiating the prevalence of dental disease on the basis of sex is also essential if gender differences are to be established. These differences, when put into context, e.g. access to diet or status of the person in the population, allow inferences to be made more easily. Lukacs (1989) also advocated the use of the Dental Pathology Profile to indicate general differences in dental pathology between different subsistence groups, but for comparisons to be made the demographic profile must be similar. As Buikstra and Mielke (1985) have indicated, differences between subsistence groups and urban and rural environments will affect the demographic structure of the population and hence its propensity to develop not only dental disease but also other pathological conditions to be discussed in the following chapters.

CHAPTER 5

Trauma

The Chapter of accidents is the longest chapter in the book.

(John Wilkes 1727–97)

INTRODUCTION

Trauma can be defined as any bodily injury or wound. It can be further subdivided into four categories (Ortner and Putschar, 1981: 55): partial or complete break in a bone (fractures); abnormal displacement or dislocation of a bone; disruption in nerve and/or blood supply; and artificially induced abnormal shape or contour (e.g. deliberate skull deformation; Fig. 5.1). Fractures and dislocations will be considered for the purposes of this chapter. The evidence for trauma in a population may reflect many factors about the life style of individuals, e.g. their material culture, economy (hunter-gathering versus agriculture), living environment (urban versus rural), occupation and interpersonal violence, and the state of healing of the injuries may indicate dietary status, availability of treatment and the occurrence of complications. Trauma (especially fractures) is one of the most common pathological conditions seen in human skeletal remains, along with the dental and joint diseases, and it appears regularly in the palaeopathological literature (Steinbock, 1976; Brothwell, 1981; Ortner and Putschar, 1981; Merbs, 1989a). Susceptibility to injury is a characteristic of all life forms. The increase in the complexity of life, both in biological and in social terms, results in an increase in susceptibility to, and complexity of, the injuries. For example, road-traffic accidents are a major cause of fractures today.

The bones of the skeleton are important as they provide a supporting framework, store minerals, make blood cells, allow movement and protect the delicate areas of the body. Damage to the skeleton will therefore affect these functions. What is of interest to the palaeopathologist is not merely the presence of isolated traumatic features but the change that has occurred in the pattern of human trauma with the passage of time. The site, degree and precise morphological characteristics of these traumatic features indicate the cause and clinical severity of the injury. They may throw light upon the lifestyle of the afflicted individual. The palaeolithic hunter, the medieval farmer and the modern factory machine operator will all exhibit traumatic evidence of their trade. Young and old alike are subject to injury characteristic of their age group. Trauma may

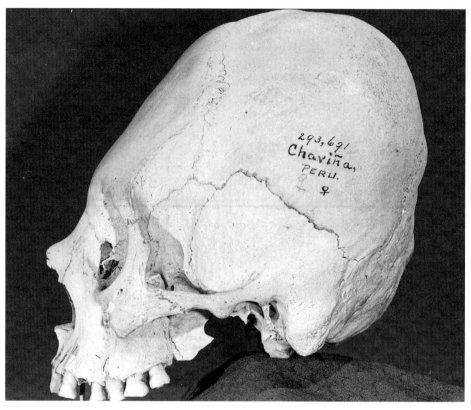

DON ORTNER

5.1 Skull deformation: NMNH 293691, adult female, probably prehistoric, Chavina, Peru

not, of course, be accidental, whether domestic or industrial. Notwithstanding the suggestions of some that people are not innately aggressive, warfare on an ever-increasing scale and complexity seems to have been a recurring theme throughout history. The Neolithic arrowhead, the medieval battleaxe and the later musket-ball may leave their evidence in the palaeopathological record. Surgical practice does, of course, result in inflicted wounds, albeit without aggression, and the primitive orthopaedic and neurosurgeons of antiquity also left their mark in the record.

Before considering the bone injuries themselves, it must be appreciated that the palaeopathological evidence of trauma is but a small part of the total spectrum of injury affecting populations. By and large it is the gross injury which is in evidence; the multitude of the commonplace cuts, abrasions and bruises so familiar to us all are lost in the archaeological record. Evidence of soft-tissue injury is sparse and merely inferential in osteoarchaeological terms, although more obvious in fleshed remains. For example, trauma, in the form of strangulation, is often seen in association with the 'bog bodies' of north-western Europe, where a ligature may be found around the neck (Brothwell, 1986). For the recognition of soft-tissue injury in skeletal remains, it is necessary for calcification or new bone formation to have occurred within the damaged soft tissue. Such an example is seen on the pelvis of a seventeenth-century Royalist soldier in whom a severe muscle tear must have occurred (Fig. 5.2) (Manchester, 1978b). Clearly, any injury that penetrates bone must also involve the surrounding soft tissues, even though the damage to these cannot be seen in skeletal remains. One can also infer damage to soft tissues by examining the location of the injury closely. Some fractures at specific sites in the body may lead to damage of blood vessels or nerves. For example, a fracture to the mid-shaft of the humerus (upper arm) often damages the radial nerve (Shaw and Sakellarides, 1967); obviously this would have implications for the individual's normal function.

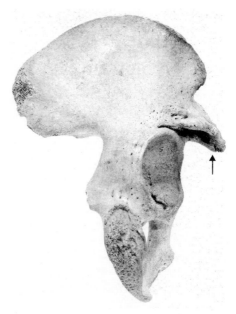

5.2 Soft tissue injury. Ossification following injury to muscle. Male 18–20 years, Sandal Castle, Yorkshire, UK

FRACTURES: POST-CRANIAL

It is with the damage to bone that the palaeopathologist is mainly concerned. Except for small accumulations of blood that become ossified beneath the periosteum, recognized as fairly circumscribed swellings on the bone surface, the results of minor trauma in skeletal material are bone fractures. A fracture can be defined as the result of any traumatic event that leads to a complete or partial break of a bone. In theory, then, injuries to the skull caused by a bladed weapon, piercing injuries and surgical procedures, such as trepanation, to bone are all classed as fractures under this definition. The fractures that occur a short time before death or maybe coincident with it, and which show no evidence of healing, are very difficult to distinguish from post-mortem breaks of bone. Therefore it is with the healed fracture or the ununited but healing fracture that the palaeopathologist is concerned, and the majority of fractures observed from archaeological contexts are healed.

All fractures belong to one of two categories, closed or open. Closed fractures are those in which there is no connection between the outer skin surface and the fractured bone itself. Open fractures are those in which there is an open connection between the fracture site and the skin surface. This connection is a ready opportunity for bacteria to enter the bone from outside the body, and therefore potentially all these fractures can be infected, a problem even in modern medical practice. Such an infection in a severely injured person in the past, without the benefit of antibiotics, was probably often fatal in many cases. Those individuals fortunate enough to survive may have been left with a chronic discharging osteomyelitic bone. The absence of soft tissues in skeletal remains clearly means that in osteoarchaeological terms, the placing of a fracture in one or other category is largely inferential unless clear evidence of infection associated with the fracture is present. Skeletal evidence for an open fracture is the superficial infection, the osteitic pitting and irregularity of bone surface around the fracture site, or osteomyelitis; however, care should be exercised in inferring an open fracture when infection may have been present before the fracture occurred.

CAUSES OF FRACTURES

There are three major causes of fractures: acute injury (e.g. the skiing accident in a modern context); underlying disease, which weakens the bone and makes it more susceptible to fracture (e.g. tumour of the bone); and repeated stress, e.g. in an athlete today (see Resnick and Niwayama, 1988: Table 74–3 for stress fractures and associated activity). In stress fractures there is often no history of direct injury and pain will increase if the activity continues. Many stress fractures are hairline in nature and are difficult to diagnose, even by radiography; once they heal there may be no evidence left to see, and in an archaeological context

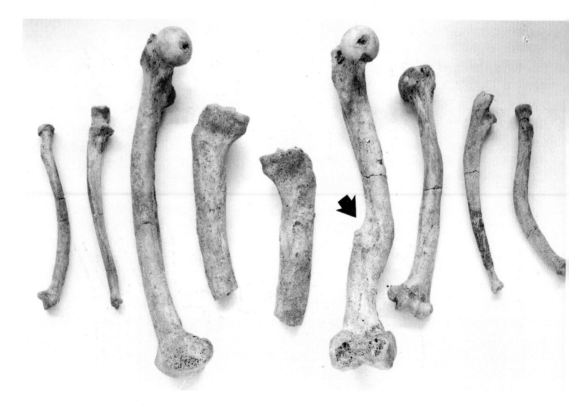

5.3 Fractured femur with underlying Paget's disease (Jarrow, Northern England, Anglo-Saxon)

identifying these types of fracture may be difficult, if not impossible. Pathological fractures may be induced by general or local disease in the body. Osteoporosis (decrease in bone quantity) may affect the body generally and a tumour may affect an individual bone in the skeleton, but both lead to a weaker structure and fracture. An archaeological example from Jarrow (Wells and Woodhouse, 1975), an Anglo-Saxon cemetery in the north of England, revealed Paget's disease and fracture to the femur (Fig. 5.3) but how can one be sure that the disease was present before the fracture occurred?

A further subdivision of fractures, and one that throws light on the cause of the injury, is the type and direction of the break in the bone (Fig. 5.4). The simplest fracture in mechanical terms is transverse, which is a horizontal break across the diameter of a long bone. A force applied at right angles to the bone, either by accident or by direct blow, is necessary to create this fracture. The spiral or oblique fracture is due to indirect and/or torsional force. In the young, immature bone, transverse fractures may be incomplete and are termed greenstick. A further feature of fractures may be the multiple splintering of the broken bones. These comminuted fractures (i.e. more than two fracture fragments) are common in road-traffic accidents today and are less likely to heal in a functionally satisfactory manner. A rather special type of fracture is the crush fracture of a vertebra (Fig. 5.5); crush or compression fractures are also commonly found at the joint surfaces. Often

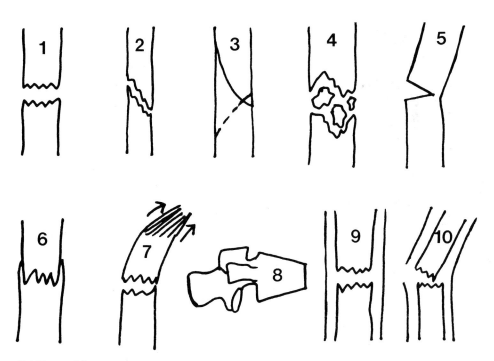

5.4 Types of fracture
1. Transverse 2. Oblique 3. Spiral 4. Comminuted 5. Greenstick 6. Impacted
7. Traction/avulsion 8. Compression 9. Closed 10. Open

associated with osteoporosis causing weakness of the bone structure, the individual vertebra collapses in a wedge-shaped manner. Impaction fractures result in the two fractured ends being forced together, producing a rather stable fracture which may heal readily, even though some length may be lost on the affected limb. A traction/avulsion fracture is the result of a sudden or violent contraction of a muscle associated with a bone. A good example is in the patella where, instead of the quadriceps muscle rupturing in a traumatic incident, the patella fractures.

HEALING OF FRACTURES

Once fractured, the healing process normally begins and consists of three phases of differing duration. In general terms, the time taken for a fracture to heal depends on the bone element fractured and type and position of the fracture, severity, apposition of the fractured fragments, stability of the fragments during healing, age and nutritional status of the individual, presence or absence of infection or other pathological process, a good blood supply and access to treatment. For example, fractures in young individuals tend to heal faster and more efficiently than in older adults.

The three phases of healing are: circulatory or cellular, metabolic and mechanical. The first phase begins with closure of the fracture and formation of primary callus or woven, immature new bone (Latin: *callum*, or hard). Blood seeps out from the fractured ends of the bone and forms a haematoma or collection of blood around and between the fracture (Sevitt, 1981). Severed blood vessels contract and become sealed with blood clots; this occurs within 12 hours of the fracture. Bone adjacent to the fracture dies, or necroses, and fibrous granulation connective tissue forms through the action of fibroblasts (Ortner and Putschar, 1981: 62); the haematoma is eventually absorbed. Fibrous union of the fracture occurs by about 15 days. The blood supply to the fractured area develops, the granulation tissue matures and fibroblasts are transformed into osteoclasts and osteoblasts which create an unmineralized intercellular matrix of collagen and carbohydrate (osteoid) by about 21 days. Calcium salts impregnate the tissue and this leads to the formation of callus by about 21–30 days. The callus occurs between the fracture at the cortex, endosteum and periosteum, and its quantity is determined by the type and level of the fracture, associated soft-tissue damage and deformity present, for example.

The metabolic phase involves replacement of the immature bone of callus with more mature lamellar bone.

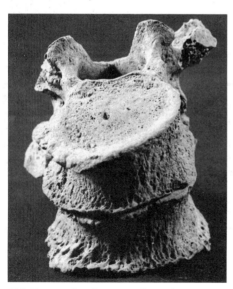

5.5 Compression fractures of vertebrae (medieval France)

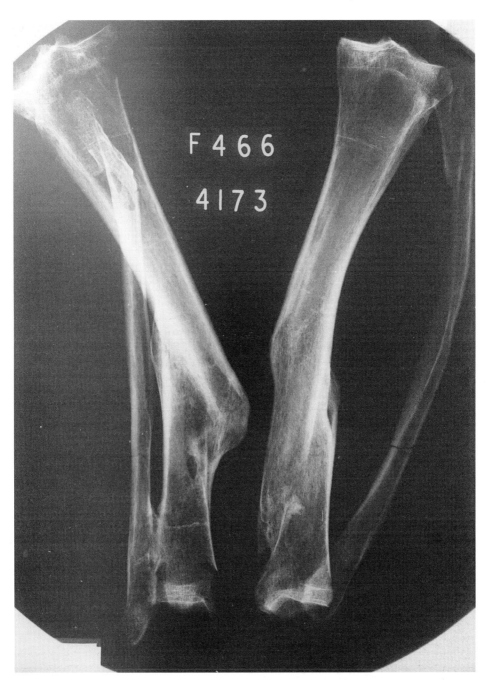

5.6 X-ray of a fractured tibia showing angulation deformities and other associated fractures

The final mechanical phase contributes over two-thirds of the total healing time and involves realignment and remodelling of bone along the lines of stress. Remodelling occurs over many years, with eventual restoration of the normal architecture of the bone to its original appearance, even on radiography. The healing process is completed at different times for different bones of the body. Radiography aids considerably in the interpretation of fractures (Roberts, 1989a), particularly to assess the mechanism behind the injury (type of fracture), and the state of healing of the fractured bone (Fig. 5.6). In archaeological contexts, taking accurate measurements of angulation, apposition (how much of the fractured fragments are apposed to each other) and overlap of the fragments is possible using radiographs.

FRACTURE COMPLICATIONS

There are several fracture complications which can occur at the time of the injury or years later, some of which can be determined by analysis of skeletal remains. Compound fractures can lead potentially to infection of the fracture site and cause delay in healing. If a fracture is not adequately reduced, i.e. the bone ends are not pulled apart and 'set' in the correct anatomical position, shortening of an affected limb and malalignment are possible, which could lead potentially to adjacent joint degeneration and osteoarthritis. Associated damage to the soft tissues, including blood vessels and nerves, often occurs specifically in relation to fractures in certain parts of the body. For example, a fracture to the neck of the femur can affect the blood supply to its head and cause problems with the normal healing process.

In archaeological contexts many of these fracture complications cannot be observed directly and are only surmised from the position of the fracture. For example, in some fractures fat globules can be released from the medullary cavity into the bloodstream and may lead to obstruction of vessels in the brain or lungs. Non-union of fractures in antiquity have been observed but care must be taken in differentiating between true non-union and non-union at the time of death, i.e. the latter suggesting that there had been insufficient time for the fracture to heal. Non-union is commonly seen in fractures to the femoral neck, and in the shafts of the forearm bones. The most frequent bone to suffer from non-union is the ulna shaft, probably because of imperfect immobilization (Crawford-Adams, 1983: 159) but other bones can be involved (Fig. 5.7). In antiquity recognition of non-union is possible, with fracture fragments displaying some opacity of the fractured ends on radiography, indicating attempts at healing. Stewart (1976) and Jurmain (1991) have described non-union of fractures in New World populations; it is, however, likely that many cases of non-union of fractures are not identified and are mistaken for post-mortem breaks.

LIMITATIONS OF TRAUMA STUDY

However, there are a number of limitations in the interpretation of fracture data. Whereas modern population studies can look at the real age distribution of fractures, in archaeological groups even though an individual died at a certain age

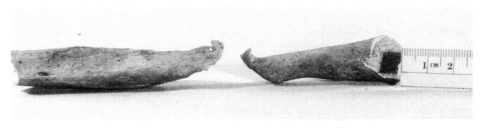

5.7 Non-union of fractured radius from Ala-329, San Francisco Bay, California (500 BC–AD 1700)

and had a healed fracture, this does not mean that it was sustained at that age; the fracture could have occurred many years before the death of the individual. Therefore it is not possible to look at age and susceptibility to fracture unless the fracture occurred around death and illustrates the very early stages of fracture healing. In addition, very few fractures are seen in the young, i.e. juvenile individuals; this cannot be accepted as the true prevalence of fractures in this age group. It is likely that many of these fractures are invisible to the palaeopathologist because they were probably greenstick fractures which healed so efficiently and quickly that they are not even visible on radiography. There are also problems in identifying peri-mortem (around death) fractures if there had been no time for healing to start to take place when the individual died; these fractures may appear to be post-mortem breaks and are not identified as ante-mortem injury. Examining the patterning of fractures and comparing the pattern observed in modern cases may help to identify these peri-mortem fractures. For example, the pattern of injury in child abuse is characteristic, with fractured ribs and localized new bone formation on some bones of the skeleton. Indeed, some biological anthropologists have started to identify this patterning in archaeological contexts (Walker, 1994b).

FRACTURES: MODERN POPULATION STUDIES

Fracture prevalence rates in both ancient and modern populations reflect both intentional violence and accidental injury. Technology has changed through time and today many more severe fractures are related to high-impact road-traffic accidents. Many fractures may be directly the result of repetitive occupationally induced stress or pure accidents such as falling. The type of information which potentially could be extracted in a study of trauma includes evidence for warfare, the type of weapon used to create the injury, general health status (i.e. was the body healthy to ensure rapid and efficient healing?) and evidence for treatment. In addition, prevalence rates compared between urban and rural, and hunter-gatherer and agricultural groups (Cohen and Armelagos, 1984) may help to highlight the living environment and stresses those populations experienced.

Age and sex determine many of the fracture patterns seen in modern populations; for example, older individuals, especially females, suffer fractures with underlying osteoporosis. Population studies of trauma in modern contexts reveal age and sex distribution of fracture prevalence in defined populations (Fife *et al.*, 1984; Sahlin, 1990; Prince *et al.*, 1993) and compare data from different environments. For example, Jónsson *et al.* (1993) studied lifestyle and fracture prevalence in Swedish populations from urban and rural environments and found a lower fracture rate in the urban environment; this was explained by the increased risk rural populations would have been exposed to during their everyday activities. However, another study (Jónsson *et al.*, 1992) showed the opposite result; the lower rate in the rural population was explained by the maintenance of physical activity in that population and its preventative effects against osteoporosis development and fracture. Osteoporosis-related fractures are a major concern confronting contemporary populations, although in antiquity it is unknown how common osteoporosis was, and whether it predisposed to a high frequency of fractures. What can be observed is that the classic sites in modern populations for osteoporosis-related fractures, the hip, wrist and spine, are affected. For example, Mensforth and Latimer (1989) recorded the prevalence of fractures of the distal radius, hip, spine and sacrum in 938 individuals in the Hamann–Todd Collection (a modern documented skeletal collection). White females were most frequently affected by fracture at all sites compared to White males and both Black males and females; osteoporosis was probably the main underlying cause.

In all the modern studies published, each fracture represents one individual and rates of fractures per 100,000 individuals are often produced. In an archaeological context, fracture rates are usually calculated as a percentage of the total bones examined. Presenting data as a percentage of individuals affected is unwise because it assumes complete survival of all the skeleton. Studies of trauma in archaeological population groups are more limited, comprising analyses of fracture prevalence in particular cemeteries and assessing the aetiological factors behind those fracture patterns.

FRACTURES: PAST POPULATION STUDIES

Notable studies of trauma in past populations are seen in the work of Angel (1974), who considered rates of fractures through long periods of time in Greece and Turkey (seventh millennium BC to second century AD). The prevalence of fractures for males and females (i.e. the number of individuals affected) was given; males were affected more than females in all periods and the prevalence rate ranged from 1.0 to 3.6 per cent. Jurmain's study (1991) of a prehistoric central Californian population examined 248 adult individuals represented by 2,047 long bones; 36 (1.8 per cent) of the bones were fractured, particularly in the forearm. Lovejoy and Heiple's study of the Libben site in Ohio (1981) revealed a 3.0 per cent fracture prevalence rate (72 of 2,383 bones) and they indicated that most of the fractures were accidental rather than due to interpersonal violence; again, most of the fractures occurred in the arm. A recent study (Grauer and Roberts, 1995) examined the fracture prevalence rates from medieval British sites and found very similar rates between them

(Table 5.1), ranging from 0.3 to 6.1 per cent. All the cemetery sites served urban communities; those with the highest prevalence rates were from St Nicholas Shambles, London, and the medieval hospital cemetery from Chichester. It is likely that the higher rates in London can be explained by the small number of bones available to examine, or that this prevalence represents the hazards of urban living. The rate for the Chichester group may reflect its use as a hospital and, therefore, the likelihood of people being admitted for care following fracture.

Table 5.1 Fracture prevalence in six British medieval populations

	Fracture no.	Total bones	%	Ref.
Whithorn, Scotland	27	9563	0.3	1
Blackfriars, Gloucester	11	1861	0.6	2
St Helen-on-the-Walls, York	41	4938	0.8	3
Fishergate, York	26	3235	0.8	4
Chichester, Sussex	41	1554	2.6	5
St Nicholas Shambles, London	18	296	6.1	6

References: 1. Cardy (1993); 2. Wiggins *et al.* (1993); 3. Grauer and Roberts (1995); 4. Stroud and Kemp (1993); 5. Judd (1994).; 6. White (1988).

Examination of the pattern of fractures in the skeleton for these sites reveals that the arm (especially the radius and ulna, Table 5.2) is the most frequently affected limb, except at Whithorn, Chichester and Fishergate where the fibula rate is higher. Rates for the femur are particularly low in all groups; today, fractured femurs at the neck or trochanteric region are common in elderly females, i.e. 60 years plus, who usually have underlying osteoporosis (Crawford-Adams, 1983), and fractures in the shaft of the femur follow severe violence (for example in a road-traffic accident). This latter probably explains their relative absence in the fracture prevalence record for antiquity, when motorized vehicles and people living into old age were not the norm. Fractures to the tibia are also rare in all groups. In Britain today motor-cycle accidents are 'by far the commonest single cause of major fractures to the shafts of the tibia and fibula' (Crawford-Adams, 1983: 251), causing an angulatory/ rotational force. The low frequency of such fractures in ancient populations could be explained again by this lack of technological advance. In modern studies fracture prevalence rates for different parts of the body vary (Table 5.3), but there are larger numbers of fractures to the bones of the leg, while the radius and ulna together contribute significantly to the fracture prevalence rate. The problem with comparing fracture prevalence between ancient and modern populations is that for modern groups all the bones of the skeleton are present to observe, whereas in an archaeological population they are not. For example, it is difficult to know whether, if an individual has a fractured radius, there was an associated fracture to the ulna if this bone has not survived burial to be examined.

Table 5.2 Fracture prevalence (%) by bone element for seven medieval British sites

	1	2	3	4	5	6	7
Humerus	0.8	5.3	0.3	0.4	0	4.2	0
Radius	1.3	8.8	1.4	0.8	0.5	3.2	0.5
Ulna	1.5	8.2	0.5	0.8	0.1	2.8	0
Femur	0.1	3.8	0.5	0.2	0.2	0.4	0.8
Tibia	0.7	6.0	0.5	0.5	0.4	2.3	0.2
Fibula	0.8	4.1	0.3	1.7	0.8	7.2	0.2

1. St Helen-on-the-Walls, York (Grauer and Roberts, 1995).
2. St Nicholas Shambles, London (White, 1988).
3. Blackfriars, Gloucester (Wiggins *et al.*, 1993).
4. Fishergate, York (Stroud and Kemp, 1993).
5. Whithorn, Scotland (Cardy, 1993).
6. Chichester, Sussex (Judd, 1994).
7. Jewbury, York (Lilley *et al.*, 1994).

Table 5.3 Fracture prevalence for bone element in three modern population studies (individuals affected)

	1		2		3	
	No.	%	No.	%	No.	%
Humerus	941	20.6	194	15.2	46	14.0
Radius and ulna	1173	25.7	679	53.2	135	41.2
Femur	631	13.8	229	18.0	45	13.7
Tibia and fibula	1821	39.9	173	13.6	102	31.1

References: 1. Buhr and Cooke (1959); 2. Garraway *et al.* (1979); 3. Fife and Barancik (1985).

Fractures to other parts of the skeleton are also observed in ancient groups. However, fractures to the hands and feet are particularly infrequent; this may be explained by the relatively poor survival of these bones in archaeological contexts. Fractures involving the pelvis are also rare, probably because today they occur most frequently following high-impact road-traffic accidents. Sternal (especially associated with anterior rib fractures) and scapula fractures are rare, but when seen in an archaeological population they may indicate the results of a blow to the back or chest of the individual and interpersonal violence. Unfortunately, the scapula is often damaged, especially in the blade area (where the majority of fractures occur) during burial or excavation, and therefore the frequency of this fracture is probably underestimated for past populations. Fracture to the acromion of the scapula has been recorded in archaeological contexts (Miles, 1994) but confusion has occurred between a true fracture (and non-union) or non-fusion of the acromial epiphysis – os acromiale (see Chapter 6), perhaps because of activity (Stirland, 1986). In Miles' population from Ensay, Scotland,

11 examples of separation of the acromial tip were recorded in 220 scapulae (10.0 per cent), and Stirland (1986) recorded 13.6 per cent prevalence in the group of individuals from the Tudor warship the *Mary Rose*. In the latter case it was suggested that non-union was the result of the movements necessary for archery practised at an early age preventing fusion of the epiphysis.

Fractures to the shaft of the ulna (the Parry fracture) may represent interpersonal violence, i.e. defending a blow to the head; fractures to the radius, often with underlying osteoporosis, may have been the result of falling on the outstretched hand. Fractures of both these bones are commonly identified in archaeological contexts (see above). The clavicle is usually broken in accidents involving falling and is also seen regularly in palaeopathology. Along with rib fractures (again, commonly observed), even in modern contexts, clavicle fractures are often left to heal without therapeutic intervention. The ribs are fractured as a result of a fall or a direct blow to the rib cage.

Vertebral trauma in the thoracic and lumbar spine can result from compression fractures caused by a vertical force induced hyperflexion injury, leading to scoliosis and kyphosis (Crawford-Adams, 1983: 98); often, underlying

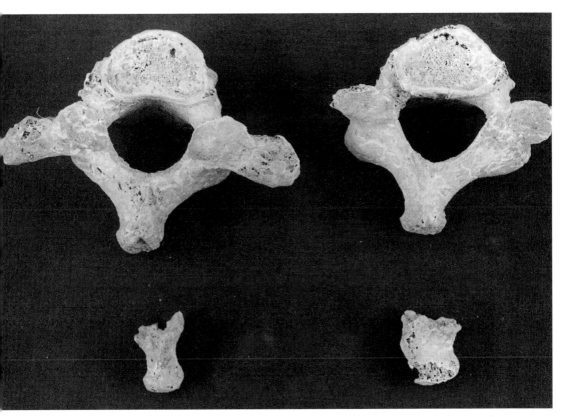

5.8 Clay-shoveller's fractures of 7th cervical and 1st thoracic vertebrae spinous processes with non-union (4th century AD, Baldock, Hertfordshire, England)

osteoporosis may lead to weakness and fracture. Merbs (1983) reported that thirty-six of eighty adult Sadlermiut Eskimo vertebral columns suffered from vertebral compression fractures from the third thoracic vertebra down to the fifth lumbar vertebra. The frequency was higher in females; the suggested reason was that females rode on sleds and toboggans over rough terrain, allowing compressive forces to be transmitted through the spine, females also carried their offspring on their backs, and older females may have had underlying osteoporosis. Compression fractures can also occur in the cervical spine and, although less frequent, are more serious (Crawford-Adams, 1983: 86); they are often associated with subluxation or partial dislocation and there is an increased risk of damage to the spinal cord at this level. Fractures to the odontoid process of the atlas and the axis arch are termed hangman's fractures; unhealed examples of these fractures in the past may be helpful clues to the cause of death. Fractures to the spinous and transverse processes also occur. Fractures at the levels of the seventh cervical and first thoracic vertebrae are termed 'clay-shoveller's fractures'. Figure 5.8 shows an unhealed example from the Romano-British site at Baldock, Hertfordshire, England. The combination of the actions of the trapezius and rhomboid muscles initiate this fracture and may help identify occupation, although there have been few reports to date in palaeopathology.

A rather special type of vertebral fracture, which is particularly common in all periods of antiquity, may have its roots in a congenital weakness of a small area of bone. This condition, known as spondylolysis, is recognized in skeletal remains as the separation of a single vertebra into two parts. The congenital weakness of the bone is present at the position between the upper and lower joint surfaces on the neural arch, that part of the vertebra lying behind the solid central body and surrounding the spinal cord. It is suggested that the recurrent stresses and strains of bending and lifting in the upright posture create a gradual series of small

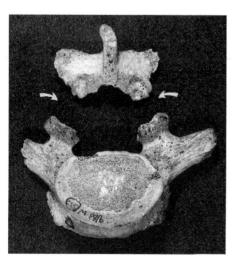

fractures at the site of weakness (Fig. 5.9); it is probably caused by stress or fatigue at the site but also acute injury. Ultimately the bone at that site fractures partially or entirely and the neural arch may separate from the vertebral body. The only attachment remaining is by ligament and fibrous tissue. Generally speaking, healing of these fractures does not take place, probably, as Merbs (1989b: 170) suggests, because of continual stress at the site, although evidence of attempted healing has occasionally been found (Eisenstein, 1978). Most cases of the condition occur at the fifth lumbar vertebra, less commonly at the fourth, and much less commonly elsewhere. The modern incidence of the condition

5.9 Spondylolysis of 5th lumbar vertebra (4th century AD, Gloucester, England)

is around 3.0 per cent of Caucasian populations (Merbs, 1989b), but there is considerable racial variation. The incidence in Eskimos may be up to 50 per cent, a feature that is attributed to their physically arduous existence. It appears to be a condition associated with some activities such as gymnastics. Jackson *et al.* (1976) found an 11.0 per cent incidence in 100 female gymnasts, and many had associated spina bifida occulta.

Apart from slight, constant, low back discomfort, the condition causes no symptoms unless it is associated with a dislocation of the now unstable vertebral body. This condition, termed spondylolisthesis, is a serious abnormality which may therefore justly

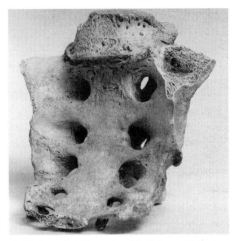

5.10 Spondylolisthesis with fusion of 5th lumbar vertebra to sacrum (6th–8th century AD, Eccles, Kent, England)

be regarded as a complication of trauma. Although uncommon, it was no doubt present in the past. The recognition of the abnormality in disarticulated skeletons from archaeological sites is difficult and rests upon the observation of bone formation along the rims of the displaced vertebral bodies (Congdon, 1931). Fusion by bone of the displaced vertebra upon its neighbour may occur. A rare case of spondylolisthesis (Fig. 5.10) shows the condition in an Anglo-Saxon individual from Kent, England, in which bony fusion between the displaced vertebra and its neighbour has occurred (Manchester, 1982). This natural process of antiquity has achieved, albeit in a poor position, what modern orthopaedic surgical practice endeavours to do.

HEAD INJURIES

In the twentieth century we are all familiar with aggressive society. Even within a single population group, one section of a society may live in peace with only sporadic infrequent episodes of aggression, while in a neighbouring area an undercurrent of continuous violence may be the norm. Often the most dramatic injuries are to the skull as, certainly in interpersonal/intergroup violence, the head is often the main target for blows; if head protection is not worn then the skull may suffer injury. In crime scene investigations where the cause and manner of a victim's death are being evaluated, it is usually the head and neck which reveal most of the trauma identified. As Knight (1991: 156) states, it is the head which is usually the target for violence as the brain and skull are the most vulnerable areas of the body when damaged. In addition, if a person falls to the ground the head is usually damaged.

Since, as noted, skull injury probably represents intentional blows, the enumeration of such injuries may indicate the peace or otherwise of communities.

Although injury in general is often more common in the male (e.g. Bennike, 1985: 101 in multiperiod Danish skeletons; and Wells, 1982 in a Romano–British cemetery), the sex difference in skull injury is perhaps the most striking. Assessing gender differences in the study of disease and injury may provide insights into social organization, occupational roles, and interpersonal and intergroup violence. Generally speaking, males, both today and in the past, often performed heavy manual work and composed a society's fighting forces; therefore their risk of injury may have been greater and so a sex difference may be expected in the study of trauma.

What is common to many past societies is injury to the skull. Injuries to the skull may be the result of hand-to-hand fighting with the opponents facing each other, resulting in injuries to the frontal and parietal bones. Only occasionally are blows delivered from behind and, accepting that 90 per cent of the world's population is right handed, an occipital bone injury at the back of the head on the right side would be expected. Not that this is invariably the case. The skeletal material from the Battle of Wisby showed frequent occipital wounds, suggesting that blows were delivered to a fleeing enemy (Courville, 1965). Wounds of the facial skeleton (excepting the nasal bones) are also infrequent, suggesting that blows to the skull which are observed in past groups were purposefully delivered to the cranium to produce maximum damage; it may be, however, that the facial bones, being commonly damaged during burial, do not survive well or often enough to identify injury to this part of the body. Nasal injuries are fairly common in antiquity and these, no doubt, are due to fist-fighting, an age-old and continuing method of solving minor disputes. Many cranial injuries are found on the left side of the skull. A blow from a right-handed aggressor engaged in face-to-face and hand-to-hand combat would result in a left-sided head injury. It has also been demonstrated at the Battle of Wisby (Courville, ibid.) that the majority of cutting wounds are the result of obliquely downward blows. Less frequent is the vertically directed blow and, even more rare, a horizontal blow. This merely reflects the ease with which a heavy sword or axe is wielded. As would be expected with fatal wounds obtained in combat, many cranial injuries consist of a single cut. In those skulls possessing several cuts, the direction of the blows is often variable, but recent work using the scanning electron microscope on skull wounds has been able to suggest the order and direction of injury in individuals from an Anglo-Saxon cemetery from Kent, England (Wenham, 1987).

The type of skull fracture sustained may indicate the direction and type of force needed to create that type of fracture (Polson et al., 1985; Leestma and Kirkpatrick, 1988; Merbs, 1989a); each fracture may be caused by direct injury (e.g. blow to the back of the head) or indirect trauma (e.g. jumping from a height, leading to skull fracture). Velocity, size, shape of and energy expended by the object causing the wound determines the resulting fracture (Gurdjian et al., 1950). In addition, and often forgotten in archaeology, the characteristics of the skull, hair and scalp, will also affect the ultimate fracture pattern (Gordon et al., 1988). Forensic experiments conducted on cadaveric material have produced useful data on the type of cranial fracture pattern produced when forces are applied from different directions (Gurdjian et al., 1950); this work is important

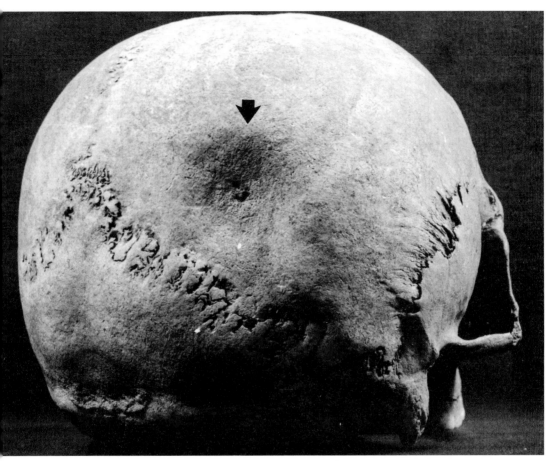

5.11 Depressed skull fracture on right parietal bone (medieval France)

for archaeological application. Probably the most commonly seen types of head injury in archaeological contexts are the depressed fractures (Fig. 5.11), where the surface of the skull is depressed inwards, and the linear fracture, often caused by a blade injury. The resulting brain damage, always a potential problem in head injury, will vary according to the fracture type. Depressed fractures often lead to brain damage, both directly underneath the fracture and at a distance from the site, and a linear, blade injury has potential for causing brain damage directly below the fracture. Of course, brain tissue is, in the majority of archaeological contexts, not preserved, and therefore the extent of brain damage can only be inferred on the basis of the type, pattern and position of the fracture on the skull. Brain damage may include necrosis of some of the tissue; this is due to increased pressure from a collection of blood inside the skull leading to lack of oxygen to the tissue (subdural or extradural haematoma). Infection of the brain is also a potential hazard in cranial trauma, and would have been a problem in antiquity; it is probable that individuals in the past who suffered infection of the brain tissue would have died before bony change had time to develop. Skull fractures usually heal with fibrous union, but bony union is occasionally found. Bone formation during the healing process is present but is less important than in fractures of the postcranium (Sevitt, 1981: 231).

Not only do cranial wounds throw light on the actions of the fighter, but they may also give an indication of the type of weapon used. A sharp blade will produce a clean cut, usually with smooth, straight polished edges, and a blunter type of instrument may cause splintering of the edges of the wound. The battle-hammer or the mace tends to produce depressed fractures (Moodie, 1927; Wells, 1964a). One of the most malicious hand weapons of all times was the medieval 'morning star' or 'holy water sprinkler'. This flailing weapon was a wooden ball with protruding metal spikes.

Of course, the cranial wound may be healed (Fig. 5.12) or unhealed, the latter suggesting that the wound contributed to the cause of death. Healing, identified as rounding of the wound edges, indicates survival of the person following the injury, but little can be said of what complications were present. Distinguishing ante-mortem or peri-mortem unhealed injury from post-mortem breaks may be difficult and requires quite sophisticated methods of analysis. The weapon used may also be interpreted from the injury observed, but only rarely is the weapon found *in situ* in its wound. In this instance, the moment of death is captured and, as it were, fossilized. Cranial wounds were often fatal and the presence of the weapon probably adds little to the reconstruction of

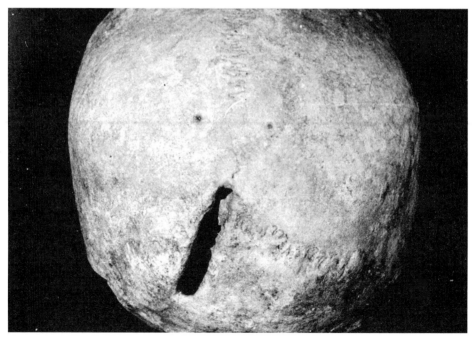

5.12 Healed wound to occipital bone (medieval St Helen-on-the-Walls, York, England)

events. With the weapon *in situ* it may be possible to surmise the direction of flight. Armed with this knowledge, and with a knowledge of anatomy, the soft tissue and skeletal damage can be assessed. Hence the clinical effects of injury can be reconstructed.

Consider, for example, the Neolithic arrowhead *in situ* in the anterior aspect of the body of a lumbar vertebra (Wells, 1964a). This weapon, entering the body of the victim from the front, would, on reaching the abdomen, perforate the gut and transfix the aorta, the largest artery in the body, lying immediately in front of the vertebra at this level. The resultant haemorrhage would have been catastrophic and death would have ensued within minutes or less. In contrast is the Anglo-Saxon example of an arrowhead which came to rest on the posterior aspect of the third lumbar vertebra (Fig. 5.13; Manchester and Elmhirst, 1980).

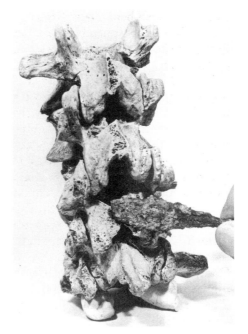

5.13 Lumbar spine with iron arrowhead on the 3rd lumbar vertebra (6th–8th century AD, Eccles, Kent, England)

Clearly, its horizontal position suggests that the arrow was shot at the upright victim, probably from fairly close range to his right. The injury did no more damage than create great pain, some bleeding and, in this instance at least, a minor opening in the spinal canal. This was insignificant because the victim shortly became subject to a tremendous blow to the right side of the back of the head.

From an examination of skeletal remains, therefore, it is potentially possible to reconstruct the cause and manner of death as is undertaken in forensic anthropology. From Denmark (Bennike, 1985) there is similar evidence for *in situ* weapons in the pelvis, palate, cervical vertebrae and sternum in skeletons of various dates from the Neolithic (4200–1800 BC) to the Viking period (AD 800–1050); all of them have no evidence of healing and the presence of the weapon suggests that these injuries contributed to the deaths of the individuals. Rarely in archaeological contexts is there evidence for bullet wounds, so commonly seen in forensic investigations (Madea and Staak, 1988), but an interesting case from a post-medieval cemetery excavated at Glasgow Cathedral (King, 1994) revealed four lead-shot balls associated with a skull with evidence of bullet holes.

The medieval knight encased in metal armour from head to toe may be the classic, or rather popular, soldier of antiquity (e.g. see Gurdjian, 1973 for a discussion of head protection through time). The rank and file, the ancestors of the twentieth-century 'cannon-fodder' were rather less fortunate. Body and skull protection for these people may have been no more than leather garments, although there are more sophisticated examples. But even these afforded some protection against an aggressive blow. The protection or otherwise of the victim must be borne in mind when examining the corporate remains of battle injury.

Specific studies of cranial trauma reveal interesting information both temporally and geographically. Walker (1989), studying 774 crania from the North Channel Islands in southern California, identified 144 individuals (19.3 per cent) with one or more fractures to the cranium; they were commonly seen on the left side of the head and on the frontal and parietal bones. Males were more affected than females (12:5), with the differences being highly significant. More injuries were seen on the island groups (perhaps because of competition for scarce resources) than on the mainland, and frequencies increased through time (possibly the result of increased population density). Both accidental and interpersonal injuries were identified. Injury was rarely seen on the occipital bone, suggesting that interpersonal injuries were sustained by 'frontal' combat, not during flight.

Healed and unhealed cranial injuries are regularly identified in archaeological contexts and vary in prevalence. Two sites in Britain with particularly high

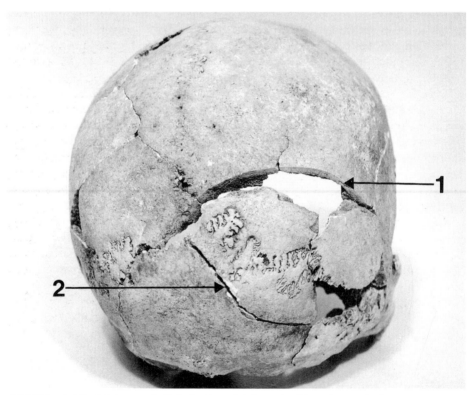

5.14 Unhealed blade injury to skull. 1. Incision of right parietal bone due to edged weapon. 2. Probable fracture line from withdrawal of weapon (6th–8th century AD, Eccles, Kent, England)

prevalence rates of unhealed cranial blade injuries come from Eccles, Kent (Manchester and Elmhirst, 1980) and Fishergate, York (Stroud and Kemp, 1993). Eccles, dated to the sixth to eighth centuries AD, revealed seven individuals with unhealed blade wounds suggesting interpersonal violence (Fig. 5.14); some of the victims also sustained postcranial injuries. At Fishergate a total of sixteen males had similar injuries, many multiple, with some also having traumatic lesions to the spine and limbs. Most of the injuries occurred on the left side of the body and mostly to young individuals. Another type of blade injury is decapitation; evidence for this activity can be identified either from cut marks on the cervical vertebrae or from the context of deposition of the body, although the former is safer. The latter may involve a buried body whose skull is placed elsewhere in the grave. At Cirencester, a Romano-British cemetery in Gloucestershire, England (Wells, 1982), six individuals had been decapitated through their cervical vertebrae; the crania were excavated in the correct anatomical position and, as suggested, this may represent partial maintenance of the soft tissues around the neck, following severance of the head.

SCALPING

Another practice resulting in cut marks to the skeleton (and, in particular, the head) involves scalping, or 'the forcible removal of all or part of the scalp' (Owsley, 1994: 335), using a sharp implement and leaving short, straight or slightly curved cut marks on the frontal and parietal bones of the skull; in some cases fragments of the implement may be identified in the wound (Olsen and Shipman, 1994). To perform scalping the periosteum and covering skin were removed from the skull, usually across the forehead, thus depriving the skull of its periosteal blood supply. This resulted in death of the outer table of the skull and production of new bone, leaving a depression in the area of scalping (Steinbock, 1976: 27). Scalping has a long history and often was undertaken to collect human trophies in order to emphasize bravery in warfare (Owsley, ibid.: 337). However, for some victims it was carried out as a therapeutic measure or for supernatural or religious significance. The amount of scalp removed varied, but it was usually taken and used as an amulet to protect against evil. It is clear that some victims survived this ordeal; this is displayed in the evidence for healing of scalped victims in the form of pitting of the bone surface and new bone formation. Owsley (ibid.: 338), however, notes that in some societies people who did survive were deemed 'not quite a man', isolated and attributed supernatural powers. Scalping was practised in many countries world-wide, and evidence in the New World suggests that the practice was present by AD 600 (Owsley, ibid.); it was also described by Herodotus in the fifth century BC. The majority of evidence for scalping comes from the Americas and indicates scalping being practised on both dying or dead individuals.

INFANTICIDE, CANNIBALISM AND DEFLESHING

Elsewhere on the skeleton, the presence of cut marks may represent other ritual practices, such as infanticide, cannibalism and defleshing, and distinguishing ante-mortem and peri-mortem from post-mortem cut marks in all these possible scenarios is important. Infanticide has also been suggested following the interpretation of the age at death distribution for perinatal individuals from archaeological sites and their deposition context (Smith and Kahila, 1992; Mays, 1993). Defleshing of soft tissue from the skeleton may also leave marks on the bone; distinguishing between scalping and defleshing may be undertaken by examining the distribution of cut marks. Cut marks located on the skull may be attributed solely to scalping, and cut marks located more widely over the body could be due to defleshing, the latter indicated by cut marks around the joint surfaces indicating disarticulation. A complicating factor may be post-mortem erosion of areas of the skeleton with cut marks before and after defleshing which may indicate that the body had been exposed prior to mutilation (Olsen and Shipman, 1994).

Cannibalism as a cultural practice has also to be differentiated from defleshing as part of secondary burial. Turner (1993) provided useful criteria for identifying cannibalism in the archaeological record, based on an assemblage of eight Anasazi individuals from Chaco Canyon, New Mexico. Peri-mortem cranial and postcranial bone breaks, cut marks, anvil-hammerstone abrasions, burning, bone fragment end polishing and missing vertebrae were suggested as evidence of cannibalism.

TRAUMA AND CAUSE OF DEATH

Usually it is not easy to establish cause of death when faced with the examination of a skeleton from an archaeological site. However, the presence of a weapon *in situ* in a bone, an unhealed injury, and decapitation will, at least, suggest the manner of death (i.e. how the death came about), if not its cause. Of course, the preservation of a body will allow a more specific attribution of cause of death to be made, purely because of the presence of soft tissues. For example, many of the north-western European bodies buried and preserved in anaerobic acidic peat bogs suggested that asphyxia had been the cause of death (Brothwell, 1986). Lindow Man, the Iron-Age body discovered in a Cheshire peat bog in England in the 1980s, revealed a sinew thong around his neck with the knot in the sinew biting deeply into the soft tissues; two of the cervical vertebrae were fractured and the throat had been slit. In skeletonized individuals strangulation, hanging, or severe trauma to the neck may be revealed in fractures to the hyoid bone or calcified thyroid and cricoid cartilages, all located in the neck region. In archaeological contexts these structures are rarely retrieved, either through poor preservation or non-recognition in the grave excavation. Often in forensic contexts it is the ossified thyroid cartilage which is fractured in strangulation and, hence, reveals cause of death (Ubelaker, 1992). Associated with fractures to these structures, the cervical vertebrae can be fractured in hanging, especially the odontoid process of the second cervical vertebra if the 'drop' is long. Although hanging and strangulation are only two causes of death, the preservation and retrieval of the hyoid bone and neck cartilages may aid in reconstructing a little-known fact for archaeological populations, that is, cause of death. However, the method of burial may also help.

Evidence for live burial, deduced from the examination of bodies during excavation, has been produced in the Danish 'bog burials' (Glob, 1973). Evidence based on skeletal posture has been revealed in the UK (Rahtz, 1960; Hawkes and Wells, 1975; Manchester, 1978a; Powlesland, 1980). In the case of live burials, the posture of the skeleton within the grave fossilizes the moment of death, with the individual struggling to free himself or herself from certain asphyxiation. Selection of the method of dispatch must surely have been dictated by the cultural attitude of society to pain and death. In the absence of documentation the reasons for judicial executions in antiquity are forever unknown. Finally, an unusual possible cause of death may be attributed to a skeletonized individual from Israel, where the right calcaneum (heel bone) had an 11.5 cm iron nail through its body, which also incorporated traces of wood (Zias and Sekeles, 1985). It was hypothesized that this was evidence for crucifixion; a likely scenario of the use of ropes to suspend the upper body from the horizontal part of the cross, and nailing the feet to the vertical part of the cross was proposed, with asphyxia suggested as the cause of death.

Dislocation

Another traumatic lesion is that of dislocation, where there is loss of contact between two osseous surfaces which are normally a joint. This may be total or partial (subluxation) and, in archaeological contexts, is recognizable only if the bones remain unreduced, i.e. out of alignment; this may be why few dislocations are recognized in palaeopathology. The cause of dislocation may be congenital (see Chapter 3) or acquired, the latter involving trauma or another disease, e.g. the metacarpophalangeal joints of the hands (knuckles) in rheumatoid arthritis. The hip and the shoulder are the most commonly affected joints, but potentially any joint could be affected. Often a joint may reduce itself, often seen in the shoulder; however, the shoulder, being a less stable joint anatomically, tends to dislocate freely and frequently in modern humans.

Osteochondritis dissecans

Apart from the obvious case of trauma-induced fractures, there is another relatively frequently occurring condition in skeletal material, that of osteochondritis dissecans. It is classified with other, so-called osteochondroses, such as Scheuermann's disease of the spine, Osgood–Schlatter's disease of the knee and Perthes disease of the hip. All these conditions involve fragmentation and collapse of the joints of the skeleton. They all affect young individuals, especially males in their first decade of life, and are the result of death of bone tissue from significant obliteration of the affected area's blood supply. The knee is affected in 80 per cent of cases, usually with an underlying traumatic aetiology. The necrotic fragment of bone separates and may remain loose in the joint, may become absorbed or may heal back into the defect (Fig. 5.15). There are few specific reports on osteochondritis dissecans in the palaeopathological literature (Wells, 1974a; Loveland et al., 1984). It is important to appreciate that there are defects in the joints which may be mistakenly attributed to osteochondritis

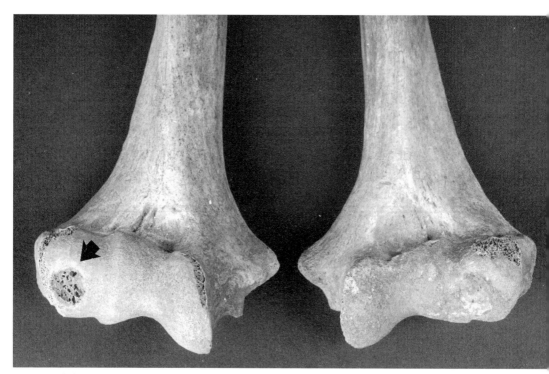

5.15 Osteochondritis dissecans in distal humerus joint surface (medieval France)

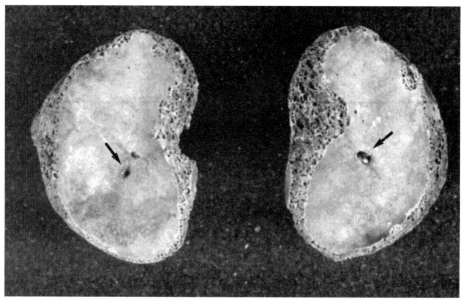

5.16 Joint lesions which may be confused for osteochondritis dissecans (proximal articular surfaces of 1st metatarsals)

dissecans (Fig. 5.16) and there is a danger of overinflating prevalence rates. A true osteochondritic lesion consists of a well-defined, porous, often circular, defect, usually lower than the normal joint surface.

TREATMENT OF TRAUMA

Trauma is painful, visual and debilitating; today people afflicted with trauma try to seek help and have their injuries treated. Fractures, like childbirth, have faced all societies in the past and may have presented problems. But the treatment of a broken leg with a simple fracture by reducing and splinting just needs a little common sense. The evidence for the treatment of trauma is plentiful in historical data but direct evidence on the skeleton is more rare. To be able to treat trauma and disease today needs some knowledge of the anatomy and physiology of the human body; this knowledge was not always evident in past communities and was often based on dissection of animals. In fact, over much of the past, dissection of the human body was not allowed (for example, the Church in Europe banned dissection for a long period of time). The discovery of the shape, structure and physiology of the brain took some time to master and was rather neglected until Vesalius, working in the sixteenth century AD, described the surface anatomy of the brain. Aristotle believed that the brain cooled the heart, the latter being the seat of intelligence (Backay, 1985). Likewise, today, many developing societies often rely on applying knowledge of animal anatomy to human problems (Lucier *et al.*, 1971). However, in some cases very detailed anatomical knowledge allowed the development of what would be recognized today as very successful methods of treatment. It was not until the work of artists such as Leonardo Da Vinci, Vesalius and Michelangelo, during the fifteenth and sixteenth centuries AD in Europe, that the study of anatomy was placed on a firm foundation of observations. As dissections became more commonplace, and illustrated anatomy texts more freely available and disseminated, there were advances in anatomical research (Schultz, 1985: 23). Recognition that anatomy needed to be learned was emphasized by Guy de Chauliac, a fourteenth-century French surgeon, who said, 'the surgeon who is ignorant of anatomy carves the human body as a blind man carves wood' (MacKinney, 1957: 402).

Amputation

Although evidence for treatment of disease and injury in the past does exist in written and artistic form, the direct evidence consists of amputation, splinting of fractures and trepanation of the skull. Amputation of limbs has been carried out since very early times and for various reasons. Apart from the traumatic amputation of a limb during battle or domestic accident, the deliberate removal of part or the whole of a limb has been carried out as a surgical procedure for the treatment of disease, such as infection, or injury, or for punishment. A particularly macabre reason for amputation in early Egypt was for ensuring statistical accuracy. Introduced in the XIX Dynasty and certainly pictorially portrayed in the Temple of Rameses III, is the practice of hand amputation of prisoners of war. Apparently this was carried out to assist in the counting of

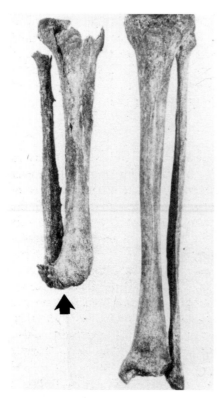

5.17 Amputation of tibia and fibula with evidence of healing

numbers of prisoners (Brothwell and Møller-Christensen, 1963). One of the earliest examples of amputation, dated to the IX Dynasty, but one which has nevertheless been disputed, is the loss of the distal half of the right radius and ulna (Brothwell and Møller-Christensen, 1963). For this case a bridge of bone between the stump ends and obvious healing and remodelling of the ends indicates that the individual survived the surgical operation of amputation. A less successful example of the operation in the past is of a lower limb of unknown date from Yorkshire (Gee, personal communication, 1975). A clean-cut end of the femur with a terminal end-saw splinter shows no evidence of healing. The specimen probably represents an operative or early post-operative death.

Evidence for amputation is rare in the archaeological record (Fig. 5.17) probably because unhealed amputated limbs could be mistaken for post-mortem breakage of bones. In both cases, whether amputated or damaged post-mortem, there would be no evidence of healing, i.e. in the former the person died at or very soon after the amputation, probably due to massive uncontrolled haemorrhage. Another differential diagnosis for bones which may appear to have been amputated is a fracture where there has been no attempt (or very little) at healing, i.e. an ununited fracture; if the distal fragment is missing an incorrect diagnosis may be made. Microscopic examination of the cut surface of the unhealed bone may reveal marks indicative of the instrument used, thus differentiating between post-mortem breakage, an unhealed fracture and an unhealed amputation. It is possible to extend the diagnosis of amputations by assessing the rest of the skeleton and observing abnormal bone change. If a limb has been amputated, a particular scenario could be envisaged. A person will not be able to use the affected limb, with resultant disuse atrophy, i.e. reduction in the size of the limb compared to the opposite, unaffected side, associated with reduction in the prominence of muscle attachments. Lazenby and Pfeiffer (1993) describe overall size, cross-sectional geometry and mid-shaft histological features in an historically identified nineteenth-century below-knee amputee, thus supporting the scenario described. Individuals may also have had a false limb and crutches; although these artefacts are generally lost to the palaeopathologist, they are described and illustrated (e.g. Epstein, 1937).

The osteoarchaeological record of amputation is scant, but such record of trepanation is abundant, albeit geographically biased. When the surgical risks of the two procedures are compared, it is perhaps surprising that, on the evidence available, trepanation appears to have been a more common surgical manoeuvre than amputation. The figures may be clouded by the ease of recognition of trepanation and the likely difficulty of recognition of amputation.

Trepanation

Trepanation is a practice known since very early times and is seen today in developing countries (Ackerknecht, 1967). The operation involves, for whatever reason, incision of the scalp and the cutting through and removal of an area of skull (Fig. 5.18). The result is the exposure of the membranes (dura) covering the brain. Survival of the patient, for patient he or she must be regarded in this surgical operation, probably depended upon the skilful avoidance of perforation of these membranes and the avoidance, either by luck or good judgement, of the major blood vessels within the skull. It should be noted that the proportion of survivors of this operation in antiquity was high (Piggott, 1940). The evidence for survival is, of course, the healing and remodelling of the bone around the operation site. Several examples exist of individuals having undergone more than one trepanning operation, having survived a preceding one. A notable specimen, the Cuzco skull from Peru, shows no less than seven trepanned holes, all showing signs of healing (Oakley et al., 1959). Perhaps equally surprising are the size of trepanned areas, particularly where survival has occurred. For example, a Neolithic skull from Latvia possessed three trepanning defects in the skull. The largest single hole measured 68 × 55 mm, and all three merged to produce an opening 120 × 60 mm in size. Surprisingly, this individual survived his horrific surgical trauma and died over 1 year later, possibly from some other disease unrelated to the trepanation (Derums, 1979).

Ancient examples of trepanation number well into the thousands and their distribution is world-wide. Perhaps because of the excellence and extent of archaeological excavation and post-excavation skeletal analysis, Europe affords many of these examples (e.g. Bennike, 1985), and Piggott (ibid.) suggests that central and northern Europe may be the original home of trepanation. The Americas (Stone and Miles, 1990), Australia (Webb, 1988), Asia, Africa and Melanesia have also produced examples. A late palaeolithic origin has been claimed and certainly in the Neolithic period it was an active practice. Although flourishing in the Neolithic period in Europe, perhaps more than at any other time, the operation has been performed during all periods since.

The technical object of operation was clear, but the actual surgical procedure adopted was variable. Dependent upon the era and the technologies available, the operation may have been carried out with a flint scraper or blade, or a metal implement which may or may not have been adapted specifically for the purpose. Recent work has provided evidence for the type of instrument used. Stevens and Wakley (1993) used scanning electron microscopy to examine a trepanation and, by experimental analogy, suggested that the implement used had been a shell. Initial incision of the scalp is a very bloody procedure, but the haemorrhage can

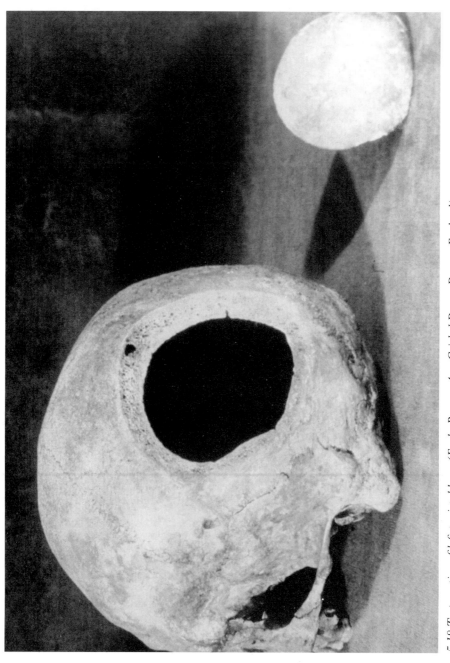

5.18 Trepanation of left parietal bone (Early Bronze Age, Crichel Down, Dorset, England)

be minimized by turning back the scalp flaps created; no doubt this was realized and carried out by early surgeons.

After cutting the soft tissues, the outer skull surface was exposed. At this point the pattern varied. Five types of trepanation have been identified from skeletal material world-wide. The scraped type involved the bone surface being removed and bevelled edges to the wound were created towards the central hole in the skull. The gouge method removed a larger piece of skull by delineating a circular area on the skull and gouging the area with an implement. The bore and saw method usually involved the use of a drill-type implement in which a series of holes were made in a circle between which saw marks were subsequently made. The saw method consisted of the creation of four saw marks in a square to enable a piece of bone to be removed from the skull. The final method involved the creation of a small hole with a drill (which can strictly be called a trephination).

These types of trepanation appear in differing frequencies in different parts of the world and eras. For example, the scraping method appears more frequently in Europe and the sawing method in South America. Studies of the site of trepanation indicate that many were performed on the left side of the frontal and parietal bones; rarely were these operations performed over the skull sutures. Hippocrates, writing in the fifth century BC (and many other authors), recommended not to trepan over the sutures for fear of lacerating a major vein (Lisowski, 1967). One can imagine the agony suffered by the patient in antiquity. Such agony may not have been physical, since after cutting the soft tissues the operation is relatively painless, particularly if pain relief is assisted by alcohol or by herbal preparations; drugs such as opium, henbane and mandrake have all been quoted as herbs used for inducing anaesthesia and analgesia in particular population groups.

During all of these processes the bone dust created may have been collected. In more recent periods human skull dust has been used among developing societies as a magical remedy (Janssens, 1970); it is known that trepanation was also undertaken to produce amulets. Whatever method was employed by whichever society, the end result was the removal of a piece of skull and the exposure of the membranes covering the brain. The post-operative care of this bloody and potentially infected area of operation is equally impressive, particularly in view of the survival of many victims. A study by Stewart (1958a) found that over 50 per cent of 214 skulls with trepanation from Peru had healed. In Britain it is apparent that the scraping method was accompanied by better survival than the other methods. Perhaps the gradual scraping of the skull allowed more precise and controlled penetration of the inner table of bone and hence less likelihood of brain injury. Osteitis and bone scarring surrounding the hole in the skull has been attributed to chemical irritants applied post-operatively. These features are, however, more likely to be due to sepsis of the wound (Stewart, 1958a). Doubtless some closure of the skin wound must have been made, either by drawing together the skin flaps or by the application of a pad, possibly of vegetation. It was noted, for instance, in historic times in Melanesia that the operation site was covered with materials such as wood bark, banana leaf and coconut shell.

The technique of operation is plain to see. The motive for the operation is not known for certain in most cases, and most likely lies in the culture of the societies who practised this operation. The popular and somewhat romantic notion that trepanation was carried out solely for magico-ritual reasons is hardly credible. Such a reason there may have been for carrying out the operation on a corpse, and this undoubtedly did occur. In these cases no healing would be expected and post-mortem damage may be implicated for the lesion. The absence of documentation from the long periods of prehistory permits only speculation. It is difficult to imagine living people submitting themselves willingly to such an horrific operation with a high mortality merely for ritual reasons, although they may have had no choice. And yet, as Oakley *et al.* remarked (1959), so many trepanned skulls have been found in the chambered tombs of the Seine–Oise–Marne area of France that it is probable that the operation had some ritual significance; roundels of human skull bone have been found in early prehistoric graves, suggesting that such objects were treated as fetishes by prehistoric people.

To the contemporary mind, however, the bizarre behaviour of the schizophrenic, the strange uncontrollable fits of the epileptic, and the incapacitating head pain of migraine may have seemed sufficient justification to 'let the evil spirit out of the brain'. These illnesses are without skeletal manifestation and must, therefore, remain speculative. There is clear documentary evidence, at least from Hippocratic times, that the operation was also carried out for justifiable clinical reasons, even by modern standards. Hippocrates recommended trepanation for wounds of the head and haematoma. Celsus also proposed the operation for cranial injuries (Lisowski, 1967). It has been noted in many examples that trepanation may be related to the site of cranial fracture (Haneveld and Perizonius, 1980; Wells 1982; Parker *et al.*, 1986), and recent evidence suggests infection of the sinuses may have initiated trepanation (Zias and Pomeranz, 1992), where a skull with two healed and one unhealed trepanations also had evidence of frontal sinusitis and intracranial infection.

Whatever the ailment being treated in the past, it is certainly clear that the association of increased intracranial pressure and head wounds was recognized. There are several other lesions of the skull that may be considered in a differential diagnosis for trepanation; thinning of the parietal bones resulting in a hole (usually in old age), tumours producing holes in the tables of the skull, enlarged parietal foramina and post-mortem damage. However, with the advent of the use of sophisticated methods of analysis such as the scanning electron microscope, these differential diagnoses should be easily eliminated.

Treatment of fractures

Satisfactory healing of fractures in adults is a long process taking perhaps many weeks, during which time total rest of the injured part is essential. This may not have been too difficult to do in the case of an upper limb fracture in the past, when the afflicted individual would have been able to perform some tasks with the opposite limb. It would have been much more difficult in the case of a person from a small community who fractured a lower limb bone. There must have been little room for 'passengers' in the work-centred groups of the past, particularly in hunter-gatherer populations. In such cases the injured, if he or she survived, would have been dependent for welfare upon kinspeople. And what reorganization of lifestyle of the group would be required if the injured was a member of a nomadic group, for surely he or she would be totally incapacitated for perhaps 3 months with a badly fractured femur? Bone fractures healing in a position of poor alignment are a common finding in skeletal remains from the past. The large bones such as the femur, which are surrounded by powerful muscles which will contract strongly around the site of fracture, are the most common sites for this malalignment. Satisfactory bone healing in a position of good alignment is even less likely in the case of the comminuted fracture. Add to the intense pain of the leg fracture, the long period of total immobility and dependence upon others and the subsequent crippling due to a grossly shortened leg, and it may be possible to gain an insight into the sufferings of the injured victim of antiquity. This is not to say that all fractures of the past healed with such appalling results.

The successful treatment of fractures is suggested in both art and written records contemporary with many historically documented populations world-wide. This is in contradiction to the statement by Wells (1974b: 220), 'with very few exceptions they [Anglo-Saxons] made virtually no difference to what the natural healing powers of the body would have achieved unaided'. The study of developing societies also supports the fact already discussed earlier, that treatment of fractures by reduction and splinting is a very simple and logical knowledge to acquire. Reduction by manipulation, or sometimes traction, and splinting of broken bones with natural products such as bark, reeds (Fig. 5.19), bamboo (Carroll, 1972), animal skins (Fortuine, 1984) and clay are observed in some societies, suggesting that, at least, some thought is being channelled into caring for the injured. Herbal concoctions and bandages, and the use of animal hair and plant fibres, comprise methods of treatment of associated wounds. The Yoruba of Nigeria today (Oyebola, 1980) are conversant with the clinical features of fractures (pain, swelling, deformity and loss of function) but, having no radiography facility, they may miss the diagnosis of crack and greenstick fractures, identifying only the major breaks. Herbal dressings and splints are applied and reapplied daily following hot fomentations. The results vary but observations suggest that

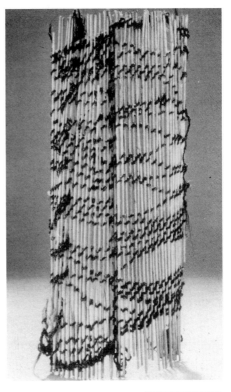

WELLCOME INSTITUTE

5.19 Reed splint used in developing communities to stabilize fractures once reduced

patients are mobilized too early, reduction is not maintained consistently and that this delays healing. However, despite these shortcomings it is clear that relatively effective treatment is practised in this and other developing societies and there is no reason to suggest that this was not the case in past communities.

Hippocrates had an intimate knowledge of the bones and joints, and described methods of treatment of dislocations and fractures, some of which are still used today. Reduction and splinting of fractures and maintaining the fracture in reduction with pads and bandages reinforced by clays and starches, including the adjacent joints in the splint using the other elements of the limb to anatomically splint the broken bone, e.g. radius/ulna and tibia/fibula, were all recommended methods of treatment for fractures by Hippocrates. He also suggested a healthy diet. During later eras in Europe similar fracture treatment methods were advocated by surgeons such as Guy De Chauliac (1300–70, France), who was the first to reduce fractures by traction (Clark, 1937: 53), Ambroisé Paré (1510–90, France) and Hieronymus Brunschwig (1450–1533, Germany).

Apart from surgeons, who would have become involved with the treatment of fractures, bonesetters were a group of people who developed specifically for this purpose; they appear to have been present in many countries around the world, particularly in the sixteenth and seventeenth centuries AD. The 'natural' bonesetter was the forerunner of the orthopaedic surgeon. He or she met the needs of the majority of the population when they had an illness involving bone, joint or muscle. The bonesetting skill was believed to descend in families. Herbal remedies such as comfrey ('knitbone') and 'bonewort' (violet/pansy) mixed with egg white were also recommended for fractured bones (Bonser, 1963) in early medieval England, but the treatment of wounds associated with fractures varied from the relatively sensible (wine, honey) to the need to make the wound septic (the 'laudable pus' of Galen; Knight, 1981). Stitching wounds was practised, the earliest evidence dating to 1100 BC in an Egyptian mummy (Black, 1982: 620), and linen, catgut, silk, wool and metal clips were also used, in addition to less conventional wound treatment in the form of cautery (application of hot irons) being used at times.

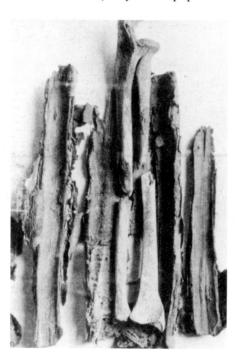

5.20 Tree-bark used as splints on a mummified arm in Egypt 5,000 years ago

Splints made from natural products, such as those identified in developing societies, were probably used for fracture treatment but rarely are they preserved in the archaeological record attached to fractured bones. Interestingly, most fractures found archaeologically are healed, which would preclude the need to bury a body with splints. However, some examples of splinting have been identified. Elliot–Smith (1908) described splints of bark held in place with linen bandages on broken, unhealed limbs of mummies from Egypt dated to 5000 BC (Fig. 5.20).

Although there is evidence in Egypt for limbs being broken post-mortem during the embalming process and splints being attached, it is known from documentary evidence that splinting as a form of treatment for fractures was practised at that time. Other direct evidence for treatment comes from the humeri and a knee joint of four skeletons from different sites and periods in Europe. Copper plates were found around the humerus of a skeleton of late sixteenth and early seventeenth-century date in Belgium, but with no evidence of disease underneath the plates (Janssens, 1987). Copper plates lined with ivy leaves were also found around the humerus of a medieval skeleton from Reading in Berkshire, England (Wells, 1964b) (Fig. 5.21). The final case, also on a humerus, comes from a Swedish skeleton (Hällback, 1976). The latter two cases had evidence of ante-mortem disease/trauma. The infected knee of an individual from the medieval cemetery of Fishergate, York (Stroud and Kemp, 1993) also appeared to have had copper plates applied to this area. All these cases indicate that copper was probably known to have a therapeutic effect.

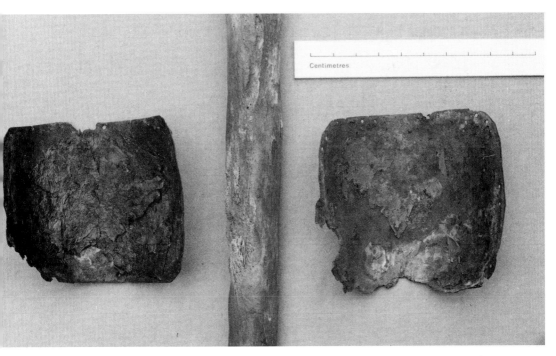

READING MUSEUM

5.21 Copper plates associated with a humerus, Reading, Berkshire, UK

Any assessment of whether a society treated fractures or not in the past should be undertaken using multidisciplinary forms of evidence (Roberts, 1988a, 1991), and data should be compared with modern clinical data on fractures treated by simple external reduction and splinting. The study of skeletal remains from archaeological sites provides a large data set for considering trauma and its implications for lifestyle in the past, as shown in this chapter. Like trauma, the joint diseases were also common in the past and will be covered in the next chapter.

CHAPTER 6

Joint Disease

To each his suff'rings: all are men, condemn'd alike to groan.

(Thomas Gray 1716–71)

INTRODUCTION

Degenerative diseases are a group of separate and yet in some ways related abnormalities. Gradual deterioration with advancing age is a phenomenon of both animal and plant worlds. In long-lived organisms, there is more time for degenerative disease to appear, advance and become clinically manifest with approaching senility. Degenerative processes affect all the major body systems. The confusion and memory loss of senile dementia due to cerebral degeneration; the dizziness, 'stroke' and coronary thrombosis of arterial degeneration; and the pain, limp and stiffness of degenerative arthritis are examples of the age-related degenerative diseases. It is a phenomenon most obvious in humans possibly because, in contrast to many non-humans, people live longer, especially today. That is not to say that non-humans do not suffer from degenerative diseases; many examples of joint disease in other mammals occur in the literature (e.g. Lovell, 1990). Joint disease is a very old disease; it has even been diagnosed in the fossilized spine of a Comanchean dinosaur of 100,000,000 years ago (Karsh and McCarthy, 1960). Degeneration of joints is also observed in earlier humans who may not have lived as long as later groups (Trinkhaus, 1983). However, age is not the only factor in the development of joint disease (see below).

Of the multitude of symptoms and signs known in clinical practice today to be due to the degenerative process, only the degeneration of joint and bone are obviously recognizable in the skeletal remains of the past. The soft-tissue degenerations may, of course, be found in mummified soft tissues, but evisceration during the mummification technique may destroy this evidence. The arterial degenerations, however, have been found in Egyptian mummies through microscopical examination of their soft tissues. This disease, for long assumed to be a problem of our modern lifestyle, has thus been shown to have a history of several thousand years. Whether the inhabitants of that time suffered the same frequency of 'strokes' or coronary thrombosis, the complications of arterial degeneration, is regrettably not known. These problems of such increasing social and economic importance may not be new phenomena at all.

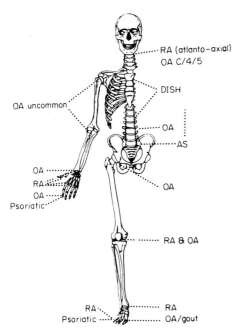

6.1 Distribution pattern of some of the joint diseases. (Reproduced with permission of Juliet Rogers)

Key
RA Rheumatoid arthritis
OA Osteoarthritis
AS Ankylosing spondylitis
DISH Diffuse idiopathic skeletal hyperostosis

The common diseases of degeneration affecting the skeleton are the joint diseases. In past (and some current) literature the terminology of these diseases does often appear confused; the simultaneous use of osteoarthrosis, osteoarthritis, degenerative joint disease, arthropathies and rheumatism is seen. Changes occurring in joints of different anatomical and functional type were often all considered as one and, hence, early descriptions of joint disease in skeletal remains were imprecise. These different joint diseases, to a large extent, have now been clarified and, using a clinical base, their characteristics, causes and clinical symptoms have been established; there is, however, still much research to be done.

Along with dental disease and trauma, the joint diseases comprise most of the evidence for disease in past human groups; 1–5 per cent of US citizens under the age of 45 years and 15–85 per cent of those older than 45 years are afflicted today, especially with osteoarthritis and rheumatoid arthritis (Cotran *et al.*, 1989: 1346), and around a quarter of all patients in the UK visit their doctor because of joint disease. The joint diseases affect one or more joints of the body, usually in a clearly defined distribution pattern (Fig. 6.1); they may destroy or form bone or promote both. The problem with diagnosing specific joint diseases in palaeopathology is that many of these numerous diseases leave identical marks on the skeleton; this means that a complete skeleton is a prerequisite to diagnosis of the different joint diseases. Even with modern technological advances in medicine, diagnosis may not be easy.

JOINT ANATOMY AND PHYSIOLOGY

The joints of the body can be classified by joint movement and by histological features. A synarthrosis is a fixed or rigid joint (e.g. sutures of the skull), an amphiarthrosis is a slightly moveable joint (e.g. the pubic symphysis) and the diarthroses are freely moveable joints (e.g. the hip). A fibrous joint may be a tooth in its socket, while cartilaginous joints include the intervertebral articulations, and a synovial joint (one whose cavity is lined by synovial membrane, and contains synovial fluid) may be the hip, knee or elbow; this latter type tends to be affected more in the joint diseases. A joint's function depends on the geometry of the bone surfaces which meet each other, its functional integrity in terms of surrounding muscles, tendons and ligaments, and the strength, resilience and elasticity of the articular cartilage covering the joint surfaces and the underlying bone; any changes to these structures may lead to subsequent degeneration. For example, damage to ligaments holding the knee stable may lead to malpositioning of the joint and degeneration.

Cartilage covers the joint surfaces and has a number of functions: transmission and distribution of loads, maintenance of contact between the bones of the joint with little friction, and absorption of shock. The first stages of joint disease usually involve the cartilage; repeated stress leads to breaking up of the cartilage structure by fissuring, flaking and pitting, and loss of cartilage leads to exposure of the bone underneath it. The joint diseases are classified in many different ways but, basically, the abnormalities observed are proliferative (bone formation), erosive (destruction of bone) or both. Table 6.1 shows one classification and includes those joint diseases to be covered in this chapter. The term 'spondyloarthropathies' can be used to define psoriatic arthritis, ankylosing spondylitis and Reiter's syndrome (not covered here), where there is a tendency for spinal involvement and the absence of rheumatoid factor, found in the blood of people with rheumatoid arthritis (Rogers et al., 1987).

Table 6.1 Classification of joint diseases

Neuromechanical	Osteoarthritis:
	     primary (with increasing age)
	     secondary (any age in a previously damaged joint)

Inflammatory*	Septic arthritis
Immune	Rheumatoid arthritis Psoriatic arthritis Ankylosing spondylitis Forestier's disease (DISH)
Metabolic	Gouty arthritis

* May also include rheumatoid arthritis, ankylosing spondylitis and psoriatic arthritis.

JOINT DISEASE: PATHOLOGICAL PROCESS

Skeletal involvement in the joint diseases potentially consists of two processes: formation and destruction of bone. Formation of bone is in the form of bony outgrowths from joint surfaces called osteophytes (Fig. 6.2); these represent the body's attempt to spread the load at the joint and compensate for the stress to

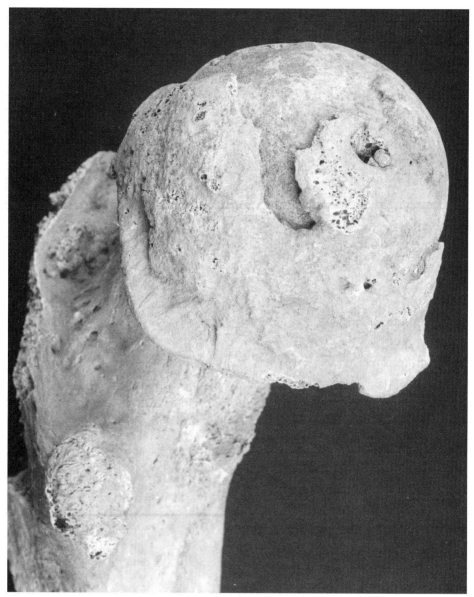

6.2 Osteophytes on joint surface and margins of femoral head (medieval France)

which the joint is being subject. Osteophytes may occur on the joint surface, marginal to it or away from it, e.g. at insertions of ligaments and tendons (entheses); in addition, new bone may form in the periosteum as a reaction to changes in the joints themselves (Rogers *et al.*, ibid.: 180). The extent and character of this new bone formation varies between and around the joint, and this may be characteristic of a particular joint disease.

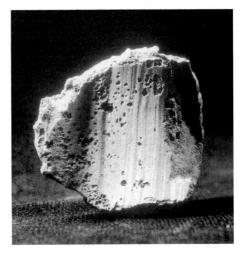

LYNN KILGORE

6.3 Eburnation of a patella (Kulubnarti, Nubia)

Once cartilage is destroyed and the individual continues to use the joint, the underlying bone can become very hard (sclerosis) and polished (eburnation – Fig. 6.3). If osteophyte formation is extensive a joint may become fused. Ossification may occur in cartilage away from the joint itself in some joint diseases; for example, the disease abbreviated to DISH (see below) usually involves ossification of costal (rib) and neck cartilages. Bone may also be destroyed in the joint diseases, on the joint surfaces themselves, on their margins or distal to the joint; the patterning and character of these lesions may aid in diagnosis. The destruction of the cartilage on the joint surface allows the bone to degenerate and become porous (Fig. 6.4). Synovial fluid can then infiltrate into the bone directly under the cartilage; the lesions formed are called subchondral cysts and are readily visible on radiographs (Fig. 6.5).

Resnick and Niwayama (1988: 1914) suggest that 'An accurate radiological diagnosis of joint disease is based on evaluation of two fundamental parameters; the morphology of the articular lesions and their distribution in the body.' The same can be said for macroscopic examination of the dry-bone lesions in the skeleton. However, comparison between archaeological and modern population groups in terms of the prevalence of osteoarthritis is difficult, largely because many of the diagnostic methods are different. For example, the occurrence of relevant symptoms, and changes on radiography, such as joint space narrowing, seen in a modern patient would not be possible to assess for an archaeological joint. It has been shown, for example, that radiography may not identify all the degenerative joint changes visible macroscopically (Riddle *et al.*, 1988; Rogers *et al.*, 1990), and that quite subtle joint changes may be missed if radiography is used for diagnosis (of course, this is not an option for modern diagnosis); this may explain, as Rogers *et al.* (ibid.) suggest, why the signs and symptoms of modern patients do not always correlate with radiographic findings.

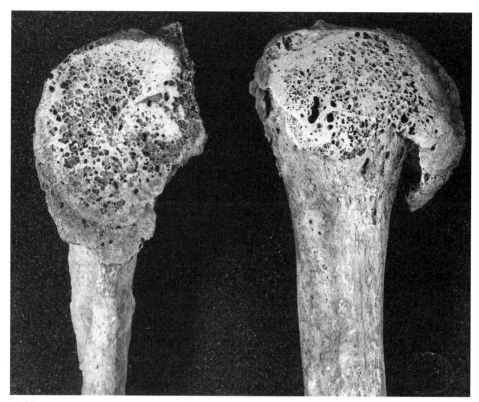

6.4 Porosity on joint surfaces of shoulder (4th century AD, Gloucester, England)

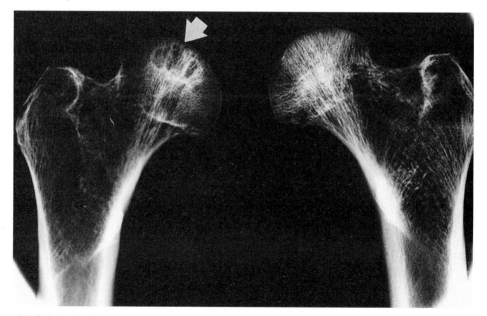

6.5 Subchondral cysts illustrated on a radiograph

OSTEOARTHRITIS

The most commonly occurring joint disease seen in archaeological human groups is osteoarthritis; this disease is non-inflammatory and affects the synovial joints (see Rogers and Waldron, 1994: 2, for the structure of a synovial joint). Diagnosis of osteoarthritis rests on the identification of the abnormalities already described, but osteoarthritis cannot be diagnosed purely on the basis of one of these features. For example, the formation of osteophytes can occur merely as a result of the ageing process. Waldron and Rogers (1991) recommend that, if eburnation is not present on the joint surface (a sure sign of osteoarthritis) then two other features of osteoarthritis must be present, e.g. osteophytes and a porous joint surface. The recording of joint disease on skeletal material has resulted in many different methods being proposed by different authors. The basic point to make is that, as with any palaeopathological lesion, recording the basic data in a standardized format is essential so that comparisons can be made. Photographs and definitions of severity must be included in reports so that another researcher can be sure that their 'severe' grade of osteoarthritis is the same as that of another study (for some examples of recording formats see Walker and Hollimon, 1989; Jurmain, 1990). Futhermore, generation of the distribution pattern of joint changes in the different bones of a joint in males and females (Fig. 6.6) may help in assessing the different loading patterns across a joint surface, how these may differ between the sexes and what the aetiological factors might have been (Merbs, 1983). What is clear is that every joint and all parts of it should be assessed to ensure a realistic picture of joint disease in groups of skeletons.

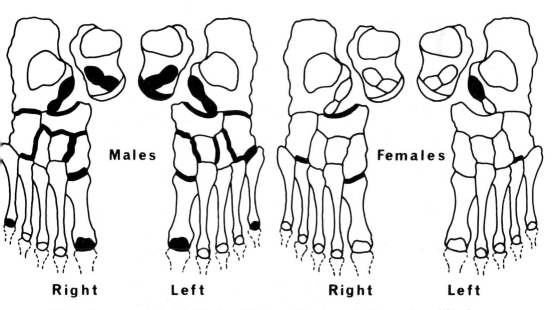

6.6 Involvement of the bones of the foot (black areas) in osteoarthritis in males and females from a Canadian Inuit population. (Reproduced with permission of Charles Merbs)

Bearing these factors in mind, it is useful to consider the study by Waldron and Rogers (1991) where people with varying degrees of expertise were given the opportunity of recording presence and absence of osteoarthritis in a series of joints. Presence and absence of eburnation, osteophytes, new bone on the joint surface, pitting of the joint and deformation of the joint contour were recorded, and the severity of lesions. There was little overall difference in agreement between beginners and experts; but there was disagreement as to whether or not the bony changes were present and their degree of severity. The presence of eburnation and new bone formation on the joint were the most agreed on criteria. Interestingly, all ten specimens had osteoarthritis according to the authors' criteria, but there were only three specimens unanimously agreed upon by the experts and only one by the beginners. This reflects the problems in recording osteoarthritis; if the basic data are not recorded accurately then any interpretations will be invalid.

Osteoarthritis is multifactorial in its aetiology. Increasing age, a genetic predisposition, obesity (leading to stress on the joints), activity/lifestyle and environmental factors such as climate may all contribute to its development. Urbanized, as opposed to rural, environments may produce different prevalence rates and skeletal distribution patterns in populations, both today and in the past. Pain, limitation of movement and deformity of joints may be clinical features associated with osteoarthritis, but some studies have shown no association between severity of joint involvement and symptoms (see above). Of course, any joint of the body can be affected, and some have characteristic epidemiologies. For example, shoulder osteoarthritis usually follows severe trauma or is related to a specific activity; it is also associated with damage to the rotator cuff soft tissues of this joint.

SPINAL JOINT DISEASE

One of the penalties paid by humans for their adoption of the erect bipedal posture is an increased susceptibility to vertebral osteoarthritis, a direct consequence of spinal stress (Bridges, 1994). It might be thought that the mechanical stress and strain upon each segment of the spine is constant in the upright posture. However, the spine is not just a straight line and exhibits a backward curve in the chest or thoracic region and a forward curve in the lumbar and cervical regions, leading to the fifth cervical, eighth thoracic and fourth lumbar vertebrae being most affected. It is suggested (Nathan, 1962) that because of these curves there are points of maximum and minimum stress, and that this is responsible for the variation in osteoarthritis in the spine.

The intervertebral discs consist of a fibrous 'capsule' containing a gelatinous internal substance. With advancing age a chemical and degenerative change occurs in these tissues. The constant stress to which these discs are subject, in the bending and lifting of everyday activity, causes the internal nucleus pulposus to invade the annulus fibrosus. The rupture of this fibrous capsule stimulates the growth of bone from the margins of the vertebral body itself (osteophytes or osteophytosis – see Fig. 6.7). This is a compensatory reaction to injury just like many other body reactions to trauma. For reasons of pure mechanics, the anterior area of the annulus and vertebral body are more liable to the process of osteophytosis than the posterior area. With increasing stress and annulus rupture, the size of osteophytes increases. At the extreme, the osteophytes from contiguous vertebrae grow together and unite, so fixing the spinal segment and preventing movement. This localized and restricted fixation, or ankylosis, is not to be confused with the more generalized diseases of spinal fixation which will be considered later. The inexorable advance of time results in all people developing the clinical symptoms and signs of vertebral osteophytosis. The intermittent backache, the stiffness and inability to touch the toes are the all too familiar features of this ageing process. Just as today, so it was in antiquity.

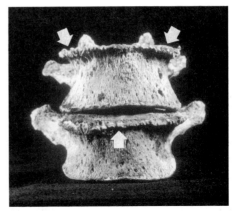

LYNN KILGORE

6.7 Spinal osteophytosis (Kulubnarti, Nubia)

In reviewing relatively modern vertebral columns, Nathan (1962) found that by the third decade of life a large proportion of individuals studied had vertebral osteophytosis, and by the fifth decade all of them had the condition. Stewart (1958b) has also used spinal osteophytes as a method of ageing adult skeletons. Since this is a mechanically induced condition there is, naturally, variation among individuals. The man or woman engaged in heavy manual work is more liable to develop osteophytosis than the sedentary worker. Quite probably, therefore, the more active lifestyle of people in antiquity will have developed their vertebral osteophytosis at an earlier age than their modern office-working descendent. Certainly the condition is almost universal in adult skeletal remains of the past, although its frequency varies between groups.

Apart from the vertebral body surfaces, the posterior apophyseal joints and transverse process joints of the vertebrae are also affected in osteoarthritis (Fig. 6.8). Associated with osteophytosis and degeneration of the intervertebral discs are Schmorl's nodes (Fig. 6.9), where the disc contents exert pressure on the vertebral body surfaces. These nodes are seen in the lower thoracic and lumbar spine and, in many cases, their specific aetiology may be unknown (Saluja *et al.*, 1986). Trauma has been implicated as one of the major causes of this condition, with underlying infection, osteoporosis and neoplastic disease weakening the bone structure, enabling Schmorl's nodes to develop (Resnick and Niwayama, 1988: 1528).

Spinal joint disease seems to be ubiquitous in past human groups of all periods (Trinkhaus, 1985) but in varying degrees of severity and distribution through the spine, perhaps reflecting the influence of lifestyle or occupation on its

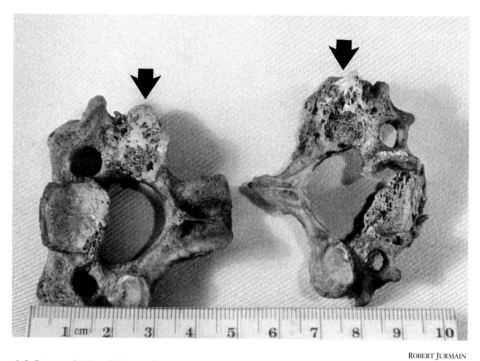

ROBERT JURMAIN

6.8 Osteoarthritis of the apophyseal joints of cervical vertebrae. Ala 329, San Francisco Bay, California (500 BC–AD 1700)

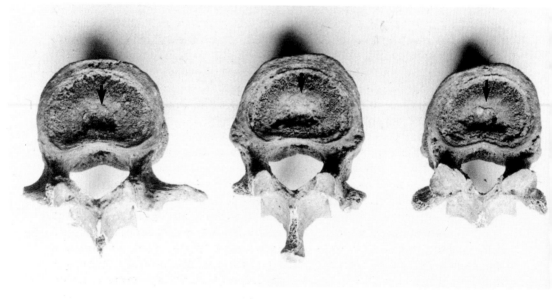

CALVIN WELLS PHOTOGRAPHIC COLLECTION

6.9 Schmorl's nodes in the superior surfaces of vertebral bodies

development. For example, Bridges (1994) reports a high frequency of neck osteoarthritis in 125 skeletons from north-west Alabama; carrying loads through use of a tumpline around the forehead is considered as a cause. A pioneering study by Sager (1969) set some precedents for recording spinal osteoarthritis for archaeological populations. Sager examined 100 cervical spines (52 males and 48 females) of a Danish modern urban population and skeletons from medieval monastic and hospital cemeteries from Denmark; the characteristic osteoarthritic changes already discussed were recorded. This study concluded that the modern material had a higher prevalence rate in all age groups than in the archaeological material. Sager's descriptions and photographic records of the stages in the disease were exemplary. A more recent study by Lovell (1994) examined joint changes in spines of individuals from a Bronze-Age site in Pakistan (4,000–5,000 years ago). The results showed that, although the pattern of arthritis in the neck vertebrae was unusual, this patterning may have been reflecting activity such as carrying heavy loads on the head. As there was no increase in prevalence with age in this study, an occupation-related aetiology was supported.

OCCUPATION AND ARTHRITIS

It is clear from modern clinical data that people practising particular occupations suffer osteoarthritis (and other changes) at certain joints, although the links are not very clear-cut. Study of, for example, osteoarthritic changes in skeletons from forensic contexts as an aid in identification has been noted, i.e. correlating osteoarthritis patterning (and changes in the robusticity of the bones) with the occupation of the individual who became the victim (Wienker and Wood, 1987). There has been a recent proliferation of work in this area as researchers try to 'put flesh on the bones'. In archaeology the study of activity-related changes in the skeleton has been used to identify differences in lifestyle with subsistence change, e.g. the transition from hunter-gathering to agriculture. Waldron (1994), however, warns of the dangers of stretching the evidence too far and the lack of correlation of bone degeneration with specific occupations in modern studies; he summarizes the potential problems inherent in an archaeological study of lifestyle, occupation and osteoarthritis. If, today, one considers the multitude of activities people are engaged in during one week of their lives, for example, each of these could affect the body. But what should be remembered is that, 'the same kinds of activities will be performed over and over again particularly if they are necessary for survival' (Merbs, 1983: 1). If a person practises a very heavy manual occupation which severely stresses the joints, it is likely that a particular patterning may occur for that specific occupation. Of course, many other factors (not least age and obesity) can influence the development of osteoarthritis and these may determine whether osteoarthritis develops and is identifiable to a specific activity. To counteract the effects of age it may be useful to study younger individuals; if osteoarthritis is seen here in a particularly high prevalence and specific patterning, it may be possible to suggest an occupationally induced osteoarthritis for this group. It is also accepted that for occupationally related changes to show, the person must start the activity young. What is perhaps safer is, in addition, to use other skeletal markers such as enthesophytes (new bone formation at tendinous and ligament insertions as a result of increase in size of associated muscles) and changes in the size and robusticity of bones, to try to suggest related activity. In addition, several 'non-metric traits' may be related to occupation (Saunders, 1989), e.g. squatting facets, and recent work has suggested that differences in bone mineral content and density may be implicated as indicators of greater mechanical loading, particularly in the dominant arm (Faulkner *et al.*, 1993). There is little direct information about occupations in the past and how they may have affected health, and much of that knowledge is based on assumption, which is then applied to skeletal populations. Whatever method of analysis is used to look at the link between occupation and arthritis, the process is not easy, and the use of comparative clinical data, ethnographic analogy and art and documentary sources is essential (Kennedy, 1989: 156).

The historical literature abounds with works on occupationally related diseases (see Kennedy, ibid. for a summary). Bernardino Ramazzini was the first author to write a treatise on diseases of workers, in Italy, in AD 1700 (Louis, 1990). Called *A treatise on the diseases of tradesmen*, it described forty-two occupations, including miners, midwives and painters, and Ramazzini was awarded the title of 'father of industrial medicine'. From this time many people became involved in looking for relationships between occupation and changes in the body. The problem with many of the associated diseases described is that a large percentage do not involve the bone. There are certainly some fascinating occupationally related diseases in the modern literature (Cherniack, 1992); 'hatter's shakes' were the result of mercury poisoning in the hatter's trade when mercury was applied to rabbit skins in the manufacturing process, and 'potter's rot' occurred when workers were exposed to silica, leading to silicosis, especially in the pottery trade. Furthermore, with the domestication of animals, populations became subject to another set of diseases. For example, anthrax is contracted by humans mainly through contact with domesticated animals and their skins; 'wool sorter's disease' was the name applied to anthrax in people working with wool in the nineteenth century (Meyer, 1964). Of particular relevance generally to occupationally induced changes in the skeleton was the law proposed in AD 1892, by a German anatomist, Julius Wolff, known as 'Wolff's law of transformation', which stated that bone will adapt to functional pressure or force by increasing or decreasing its mass to resist the stress (Kennedy, ibid.: 134); formation of bone will sustain and distribute the load. This means that if the body is involved with a repeated activity the skeleton will respond by becoming 'larger'. Enthesophytes will also develop at muscular attachments and degeneration of the joints will occur.

A number of archaeologically based studies have been published on the relationship of occupation and arthritis. They are of two types: first, studies of the generalized distribution of osteoarthritis around the body in a skeletal population, often discussed with reference to occupation and lifestyle; and, secondly, studies directly addressing the question of osteoarthritis prevalence and change in economy. Bearing in mind the premise that occupation is a difficult study area in archaeological populations, there have been interesting studies. Perhaps one of the most consulted examples of osteoarthritis and its relationship to activity is that of Merbs (1983). Osteoarthritis was recorded for both male and female skeletons in a Canadian Eskimo group. Males had more lower-limb osteoarthritis, and females had more changes in the temporomandibular joints and some of the vertebral joints. Osteoarthritis was seen more in the thoracic region in females and in the lumbar spine in males. By studying reports of accounts of meetings with the Sadlermiut Eskimos before their extinction, reports on discussions with the Aivilingmiut, who had lived with the Sadlermiut earlier, and the archaeological record, Merbs was able to reconstruct potential activities within this group of people (Merbs, ibid.: 138–9). As he said, 'this is not as good as a first hand detailed ethnographic account, but it does allow a reconstruction of the most important elements of Sadlermiut behavior'. Merbs interpreted the osteoarthritic patterning seen in the material studied as being due to the male activities of harpoon throwing, kayak paddling and lifting and carrying heavy loads, and in the females as due to making clothes, carrying children and sledding. Similar work is reported by Lai and Lovell (1992) who recorded joint disease and other skeletal changes (enthesophytes and increased bone robusticity) which may be consistent with habitual lifting, canoeing and paddling or rowing in three males dated to the Fur Trade Period in Alberta, Canada. Transport of furs, provisions and officers of the Hudson's Bay Fur Trade Company was by canoe and boat on fast-flowing rivers; some journeys lasted seventeen or eighteen hours and it is possible that this type of work induced the skeletal changes observed.

Other studies have used osteoarthritis as a means to answering questions about activity in contrasting economies, particularly in hunter-gathering and agricultural economies, and conclusions vary. Cohen and Armelagos (1984), in summing up the data for physical stress (including osteoarthritis and skeletal robusticity) in the studies in their book, suggest that there was a probable reduction in workload associated with the adoption of agriculture (ibid.: 590), but this did not necessarily imply less time spent on food production. Furthermore, many of the hunter-gatherer groups studied had greater longevity and this may have had an influencing effect on the development of osteoarthritis in these groups compared to the agricultural populations. Jurmain (1990) found a similar picture in his study of 167 skeletons from the south-eastern San Francisco Bay area, dating from AD 500 to pre-European contact. More osteoarthritis was seen than in comparative agricultural groups. Bridges (1991) also found this difference in the hunter-gatherer (6000–1000 BC) and agricultural (AD 1200–1500) groups she studied in north-east Alabama; the results, however, were not significant except for a few joints (Fig. 6.10). Multiple aetiological factors affecting a population's predisposition to osteoarthritis are suggested as the reason behind inconsistencies in results of similar studies. Bridges (ibid.) suggests that examination of bone strength and osteoarthritis may help to explain activity patterns in past populations, as these changes may be responses to different kinds of forces. Her study in 1989 showed that the agricultural population had stronger bones than their hunter-gathering predecessors, suggesting an increased workload; these findings are supported by osteoarthritis in the same populations, already discussed (Bridges, 1991). Goodman et al. (1984) also suggested significantly increased osteoarthritis in their Dickson Mound population with the

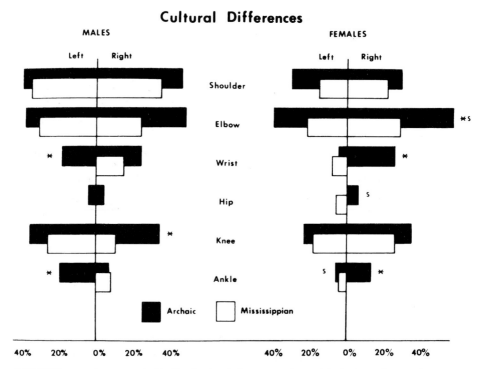

6.10 Differences in osteoarthritis distribution in hunter-gatherer (Archaic) and agricultural (Mississippian) populations. (Reproduced with permission from Patricia Bridges)

transition to agriculture, and Walker and Hollimon (1989) noted increased mechanical stress with a shift to intensive exploitation of a marine environment from hunter-gathering by southern Californian Indians in the Santa Barbara Channel area.

Related to these studies of the change in frequency of osteoarthritis in joints in populations practising different economies, there have been other supporting studies suggesting more specific activities. Molleson (1989) has described skeletal abnormalities of mesolithic/neolithic skeletons from Syria dated to around 8,000 years ago. Here, the abnormalities in the toe and ankle joints were suggested to be the result of extreme dorsiflexion of the joints of the foot in using a quernstone, and robust arm bones, osteoarthritis of the lower spine, knees and big toes also contributed to this picture. Ubelaker (1979) noted similar changes on the metatarsals and first proximal foot phalanx in a prehistoric sample from Ecuador, and suggested that a habitual kneeling posture may be implicated for the changes.

Occupation has become of great interest to biological anthropologists world-wide because assessing a person's lifestyle in the past helps to complete one more part of the complex jigsaw puzzle of past human behaviour. More specific studies of occupation should be discussed here briefly to show the range of potential in this area. The possible use of traumatic lesions (e.g. the clay-shoveller's fracture) and culturally induced dental modifications have already been described elsewhere in this book. What people specifically do for a living has been addressed by several authors. Kennedy (1986) considered the supposed correlation between auditory exostoses (bony growths in the ears) and immersion in cold water in populations from different geographic regions. The hypothesis was that low frequencies would be expected in polar and subpolar areas (i.e. avoidance of cold water because of the potential problem of hypothermia) and the tropical latitudes, where people were accustomed to warmer water. Higher frequencies were expected in people who exploited either marine or freshwater resources through diving

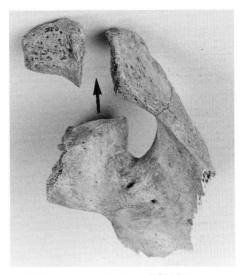

6.11 Os acromiale (medieval Chichester, England)

(ibid.: 407); these hypotheses were substantiated and the genetic predisposition for these abnormalities could not be sustained (Berry and Berry, 1967). In fact, it is now suggested that many of the non-metric, epigenetic skeletal traits described in the literature may be culturally and not genetically induced (Saunders, 1989). Stirland (1986) has considered the possible correlation between non-fusion of the acromial process of the scapula (os acromiale; Fig. 6.11) in skeletons from the *Mary Rose* which sank off the south coast of England in AD 1545. She found that of 110 individuals, 15 had os acromiale (13.6 per cent); comparison with modern dissection room frequencies of 8.0 per cent showed that there was a clear difference. The highest frequency in this archaeological group was found in the area of the ship where archery equipment was stored. Longbows were used from a very early age at this time, well before the fusion of the acromion could have occurred; a combination of this factor and possible fracture at the site may have been associated with archery. Of course, knowing the precise lifestyle of a person is useful for interpreting skeletal changes, and a study by Mann *et al.* (1991) is appropriate in this respect. Continued knee flexion, perhaps resulting from long-term paralysis, was inferred from the bony changes seen in the knees of three 'modern' skeletons. The medical histories of these individuals supported this interpretation even though a specific conclusive cause could not be supported on the evidence.

OSTEOARTHRITIS: SKELETAL INVOLVEMENT

In both archaeological and modern population studies, the hip and knee are often the most commonly affected joints of the body in osteoarthritis; these are the major weight-bearing joints. In the upper body, osteoarthritis of the elbow is rare today, except in people with particularly stressing occupations such as mining or pneumatic drilling (Resnick and Niwayama, 1988: 1406); osteoarthritis of the shoulder is also rare without a history of trauma. However, the acromioclavicular and sternoclavicular joints are affected in many elderly individuals today. The hands and feet are affected by osteoarthritis with varying rates in modern populations, with the joints of the hand (interphalangeal, metacarpophalangeal and some of the wrist bones) being commonly involved, especially in middle-aged post-menopausal women (Resnick and Niwayama, ibid.: 1398). Osteoarthritis of the ankle is rare but significant change in the first metatarsophalangeal joint (big toe) is seen frequently. Joint disease of the temporomandibular joint (TMJ) has already been discussed in Chapter 4. Its frequency in modern populations can be high and is discussed in Hodges (1991). This study examined the occurrence of osteoarthritis at the TMJ joint and its association with attrition, tooth loss, age and sex in five British skeletal populations. Only attrition and joint disease were significantly associated. Although attrition was probably a major predisposing factor to the development of joint disease in the jaw, structural abnormalities in the anatomy and physiology of the joint may also be a factor in its development.

In archaeological groups, osteoarthritis of the upper extremities is more common than for modern populations (Merbs, 1983: 99), which is surprising because increasing age is a strong correlate of shoulder and hip osteoarthritis rather than elbow and knee osteoarthritis (Jurmain, 1980: 144). If people live longer today then a higher frequency of joint disease in the shoulder would be expected. However, it is likely that osteoarthritis in the upper limb suggests a lifestyle predisposing these joints to degeneration, a lifestyle which was quite different from that of today. Skeletal studies have also shown a stronger side difference in size of upper compared to lower limbs, probably reflecting lifestyle or occupation (Constandse-Westermann and Newell, 1989).

Relatively little work has been carried out on osteoarthritis of the hand and foot in archaeological groups, perhaps because these smaller bones often do not survive burial and excavation. Hand osteoarthritis is a common finding in modern population studies, especially in females (Resnick and Niwayama, 1988) and may be related to occupation; in fact, one of the few studies of osteoarthritis of the hands suggests a similar frequency in past populations (Waldron, 1993a). Waldron and Cox (1989) also examined the hand bones of 367 skeletons from the crypt excavations at Spitalfields, London, dated to between AD 1729 and 1869. The occupations of these individuals were obtained from historical sources; twenty-nine of the males were weavers, the hypothesis being that this occupation could induce hand osteoarthritis. However, of the thirteen males with osteoarthritis in their hands, only three were weavers, and there appeared to be a strong correlation with increased age in those affected.

SEPTIC ARTHRITIS

Several other specific joint diseases deserve discussion in this chapter. Septic or inflammatory arthritis is also discussed in Chapter 7 under 'tuberculosis', but septic arthritis can also be caused by organisms other than *Mycobacterium*

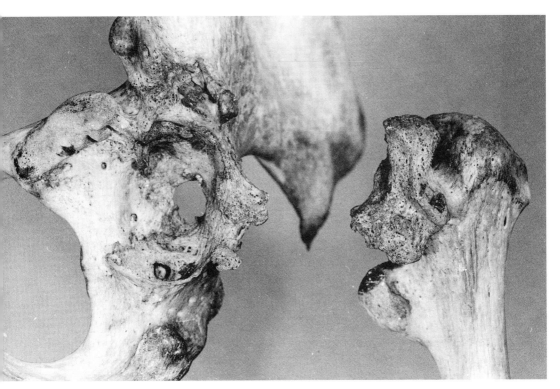

6.12 Septic arthritis of hip: NMNH 345394, Eskimo male, 20 years old, Yukon River, Alaska, ? historic

tuberculosis. Arthritis caused by non-specific infection may have two aetiological pathways. The bacteria (usually Streptococcus or Staphylococcus; Resnick and Niwayama, 1988) spread via the blood to the joint cavity, but infection of a joint can also result from spread of an infection from the bone to the joint (e.g. osteomyelitis). In a normal synovial joint the synovial fluid nourishes the cartilage, particularly with sugars. In septic arthritis the cartilage is starved of these sugars because of the competing needs of the bacteria. Septic arthritis usually affects one joint, the knee or the hip in two-thirds of cases (Ortner and Putschar, 1981: 399), but other joints can potentially be involved. When compared to tuberculous arthritis, septic arthritis caused by other organisms (although usually an acute condition) is less destructive of the joint surfaces and is characterized by erosion of the bone around the edges of the articulating area, and a reduced tendency to fusion. Whereas tuberculous arthritis primarily affects children, non-specific septic arthritis can affect all ages. Septic arthritis is an infrequent finding in archaeological material (Fig. 6.12), and distinguishing between a tuberculous and non-tuberculous aetiology is often problematic without other supporting evidence in the skeleton for tuberculosis, for example. Septic arthritis may also be complicated by non-septic osteoarthritis or other joint diseases, so that, in any one individual, a number of joint diseases may present themselves but are impossible to differentiate from one another.

RHEUMATOID ARTHRITIS

Compared to osteoarthritis, rheumatoid arthritis (RA) in the archaeological record is rarely seen. Although, in skeletal material, the palaeopathologist only sees the bony changes of rheumatoid arthritis, it is a disease affecting multiple systems of the body (Cotran *et al.*, 1989: 1349). It is a chronic inflammatory disease of connective tissue and has adult and juvenile (Still's disease) forms; it is one of the erosive joint diseases. One per cent of people in the world suffer the disease and females are affected three times more than males, especially in their third and fourth decades of life. RA is classified as an autoimmune disease (i.e. an individual develops antibodies to their own body tissues), and around 80 per cent of people with the disease have a circulating autoantibody called the rheumatoid factor. The factors initiating an autoimmune response in RA are unknown but what is certainly known is that people with RA experience more chronic symptoms in colder climates and with specific diets (e.g. including large proportions of red meat and red wine). High protein and saturated fat diets are also implicated (Buchanan and Laurent, 1990: 83). RA affects multiple synovial joints symmetrically, especially the joints of the hands and feet, wrist, elbow, knee, shoulder and cervical spine; less commonly affected are the ankle, hip and sacroiliac joints. The synovial membrane is affected first; this thickens and forms a layer of granulation tissue called pannus, which spreads over the cartilage of the joint, eventually destroying it. The bone underlying the cartilage and adjacent to it is also damaged. Ligaments and tendons associated with the joint are also affected, often leading to partial dislocation (subluxation) of some joints, especially the metacarpophalangeal joints. Bone is eroded at the joint edges and later on the joint surfaces, and there is usually an associated osteoporosis. People with the disease are weak, often have anaemia, and suffer weight loss and muscular weakness. Swollen, stiff, painful joints lead to reduced function and severe deformity in later years. Fusion of joints is less common than in other similar joint diseases.

RA has rarely been identified convincingly in the archaeological record and it is likely that the disease may be mistaken for other joint diseases. Its rarity has induced studies of joints from known RA sufferers to ensure diagnostic criteria are correct for identifying cases in the past (Rothschild *et al.*, 1990; Leisen *et al.*, 1991). Many of the examples described in Ortner and Putschar (1981), Short (1974) and Steinbock (1976) are only identified as possible cases. Short (ibid.) has argued that it is a very recent disease in terms of time. Many of the early medical writers (e.g. Hippocrates in the fifth century BC) refer to a disease which could have been RA – 'a form of arthritis generally showing itself about the age of 35, first involving the hands and feet, which become cold and wasted, and next the elbows, knees and hips' (Short, ibid.: 196). This type of description is somewhat non-specific and not very useful in tracing the history of RA. The first good description was given by Sydenham in the seventeenth century AD (Buchanan and Laurent, 1990). Paintings of people with RA also appear from the late and post-medieval periods in Europe (Dequecker, 1977). Of course, the skeletal evidence is the primary evidence for the disease.

If the cases highlighted already in the literature are accepted, then the disease appears to have been present in Egypt in the third millennium BC. Bennike (1985) describes two cases from Denmark dated to AD 200–400 (mature male) and 1800–800 BC (female adult). Ortner and Putschar (1981) and Ortner and Utermohle (1981) discuss two cases in an Alaskan male and female, the latter dated to AD 1200, and Kilgore (1989) reports on a possible case in an elderly female at Kulubnarti, Sudanese Nubia, dated to between AD 700 and 1450. In Britain, examples dated from the seventh century AD up to the nineteenth century AD have been reported, although some of these cases have now been disputed (discussed in Kilgore, 1989). The most recent report is from Waldron and Rogers (1994), who claim their case to be 'the first evidence of rheumatoid arthritis in the United Kingdom' (ibid.: 165, and Fig. 6.13). Farwell and Molleson (1993) also report on twenty-seven cases of erosive arthropathy in the Romano-British cemetery at Poundbury, Dorset, England, and ascribe possible specific diagnoses to them; fourteen cases are diagnosed as rheumatoid arthritic, out of 1,400 inhumations.

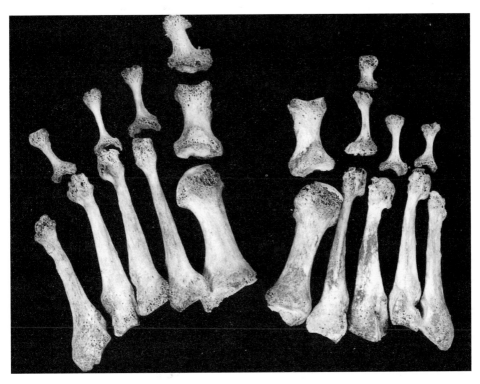

T. WALDRON & J. ROGERS/JOHN WILEY

6.13 Erosive lesions of the feet in rheumatoid arthritis (post-medieval England)

The rarity of the disease could be due to a number of factors. It may really have been a recent disease and the factors influencing its occurrence today were not present in the more distant past. However, diagnostic confusion with other joint diseases, such as osteoarthritis, may be instrumental in the perceived picture. Other suggestions could be that the more severe and chronic bone changes do not appear to occur until later in life (did people live long enough to develop the disease?), or that the palaeopathologist just does not see the survival of enough of the small hand and foot bones from archaeological excavations and therefore does not see the evidence.

The three other joint diseases that must be considered in the differential diagnosis of RA are osteoarthritis, gout and psoriatic arthritis. In osteoarthritis there are usually no lytic lesions and the distribution pattern is often more asymmetrical. Gout has an asymmetric nature, 'overhanging edge' lesions (see below), and rarely has associated osteoporosis; it also predilects for the great toe joints. Finally, psoriatic arthritis (see below) is asymmetrical in occurrence, has 'pencil and cup' deformities at the joints, associated new bone formation and involvement of the sacroiliac joints, but rarely osteoporosis. Consideration of these very clear differences in character and distribution of lesions should make diagnosis straightforward; problems occur either when there are several different joint diseases present on the same joint, or when the skeleton is not complete and/or well preserved.

PSORIATIC ARTHRITIS

Psoriatic arthritis (PA) appears in about 5 per cent of people with psoriasis, the skin disease (Cotran et al., 1989: 1361). It has an association with the antigen HLA-B27 in the blood (and people affected never have the rheumatoid factor in their blood). Although its cause is unknown, genetic, nutritional and infective factors may be instrumental in its development. The disease can affect any of the synovial joints, singly or multiply, and usually asymmetrically. Tendon and ligament attachments to bone may also be involved, with new bone formation or enthesophytes (Resnick and Niwayama, 1988: 1171). Males and females may be affected equally, but this varies, and 85 per cent have psoriasis. The phalanges of the hands and feet tend to become eroded at their surfaces and marginal to the joints, with development of 'pencil and cup' deformities, and the spine and sacroiliac joints are affected, with ossification of vertebral ligaments. New bone formation on the shafts of short bones of the hands and feet and around the joints is characteristic, and fusion of joints can occur. Few specific examples of PA have appeared in the palaeopathological literature; perhaps some cases of PA have been misdiagnosed? Farwell and Molleson (1993), however, list seven cases from Poundbury (see above). It is likely, however, that the diagnosis of PA is confused with other joint diseases.

ANKYLOSING SPONDYLITIS

Another of the autoimmune joint diseases is ankylosing spondylitis (AS), or Marie–Strumpell's disease, named after the French and German doctors who first described the disease in the 1880s. It is a progressive inflammatory disease of unknown aetiology. Like PA, affected people have the HLA-B27 antigen in their blood (in up to 95 per cent of cases – Cotran *et al.*, 1989: 1354). It affects young males predominantly, with an age of onset of between 15 and 35 years. It is seen commonly in Caucasians and native American populations but rarely in Japanese or African groups; it is quoted to have an incidence of 0.1 per cent today (Resnick and Niwayama, ibid.: 1105). The synovial and cartilaginous joints and entheses are affected and erosion and fusion of some of the joints, especially the sacroiliac joint, occurs; involvement of the sacroiliac joint is 'the hallmark of ankylosing spondylitis' (Resnick and Niwayama, ibid.: 1112). The small joints of the spine fuse, and the vertebral bodies begin to fuse from the lumbar vertebrae upwards, not only via the joints, but also through ossification of the inter- and super-spinous ligaments (Fig. 6.14), formation of vertebral syndesmophytes (thin vertical outgrowths of bone) and ossification of parts of the outer fibrous layer of the intervertebral discs. Low back pain, limitation of chest expansion, immobility, weight loss and fever are some of the signs and symptoms. The hip, shoulder, knee, ankle, wrist, hand and foot joints are the most commonly affected peripheral joints of the body (Rogers *et al.*, 1987) and appear to be affected in up to 50 per cent of people with the disease.

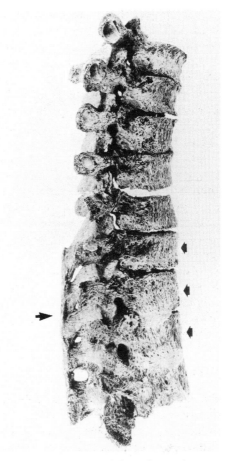

6.14 Ankylosing spondylitis of spine showing small syndesmophytes and ossification of spinal ligaments (6th–8th century AD, Kent, England)

Cases of AS in the past have been described from Egypt, Nubia, Canada, the United States, Guatemala, France, Denmark and the UK, summarized in Steinbock (1976) and Ortner and Putschar (1981). It is possible that many cases of AS are not being diagnosed because of the problem of differentiating this condition from Forestier's disease (see below). However, several features can be used to distinguish the two conditions from each other and from rheumatoid arthritis and psoriatic arthritis (Resnick and Niwayama, ibid.). AS has significant erosions of the synovial and cartilaginous joints of the axial skeleton. PA involves the synovial joints of the appendicular skeleton and the cartilaginous joints of the axial skeleton, whereas both diseases promote erosion and repair of the entheses involved. Bony proliferation and fusion with no osteoporosis characterizes PA and AS, and in RA the cartilaginous joints may or may not be affected. If a complete skeleton is available for analysis, it should be possible to differentiate these erosive arthropathies.

DIFFUSE IDIOPATHIC SKELETAL HYPEROSTOSIS

Diffuse idiopathic skeletal hyperostosis (DISH, or Forestier's disease) also affects the spine but it has very characteristic bony abnormalities elsewhere in the body that distinguish it from AS. It has been described in a Neanderthal skeleton from Iraq, dated between 40 and 73,000 years BP (Crubézy and Trinkhaus, 1992), the earliest known case. Although first described in 1950 (Forestier and Rotès-Querol) as a spinal disease, it has more recently become synonymous with

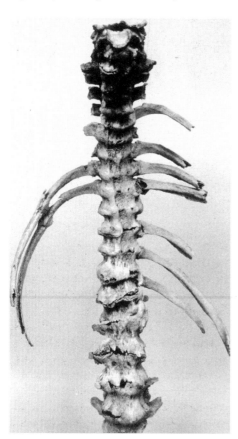

extraspinal manifestations. Its specific cause is unknown, but it appears to be associated with obesity and diabetes. Males are slightly more affected than females and the age of onset is usually over 50 years (Resnick and Niwayama, 1988: 1563). People affected are 'bone formers'. There is gradual and complete fusion of the spine (Fig. 6.15), particularly in the thoracic region, with retention of integrity of vertebral body surfaces and apophyseal joints. The anterior longitudinal ligament of the spine and paraspinal tissues ossify. The osteophytes produced are large and flow like 'candlewax'; they are especially seen on the right side of the vertebral column at the level of the seventh to the eleventh thoracic vertebrae, and are probably prevented from developing on the left side because of the presence of the aorta. Fusion of four contiguous vertebrae is necessary for a diagnosis. In addition, there are enthesopathies at tendon and ligament insertions (Fig. 6.16); it is not known whether these latter changes occur before or after spinal involvement. Cartilage also ossifies, especially the neck and rib (costal) cartilages. Pain, aching and stiffness are some of the symptoms of the disease.

6.15 Diffuse idiopathic skeletal hyperostosis involvement of the spine; note the flowing 'candlewax' new bone formation especially on the right side in the thoracic region, fusion of the spine, and ankylosis of some of ribs (Roman Droitwich, England)

Although not reported in high frequencies in the palaeopathological record to date, DISH is increasingly being seen in both monastic cemetery (Stroud and Kemp, 1993) and non-monastic cemetery groups (Waldron, 1993b). Its modern frequency is 2.8 per cent, whereas at Merton Priory in Surrey, England (Waldron, ibid.) a frequency of 8.6 per cent was indicated in the forty-two skeletons examined, dated from the twelfth to sixteenth centuries AD (Waldron, 1985). It was suggested that a rich diet and lack of exercise predisposed people in the priory to obesity and late-onset diabetes. Waldron (1993b) also reported on forty-seven skeletons with DISH excavated from the post-medieval crypt at Spitalfields, London. The majority were male and of old age. Stroud and Kemp's study (ibid.) noted seven definite cases of DISH and a further eight individuals probably suffering from an early stage of the disease. All the skeletons were associated with Period Six of the site, that is the cemetery associated with the Gilbertine Priory of St Andrew, York.

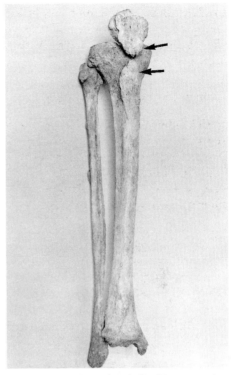

6.16 Diffuse idiopathic skeletal hyperostosis: extra spinal manifestations (new bone formation) at knee joint (Roman Droitwich, England)

It is suggested by Resnick and Niwayama (ibid.: 1600) that DISH 'may not represent a disease *per se* but rather a vulnerable state in which extensive ossification results from an exaggerated response of the body in some patients to stimuli that produce only modest new bone formation in others'.

Differentiating the bony abnormalities in DISH and AS is the first step to identifying the prevalence of both conditions in the past. DISH is usually found in older males and consists of characteristic thick, flowing spinal osteophytosis and enthesopathies extraspinally, but there is usually no fusion of the small vertebral joints or the sacroiliac joints. AS has thinner, vertically orientated spinal syndesmophytes, fusion of the small vertebral and sacroiliac joints and no extraspinal bone formation. Determining their specific aetiology in archaeological populations is more difficult than today, but the study of cultural factors at work in different populations with contrasting prevalence rates may shed light on their prevalence.

GOUTY ARTHRITIS

The final joint disease to be considered is much less common than AS or DISH. Gouty arthritis has a modern prevalence of between 0.13 and 0.37 per cent (Cotran *et al.*, 1989: 1355), and is characterized by a high level of blood uric acid (hyperuricaemia), caused by an excess of uric acid production or a reduced excretion by the kidneys. It affects males twenty times more frequently than females and occurs in older age groups (50 years +) (Resnick and Niwayama, 1988: 1619). There also appears to be a genetic predisposition. Urate crystals appear in the synovial fluid of joints and lead to inflammation and erosion of cartilage and bone. The bone may be eroded on the joint surface, at its margins, or at a distance from the joint, producing overhanging bony lesions shaped like a hook. The joints affected are mainly those of the feet, hands, wrists, elbows and knees, with the first metatarsophalangeal joint (great toe) usually involved (90 per cent of cases); joints are affected asymmetrically. Urate crystals also accumulate in tissues associated with the joint, e.g. tendons and ligaments, and also away from the joints, e.g. in the fingertips and soles of the feet; these are called tophi. It is an extremely painful condition and is intermittent in its affectation; it appears to be associated with excessive alcohol intake and gluttony. The attribution to alcohol is in part because during the distillation process a certain amount of lead was added in times long ago to improve the taste. The distillation process was also carried

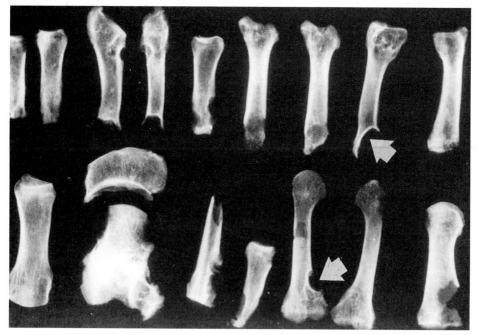

6.17 Radiograph of erosive lesions in articular and para-articular surfaces of metatarsals, and sclerosis, suggesting gout (Roman Cirencester, England)

out in leaden vessels, a further source of the metallic poison. This lead, after prolonged and repeated ingestion, caused kidney failure and a consequent rise in blood uric acid concentration. It was not the alcoholic beverage *per se* but the lead which damaged the kidneys (Steinbock, 1976: 309).

Although the literature of gout goes back to the Hippocratic School and has been prolific ever since, the palaeopathological evidence is rare. The most celebrated example of gout is an Egyptian mummy of the Christian period in which actual deposits of urate crystals were identified (Elliot-Smith and Dawson, 1924). The osteoarchaeological evidence is no more than a few cases. Three male skeletons of the Romano-British period from Cirencester, dated to about AD 150, show the destructive features in several joints. Wells (1982) considered these typical of gout (Fig. 6.17).

This necessarily brief survey of some of the more commonly occurring and recognizable joint diseases visible in skeletal remains of past humans is but a small part of the total picture of the many hundreds of joint diseases known to modern medicine. No doubt more precision on specific aspects of these diseases in the past will be forthcoming since the diagnostic criteria are now better known. The further study of the skeletal manifestations of these diseases in modern populations will aid in this goal. In addition, refinements in the correlation of osteoarthritis and occupation are desperately needed to help place a perspective on lifestyle in past human groups. What people do for a living will affect their predisposition to any disease process and this information is, in effect, instrumental in the study of palaeopathology. In the absence of modern treatment, both drug and surgical, the symptoms suffered by the elderly city dweller today are the same as those suffered by the elderly palaeolithic cave-dweller. Unfortunately for the latter, they were denied the medical relief and the creature comforts which we find so necessary in approaching old age.

CHAPTER 7

Infectious Disease

Diseases in general and infective diseases in particular were developed on the earth at a very remote epoch.

(E. Metchnikoff 1845–1916)

INTRODUCTION

In the past, the mortality, morbidity and misery wrought by micro-organisms far exceeded that of warfare and famine. Today the degenerative diseases account for the baseline of illness in Western society. In the pre-antibiotic era, the infectious diseases occupied this position in the league table. Bacteria and viruses also accounted for most of the deaths in the past. It will be remembered that these deaths occurred at a much earlier age than today and this in part reduced the importance of the ubiquitous degenerative disease of the skeleton and cardiovascular system so familiar in modern geriatric practice. Infants and young children are particularly vulnerable to acute gastrointestinal and respiratory infection, and death in these groups, even with modern care, is a high risk. It would have been so much higher in antiquity without the availability of antibiotics and without the knowledge of correct rehydration procedures. It is likely, but without proof, that many of the young people represented by infant skeletal remains from archaeological contexts died as a result of acute fulminating infection before there was a chance for observable bone change to develop.

The fearful epidemics of plague, smallpox, malaria and other rapidly transmitted infections were responsible for large numbers of deaths in their years of visitation. The ever-present and much less spectacular bacteria and viruses would have accounted for the more or less constant and unremitting death rate of the non-epidemic periods. Most of these latter micro-organisms cause infection today just as in antiquity, but the advent of penicillin and the synthetic antibiotics has largely eliminated their fatal effect. The exception, of course, is still the virus because, as yet, no universal antiviral agent comparable in efficacy to antibiotics has been discovered. In this context, however, the immunization of the young against such viral diseases as poliomyelitis, measles and rubella has reduced their incidence and has, therefore, reduced the impact of these diseases in the overall population profile of morbidity and mortality. In the current Western generation, children physically disabled by poliomyelitis are a rarity, and the congenital defects resulting from maternal rubella are no longer a problem. The significance of vaccination against smallpox in the elimination of this disease is paramount in the history of disease control (Jenner, 1801) and, as a result of this and other public health procedures, the world is now free of this scourge of antiquity. But these are measures of prophylaxis. Once contracted, the misery, morbidity and, at times, mortality due to viral infection is unchanged. There can surely be no better illustration than the spreading global infection of HIV and its attendant clinical manifestation of AIDS (Grmek, 1989; Inhorn and Brown, 1990; Sattienspiel, 1990). Perhaps overall well-being and improved health status in developed countries today reduces the mortality risk of many viral infections, but in the less fortunate and subsistence-level communities of the world, the morbidity and mortality of such commonplace viral infections as measles and influenza are considerable. Clearly, there are many factors responsible for lessening the effects of bacterial and viral infection during the passage of time and with increasing material prosperity. Doubtless the overworked and inadequately fed child living in the squalor of an early nineteenth-century industrial town was, relatively speaking, more susceptible to the respiratory and gut infections than was the child of a Neolithic village. The general tendency has, however, been one of improving living and health standards since distant antiquity.

Infective lesions of greater or lesser degree are a very common finding in skeletons from archaeological sites. If we consider the infections from which we all suffer today, it is apparent that the vast majority affect the soft tissues of the body. Even without active treatment, most of these infections resolve within a short time. Influenza, measles and bronchitis are but a few examples of this wide spectrum. More sinister, and often fatal in the absence of treatment, are appendicitis, meningitis and pneumonia. In all these examples, resolution of infection, or death of the individual, occurs fairly rapidly and long before the infective process will have spread to the bones. The infection, be it of soft tissue or bone, is associated with the pathological process of inflammation. Inflammation is a cellular reaction to the invading organism, be it virus, bacterium, or larger parasite, and is manifest in the symptoms of pain, swelling, tenderness and raised temperature. Inflammatory bone lesions are, therefore, manifestations of chronic, that is long-standing, infection. This is not to say that the micro-organisms causing the acute infections mentioned above do not cause bone inflammation under different circumstances, but that there is just not time for bone change to develop during the short course of these acute infections of soft tissues. By and large, these infective bone lesions of antiquity were created by bacterial and not viral infection, since these latter were more rapidly resolved or fatal, and did not lead to the chronic invasive process as did bacteria. There are certain characteristic infective lesions of bone that are caused by specific bacteria. The type of change noted in the bone can be ascribed to the particular bacterium, and the change is unlike that produced by other bacteria. These specific infections of tuberculosis, treponemal disease and leprosy will be considered later.

Non-Specific Infections

The pathological changes brought about by other bacteria are relatively non-specific; infection by one bacterium is indistinguishable from that of another. The bacteria commonly involved today in bone infection in the world are staphylococci, streptococci, pneumococci and, less commonly, the typhoid bacillus. Although unproven, it is likely that these were the cause of the non-specific infections of bone in antiquity. In modern pathological bone specimens such individual bacteria may be isolated and identified. Clearly, however, the micro-organisms responsible for infections in antiquity do not persist in preserved skeletal remains, although specific parasites have been identified in mummified human tissues, and advances in techniques for identification of pathological processes suggest that molecular structures of bacteria do survive in some circumstances (Salo *et al.*, 1994). It is therefore impossible to distinguish the particular bacterial cause by the examination of the non-specific bone changes from the past.

Bone infection is called osteomyelitis, a name which indicates that the solid compact wall of a bone, together with the relatively loose and bloody marrow or medullary cavity in the interior, are affected by the infection. Although not present in skeletal remains, it is assumed that the fibrous covering of the bone, called the periosteum, is also affected. Each or all of these layers, periosteum, compact bone and medullary cavity, may be involved in a bone infection. Sometimes the terms periostitis, osteitis and osteomyelitis are applied respectively to infection of these separate layers. Since bone is a single biological unit, such an arbitrary division of terms is perhaps artificial (Sandison, 1968) and it is preferable to use the single term osteomyelitis for all infective lesions of bone. However, a semantic discussion is inappropriate since both systems of description have their uses.

In osteomyelitis, the pathological process is one of bone destruction and pus formation, and simultaneous bone repair. In consequence, an individual bone frequently becomes enlarged in part or whole and is deformed from its healthy state. The bone destruction is manifest as pitting and irregularity of the bone surface and, possibly, cavity formation within the bone interior. This cavity, which is a pus-containing abscess, may gradually and progressively penetrate the compact bone wall and discharge pus into the surrounding body tissues. There is then to be found a clear and smooth passage between the surface of the bone and the internal abscess cavity. The longitudinal and transverse spread of bacteria and, hence, inflammatory process in bone is via microscopic channels known as Haversian canals and Volkmann's canals, which are found in all sites of compact bone. Thus the pathogenic micro-organisms are spread (from the initial focus) through the length and breadth of individual bones, producing satellite abscesses which may ultimately coalesce. More rarely the abscess may remain localized and contained within the bone interior and be undetected except by radiography or by bone section. Such a restricted cavity is known as a Brodie's abscess.

The bone reparative process in osteomyelitis is seen as the development of new plaques of bone on the surface. The new bone applied to the original external cortical surface is produced by bone-forming cells (osteoblasts) in the innermost layer of the periosteum. Initially the new bone lacks an organized microstructure and is termed woven bone. Later, through the complimentary action of bone absorptive cells (osteoclasts) and osteoblasts, the woven bone gradually assumes the micro-structure of mature compact bone. In unresolved and progressive osteo-myelitis the original bone may become more or less ensheathed by a cast of new bone. In such an extreme circumstance the ensheathed old bone may die. Gradually and intermittently this bone, the so-called sequestrum, may extrude with the pus to the bone exterior. In consequence the enlarged, deformed and mechanically less efficient new bone, called the involucrum, may be the sole structural support of the specific skeletal part. All of these aspects of the pathological process of osteomyelitis are seen in Fig. 7.1 and its associated radiograph (Fig. 7.2).

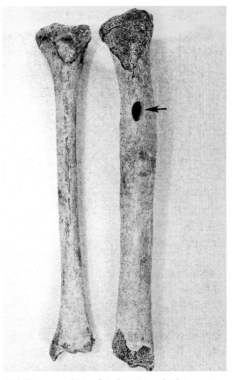

7.1 *Osteomyelitis of right tibia which is thickened and deformed. Sinus is arrowed into abscess in bone interior (6th–8th century AD, Eccles, Kent, England)*

Since these pathogenic, or disease-producing, bacteria are not normal inhabitants of bone, they must be transported to the affected bone from some other part of the body. In this, two main methods are involved. Probably the more common in pre-antibiotic antiquity was the transport of bacteria by the bloodstream from some primarily infected area and, quite possibly, this latter would have been the throat, ear, sinuses or chest. Acute bacterial infections, usually by streptococci, staphylococci, pneumococci or *Haemophylus influenzae*, of the tonsils, middle-ear cavity and bronchial tree, are common clinical conditions today and must have been so, particularly in the young, in antiquity. In the pre-antibiotic era these relatively insignificant infections of today would be followed by bacteraemia and the consequent haematogenous spread of the pathogens to more distant organs, including bone. For reasons unknown, in immature individuals, commonly only a single bone was involved in this secondary infective process. However, in adult individuals multiple bones were affected in approximately two-thirds of cases (Ortner and Putschar, 1981). Clearly, these were generalized infections only secondarily affecting bone, but commonly only a single bone was involved. No doubt, the individual so afflicted was seriously ill with fever, pain and immobility in the affected area. But, in order for the bone changes observed in skeletal remains to take place, recovery and not death from the generalized infection must

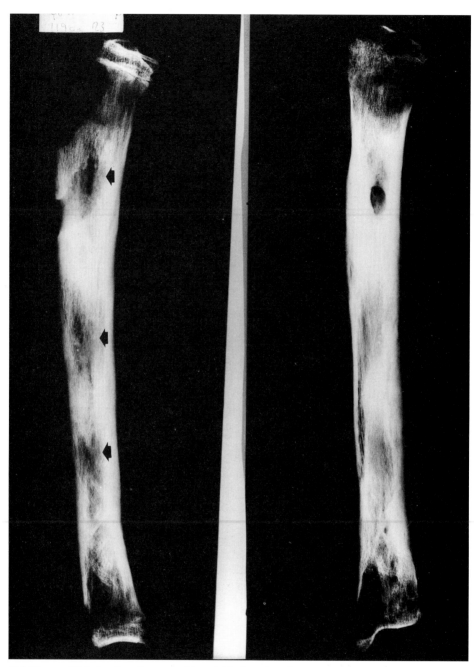

7.2 X-ray of 7.1 showing abscess cavities within bone interior

have occurred. Septicaemia, or blood infection, is a very serious problem even today and carries a significant mortality risk. The infection was much more serious before the advent of antibiotics and survival in antiquity was probably uncommon. Maybe such cases of osteomyelitis in the archaeological record testify to the survival of the fittest.

As will be noted, osteomyelitis resulting from this mode of transmission is more common in some bones, notably the femur and tibia, than others; the reason for this is obscure. The initial site of secondary infection in a long bone is frequently at the metaphysis near the growing end. This zone of the bone has the most abundant blood vessel supply and is therefore most likely to receive the bacteria and sustain the inflammatory process. Less commonly, osteomyelitis may result by the direct injection of bacteria from the skin surface during a penetrating bone injury. The normal skin surface is a regular harbour of potentially pathogenic bacteria. In this case the bone infected is the bone injured and the injury will be evident. Occasionally infection may spread from a severe and chronic skin lesion down through the deeper tissues, eventually infecting the bone surface itself. In this case of direct spread, the site is usually one in which the underlying bone is fairly superficial.

Infective lesions are common findings in palaeopathology. As with most diseases, the prevalence varies from place to place and from era to era. It was noted in an early Indian group from Texas that 18.3 per cent of adults possessed inflammatory bone lesions (Goldstein, 1957), whereas in early Anglo-Saxons in the UK (sixth century AD) the figure is about 10–15 per cent. In contrast, an analysis of 912 aboriginal skeletons from South Dakota demonstrated a prevalence of infective disease of bone of 1.75 per cent (Gregg and Gregg, 1987). It has also been shown in an examination of early American populations that the frequency of bone-infective lesions increases with an increasing population density (Lallo et al., 1978). This increased population density encouraged the rapid and extensive spread of bacteria and viruses throughout the community. Associated with an increasing population of increasing social and economic complexity there is an extension of trade networks. The area of trading increases and the frequency of trade contacts increases. Such networks act as routes for the transmission of infectious diseases between communities. Thus, the factors affecting the prevalence of infective disease in populations are multiple and varied. The immune status of the host, the virulence of the parasites, population density, malnutrition and ecological considerations are all significant.

As has been noted, not all bones are infected with equal frequency by bloodstream spread and, usually, only one bone is involved. In modern groups the femur and the tibia are the most commonly involved (Steinbock, 1976). In British societies from the Neolithic to the Saxon period, the tibia and the fibula are those most commonly involved (Brothwell, 1981).

There is one non-specific inflammation of bone which should be examined separately. Occurring in Anglo-Saxon skeletons in England rather more frequently than many other groups, there is a surface inflammation, or periostitis, of the tibiae which is not part of a total osteomyelitic process of the bone. The inflammatory process is manifest as fine pitting, longitudinal striation and,

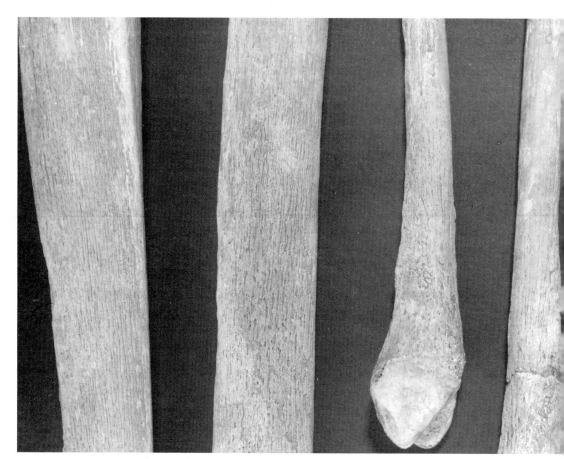

7.3 Periostitis indicated by striated new bone formation on the surfaces of tibiae and fibulae shafts (1st century BC, Beckford, Worcestershire, England)

sequentially, plaque-like new bone formation on the original cortical surface (Fig. 7.3). This shin bone lies close to the skin surface and is subject to recurrent minor injury today. Agricultural communities may have been subject to minor shin trauma. Alternatively, varicose veins, venous stasis and consequent ulceration of the lower leg may lead to chronic low-grade inflammation, but there is doubt as to this as a cause of the observed tibial periostitis. Tibial periostitis has also been suggested by many to be one of the many indicators of stress visible in the skeletal record (Goodman *et al.*, 1988). Such trauma, stress or, in some few cases, varicose ulceration may have given rise to this superficial and insignificant inflammation of the lower legs. It was unlikely to produce the debilitating and even crippling symptoms of the more severe osteomyelitis.

One feature common to all life forms, however large or small, simple or complex, is their susceptibility to predators; and micro-organisms may perhaps be considered as such. Consequently, evidence of infection has been noted in a Permian reptile from Texas (Moodie, 1923) and doubtless was a problem of previous times. Certainly infection has been a constant companion of people, but following the discovery of penicillin by Sir Alexander Fleming, the severe and chronic infective lesions of bone have now been eliminated in developed societies. The palaeopathologist of the future will find scant evidence of osteomyelitis in the skeletons of ourselves.

Paranasal sinusitis and middle-ear infection

Although bone infection induced by blood-borne bacteria was a common disease in antiquity, and bacteria had probably spread from a primary focus of infection in the throat, ear, nasal sinuses or chest, the evidence for these infections in skeletal remains is sparsely reported. The nasal sinuses are cavities within the bones of the face and are therefore difficult to inspect, the more so since they are usually full of soil on excavation. Probably, therefore, many examples of sinusitis from the past have been undetected, and the infection may not have been uncommon at all (Wells, 1964c, 1977). In the dry bone, the condition is recognized as the irregular pitting and new bone formation on the interior surface of the sinuses (Fig. 7.4). In a recent comparative study of skeletons from a medieval rural population and a contemporaneous urban population, Roberts and Lewis (1994), using an endoscopic technique, found evidence of maxillary sinusitis in 38 and 55 per cent of individuals, respectively. Certainly in the inhospitable climate of northern Europe today, the disease is common indeed; allergies, smoke, environmental pollution, upper respiratory tract infections and house dust are just some of the predisposing factors. The man or woman of the past, huddled around open hearths in the smoky, ill-ventilated houses of antiquity, would surely have been susceptible to this chronic and irritating infection. Such an environment would favour the production and stagnation of pus within the sinuses and so create the chances of inflammation. In addition, today, and perhaps frequently in the past, the maxillary sinuses may become infected by the perforation into them of a dental abscess of the upper jaw. The cause is then recognized by the open connection between the sinus and the tooth cavity (Wells, 1977). Gregg and Gregg (1987) identified dental abscesses as the predominant cause of maxillary sinusitis in a series of Crow Creek Indians.

In modern medical practice middle-ear infection, particularly in childhood, is a frequent occurrence (Daniel et al., 1988). Untreated, the disease frequently settles following perforation of the ear-drum and the discharge of pus from the abscess beneath. It must also have been common in the past. In the purely skeletal remains of the past, the delicate membranous ear-drum does not survive and the evidence of perforation is therefore lost. However, during autopsy of the Egyptian mummy Pum II, perforation of the preserved ear-drum was noted (Cockburn et al., 1975). The pain endured by this man (dated to about 170 BC) was, no doubt, relieved by this perforation from the infected middle ear.

Although there is no observable bone change associated with this acute infection of the middle-ear cavity, persistence of the infection with a chronically discharging ear induces inflammatory changes in the walls of the middle-ear cavity, and in the small bones (auditory ossicles) of the middle ear. Microscopic

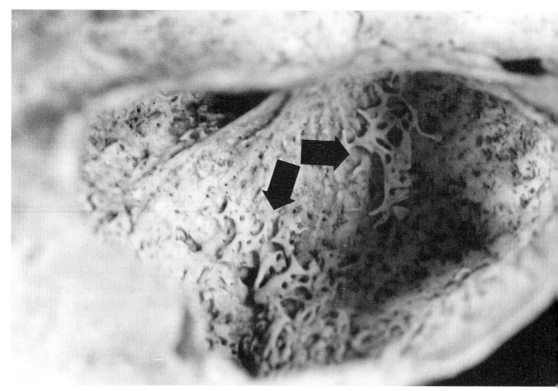

7.4 New bone formation on floor of maxillary sinus (medieval Chichester, England)

examination of these ossicles has been carried out by Bruintjes (1990) on skeletons from a medieval leprosy hospital cemetery. Erosive lesions suggesting chronic middle-ear infection were recorded in 51 per cent of ear ossicles (136 ear ossicles from 89 individuals were recorded; 69 had erosive lesions). For the general population such a frequency of middle-ear infection would, indeed, be very high and Bruintjes' findings are probably biased by the coincident infection of leprosy in the individuals examined.

Infrequently, the middle-ear abscess bursts through into the surrounding bone and produces mastoiditis. Unresolved, this infection of the mastoid bone behind the ear ultimately bursts through the bone surface either to the exterior or to the interior of the skull. This opening in the bone surface should be visible, provided that bone preservation is good. If the mastoid discharge was into the interior of the skull, the outcome was probably fatal, but if to the exterior then recovery was likely. In this disease, the infection may be recognized in archaeological material. However, this area of the skeleton is frequently damaged by burial and so the mastoid bone and its abnormal hole may be destroyed.

The disease is more common in children today than in adults. However, from an examination of skeletons from Merovingian cemeteries in southern Germany and dated to between AD 500 and 700, it was suggested that middle-ear infection was more common in older people and in the lower classes of society. On this finding, it was proposed that environmental factors of poor diet and general health in infancy predisposed to the later development of the condition in the lower social groups (Schultz, 1979). The child skull from the past is rarely well preserved because of the thinness, size and fragility of the bones and this, too, makes diagnosis of the disease in antiquity difficult. Nevertheless, the diagnosis has been made on these criteria in several specimens from Egypt, Europe and Great Britain (Wells, 1962).

The earliest recorded and most celebrated case is the skull of Rhodesian Man from Broken Hill, Zambia. It is dated to the Upper Pleistocene, possibly about 40,000 years before present (Day, 1977), and clearly demonstrates a perforation of the left mastoid area. It is tempting to imagine this man suffering from intense earache and fever unrelieved by the benefits of modern medicine. Relief only came to him with the perforation of the mastoid bone and discharge of pus. The long-term consequence was deafness, but this was preferable to the fatal alternative. Recently, however, doubt has been cast upon the diagnosis of mastoiditis in this early skull and the changes may, indeed, represent nothing more than post-mortem damage (Montgomery et al., 1994). This is a further demonstration of the difficulty of palaeopathological diagnosis. Further evidence of mastoid infection may be found from radiography of the mastoid bone, because infection induces changes in the pattern and size of the air-containing spaces contained within the bone (Gregg and Gregg, 1987: 72–4; Dalby, 1994).

Soft-tissue infection

Unfortunately, direct evidence of infections of soft tissues alone is not found in the dry bones of archaeology. A brief glimpse of these problems of antiquity comes from the detailed dissection and microscopic examination of mummies. Pneumonia, which must have been a major cause of death in the past, has been diagnosed by microscopy in Egyptian mummies and this disease must have been more common in northern climates. An examination of an Aleutian mummy has demonstrated the lung changes of lobar pneumonia in which the normal aerated lung tissue becomes solid. The bacteria responsible have been partially identified and multiple abscesses secondary to septicaemia have been seen (Zimmerman et al., 1971). By such meticulous post-mortem examination, the precise cause of death of this late seventeenth- or early eighteenth-century man was determined. A preserved Byzantine body has produced evidence of appendicitis (Rowling, 1961), which may also have been fatal. The evidence of viral infection is more rare still, and one example in the palaeopathological record classically rests upon the appearance of the skin of the mummy of Rameses V. The blistering lesions on the face, lower abdomen and thighs have been attributed to smallpox, but this diagnosis has not been supported by laboratory tests (Hopkins, 1980). A more recent study has identified smallpox in a sixteenth-century mummy (Fornaciari and Marchetti, 1986). A skin infection of bacterial cause has also been identified in a mummy of the Tiahuanaco culture from Peru (Vreeland and Cockburn, 1980). This disease, called verruga, is confined to Peru and neighbouring countries and is characterized by multiple fungating skin lesions.

As already stated, almost invariably, viral infections are fatal or resolved before inflammatory reaction in bones occurs. Direct evidence of viral infections is therefore absent in human skeletal remains, but the potential for their identification may lie in the application of modern DNA extraction methods to human remains from archaeological contexts. However, some examples do exist; an example of osteomyelitis due to smallpox has been identified (dated to the seventeenth century) (Jackes, 1983) but this, to date, is unique.

Poliomyelitis is a viral infection of the central nervous system, which is manifest clinically as the paralysis of one or more muscle groups. The disease is most common in early life, hence its alternative name of infantile paralysis. Paralysis of a limb at this early age results in muscle wasting and possible failure of growth of the bones in the affected limb. Therefore, marked inequality of bone growth in opposite limbs, a feature which will be apparent in skeletal remains, may suggest poliomyelitis. Other causes, both infective and traumatic, of bone growth arrest or muscle wasting must be considered, but poliomyelitis in recent times has been the most common cause of this phenomenon. Probable diagnoses

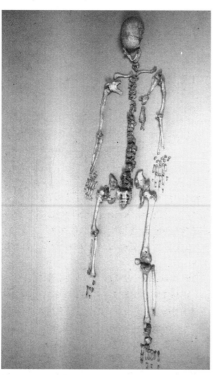

7.5 Probable poliomyelitis in an 8th–10th century individual from Raunds, Northamptonshire, England, showing failure of growth of right leg

of poliomyelitis in antiquity have been made on such features in a Neolithic skeleton from Cissbury, Sussex and a Bronze-Age skeleton from Barton Bendish, Norfolk (Wells, 1964a). The disease has also been diagnosed in Egyptian mummies, but the club foot of the Pharaoh Siptah, usually attributed to poliomyelitis, is more likely attributable to a congenital abnormality (Sandison, 1980b). Figure 7.5 illustrates a male, aged 20–30 years at death, from Raunds, Northamptonshire, England, dated to the eighth to tenth century AD, in which there is failure of growth of the right femur, tibia, fibula and foot. Although possibly associated with tuberculosis, poliomyelitis is the most likely cause of this crippling abnormality. The skeletal and mummified evidence of non-specific bacterial and of viral infection must represent only a very small part of the total spectrum of infectious disease to which people in antiquity were exposed.

In the present context of soft-tissue inflammatory disease, it is appropriate to consider the industrial contamination of the past. Clearly the problem is not infective, but the inhalation of dust particles does induce the changes of inflammation. Silicosis results from the inhalation of sand particles. It may represent the industrial contamination of a stone-worker's life, but in the Egyptian man or woman of long ago it may have been a consequence of living in a desert (Cockburn *et al.*, 1975). Only a quantitative assessment of silica content of lungs in a large number of mummies will separate those cases exposed by occupation to increased dust inhalation.

In ancient mummified human remains, carbon particles in the lungs are common findings. This element causes little in the way of physical incapacity when compared with silica. No doubt, when people enjoyed the comforts of companionship by the open fire they did expose themselves to smoke inhalation and deposition of carbon particles in their lung tissue, a problem called anthracosis. Evidence for this is, of course, missing in purely skeletal remains of the past. The dissection of mummies and the rehydration and microscopical examination of lung tissue has, however, demonstrated the changes of anthracosis (Zimmerman *et al.*, 1971). Added to the harsh, cold climate of northern Europe, deposition of carbon particles may have encouraged the chronic bronchitis so familiar to the modern medical practitioner. It should not be imagined, however, that the town residents of the past blithely accepted as inevitable the smoke of coal fires. There was agitation against this atmospheric pollution. So loathsome was it to Queen Eleanor that she felt obliged to leave Nottingham and its smoke in 1257 (Brimblecombe, 1976). It is perhaps only in the clean-air zones of the twentieth-century city that the results of at least 700 years of protest have been achieved, although many cities of the world are suffering increasing problems.

SPECIFIC INFECTIONS

Tuberculosis

A queue of afflicted people awaiting the royal touch and the gold angel is one aspect of the medieval court. Possibly originating in the reign of Edward the Confessor, this practice of the monarch touching individuals afflicted with King's Evil no doubt increased the royal claim to divine right. King's Evil was a term applied to scrofula, tuberculous infection of the lymph nodes of the neck (Wiseman, 1696).

A disease of considerable antiquity, tuberculosis increased steadily in prevalence until, by the seventeenth century, it was responsible in London for 20 per cent of all deaths in non-plague years (Clarkson, 1975). The deaths were said to be due to consumption, a term which implies pulmonary tuberculosis or primary lung infection. By modern standards, the diagnostic accuracy in the seventeenth century was probably poor. Many cases diagnosed as consumption may not have been tuberculous; these people may have been suffering from bronchitis or non-tuberculous pneumonia. However, the application of this term consumption does imply that tuberculosis at this time was a well-recognized and common disease. The London Bills of Mortality, written records of death, allow such figures to be known: doubtless other large centres of population suffered similar problems. No wonder then that Elizabeth I ordered that the weight of the gold touch piece given to sufferers of the King's Evil was to be reduced. With such an increase in tuberculous patients, England's exchequer stood to lose a great deal! It must be remembered in this context, of course, that many of the tuberculous men, women and children did not possess the manifestations of King's Evil. Cervical lymph node enlargement is merely one of the several presentations of tuberculous infection in humans.

In 1882 the German bacteriologist Robert Koch discovered the bacillus responsible for tuberculosis. Since then the bacterium has been further investigated and classified, and there are now known to be several types of this bacillus of Koch. These types, together with others of similar characteristics, including the bacillus of leprosy, belong to the genus *Mycobacterium*. The relationship between the mycobacteria of tuberculosis and leprosy may be responsible for the historical differences between the two diseases (Grmek, 1983: 198–209; Manchester, 1991: 23–35); this will be considered later. There are several closely related types of the tubercle bacillus; the 'cold-blood' type causing disease in cold-blooded animals, the avian type causing disease in birds and occasionally mammals, and the bovine and human types causing disease in the mammals including humans. These types may represent an evolutionary chain in the development of *Mycobacterium tuberculosis*, or the origin of the four types may have been from a common mycobacterial ancestor millennia ago. However, only the bovine and the human types of bacillus are of significance in human tuberculosis.

Bovine tuberculosis is, as its name suggests, a disease of cattle and other mammals, spreading secondarily to humans. It is probable, therefore, that a necessary condition for its transference from animal to human is the close association between the two. Indeed it is found in North America that the prevalence of human tuberculous vertebral lesions increases as native American populations became more settled and dependent on agriculture (Widmer and Perzigian, 1981). The close association is fostered by the domestication of cattle. A fairly close relationship existed between Magdalenian human groups and reindeer herds, but it had not been a continuous phenomenon for humans to be linked to herds prior to the Neolithic in Europe. Since domestication of animals is a feature of the Neolithic period, the advent of bovine tuberculous infection in humans may be coincident with this phase of animal husbandry. A single large centre of cattle domestication in the north-eastern basin of the Mediterranean first occurred in the seventh and sixth millennia BC (Bokonyi, 1977). Milking of cattle probably first occurred in the fifth millennium BC (Sherratt, 1981). The spread from infected cattle to humans is largely by the drinking of infected milk, and this may explain the recent predominance of bovine tuberculosis in children. It should not, of course, be forgotten that the disease may also be contracted by eating infected cattle flesh. Clearly, immediate and widespread cattle infection and subsequent human infection with bovine tuberculosis did not occur with the advent of animal domestication; such a feature is not a biological reality. Whence tuberculosis of domesticated animals came is also a problem. The earliest evidence of tuberculosis in animals is of Indian origin. There is clear evidence of the disease in elephants prior to 2000 BC (Francis, 1947) and it is known that, late in the Pleistocene period, Indian elephants extended through Mesopotamia to the borders of Asia Minor. It may be that domestic cattle infection owed its origin to these animals.

Whatever its source, and whatever its evolutionary pathway, the tubercle bacillus capable of infecting humans has created chronic, endemic and widespread suffering in human populations. In many parts of the world this suffering continues. It is a truism that the introduction of a new infection into a human population produces a disease which is severe and often fulminating. This statement usually refers to a disease that is already endemic in a different group, as for example in the smallpox devastation of the Mesoamericas at the time of Cortez, but to what extent it applies in tuberculosis, a disease totally new to humans, is of course not known. If the premise is correct, then the pathological changes of tuberculosis in very early eras must surely have been acute and of soft tissue only. The bone changes indicative of long-standing disease would have been unlikely to develop. Thus, the evidence from this time may not have survived in skeletal remains. Also, did the bovine tuberculosis bacillus spread throughout the world population from this single focus of origin in the Near East, or were there multiple foci of origin consequent upon animal domestication?

Human-type infection is spread from human to fellow human. The infected person coughs and exhales bacilli; their sputum and other excreta may contain bacilli which are capable of survival outside the body for some time. The healthy person, particularly a child, coming into contact with these vehicles of infection may become tuberculous themselves. This then is a disease of closely gathered groups; in essence an urban disease. Perhaps the human-type bacillus is a micro-evolutionary development of the bovine type and is, as it were, the end of the tuberculous chain.

The pathological changes of tuberculous infection occur in several areas and organs of the body, determined, to some extent, by the type of infecting bacillus and its portal of entry. For example, pulmonary tuberculosis is the common mode of infection by the human-type bacillus. The stomach and intestinal tract are the sites common to the bovine type, and it is noted also that bovine infection is more common in children than in adults, a fact possibly related to the consumption of milk in infancy.

The evidence for tuberculosis in antiquity mainly rests, as with most diseases, on the recognition of skeletal change. The evidence from mummified soft tissue is a significant but numerically small contribution to the picture of early disease. The skeletal features of tuberculosis are osteomyelitis which, largely because of the site in the body, is diagnostic. The areas of the hip joint and knee joint are the most commonly affected areas outside the spine. This osteomyelitic process occurs at the ends of these long bones and frequently affects the joints themselves (Fig. 7.6) producing a septic arthritis, with characteristic destruction of the joint surfaces progressing ultimately to fibrous fixation (ankylosis) of the joint. However, a diagnosis of tuberculosis made on such evidence is usually tentative and may be confused with the other causes of osteomyelitis and arthritis. Unlike the degenerative arthritic diseases, the tuberculous involvement is usually of one

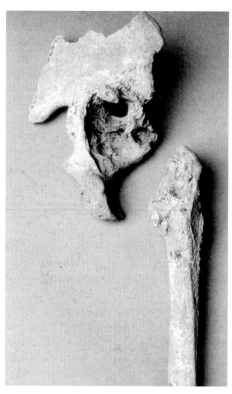

7.6 Probable tuberculosis of the hip with extensive destruction of femoral head and acetabulum with evidence of healing (medieval St Oswald's Priory, Gloucester, England)

joint only and the bone destructive process is more marked than the bone reparative process. In the context of palaeopathology, most diagnoses of tuberculosis are made on the discovery of significant lesions of the spine.

Involvement of the spine is present in 25–50 per cent of all cases of skeletal tuberculosis (Steinbock, 1976) and it is not surprising therefore that this aspect is important in palaeopathological diagnosis. The changes in the spine are usually found in the lower thoracic and upper lumbar vertebrae and between two and four vertebrae only are involved. But the involvement is severe, with abscess formation within the body of the vertebrae, perforation of the abscess into the chest or abdomen, collapse of the affected vertebrae and the subsequent bony fixation of several pieces of the vertebral column. A characteristic feature of tuberculosis of the spine is the early involvement, by destruction, of the discs between the individual vertebrae and the relative absence of change in the neural arch, the most posterior part of the individual vertebra. Although they may be confused with other diseases causing spinal collapse, such as traumatic crush fractures and malignant disease, these spinal features of tuberculosis are known as Pott's disease (Fig. 7.7). Sir Percival Pott, a surgeon at St Bartholomew's Hospital, London, described the condition in a monograph in 1779. The spinal collapse results in an angular deformity of the spine so frequently portrayed by pen and chisel as the hunchback. However, for reasons of diagnostic uncertainty, many of these portrayals may not be tuberculous. A person with osteoporosis of the spine may present a similar deformity.

If, indeed, it was as a result of cattle domestication that people were first exposed to the tubercle bacillus, then the earliest human evidence of tuberculosis might be expected to come from the eastern Mediterranean. However, just as with all other diseases, nobody supposes that the history chapter is finalized; the discoveries of tomorrow may extend both the time and the geographic perspective.

The earliest evidence of tuberculosis in human remains is from Italy, dated to the fourth millennium BC, and consists of a skeleton with the destructive and collapsed spinal lesions characteristic of Pott's disease (Formicola *et al.*, 1987). There is also a figurine of similar date from Egypt exhibiting spinal angulation and excessive weight loss typical of advanced tuberculosis (Morse *et al.*, 1964; Fig. 7.8). Perhaps more than any other form of evidence in the history of disease, such ancient figures are poignant reminders of the sufferings of our ancestors. Each prominent rib and each sunken eye suggests the profound misery of tuberculous cachexia.

Although other pre-Dynastic figurines are known exhibiting spinal angulation, no early written records from the Near East contain descriptions of tuberculosis. The Semitic Code Laws of Hammurabi of Babylon, the Ebers Papyrus (Mercer, 1964) and the Medical Papyri (Cave, 1939) do not contain references to a disease identifiable as tuberculosis. Further skeletal evidence of tuberculosis has been discovered in Early Bronze-Age populations of Bab-edh-Dhra, Jordan (Ortner, 1979).

Because the pathological changes

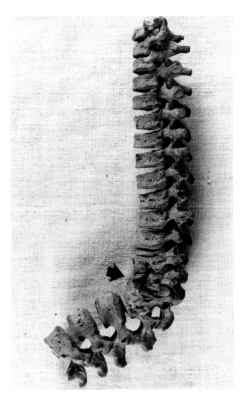

DON ORTNER

7.7 Spinal tuberculosis in a 9-year-old child: NMNH 327127, Pueblo Bonito, New Mexico, AD 950–1250

and, in relation to this earliest evidence, the spinal collapse are identical in human-type and bovine-type tubercle bacillus infection, it is not known whether these early sufferers gained their infection through ingestion or inhalation, although the former is more likely because of the infected meat or milk from domesticated cattle. Recent research (Kelley and Micozzi, 1984; Molto, 1990; Pfeiffer, 1991; Wakely *et al.*, 1991; Kelley *et al.*, 1994; Roberts *et al.*, 1994; Sledzik and Bellantoni, 1994) has demonstrated criteria for the skeletal identification of pulmonary infective lesions; although not definitive in aetiology, this work suggests that pulmonary infection by tuberculosis may cause an inflammatory response on the visceral surfaces of ribs (Fig. 7.9). In fact, in skeletal populations in the UK rib lesions are a common phenomenon; for example Chundun (1991) found 54 of 306 individuals (17.7 per cent) in a medieval hospital cemetery with these lesions.

However, a suggestion of pulmonary tuberculosis is found in the First Book of Epidemics of Hippocrates (Adams, 1849) but Hippocrates was, quite probably, writing of diseases in the early cities of the eastern Mediterranean in which population density was high and where this form of the disease would have been

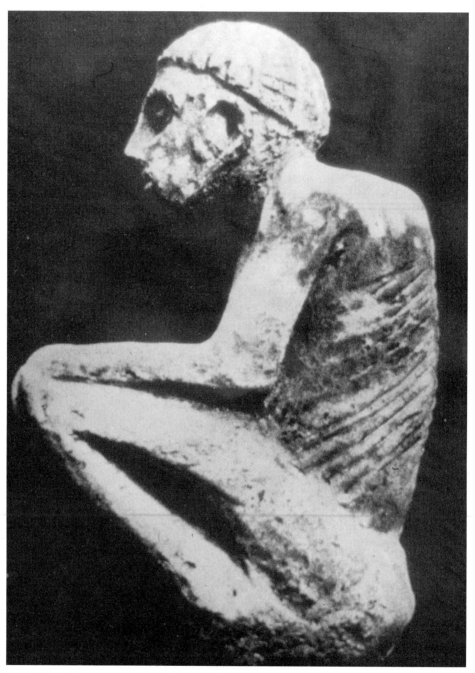

7.8 Possible tuberculosis shown in the spine of an Egyptian figurine

prevalent. From the Far East, Suzuki (1985) has identified tuberculosis in a skeleton from protohistoric Japan. Apart from the case already described from Italy, early evidence of tuberculosis in Europe also comes from Denmark and is dated to the third/second millennium BC. The skeleton exhibits spinal collapse of Pott's disease (Sager *et al.*, 1972). By the Romano-British era, tuberculosis was established in Britain (Wells, 1982; Stirland and Waldron, 1990) and contemporaneously in Continental Europe. During the early medieval period in Britain evidence of tuberculosis is sparse (Manchester and Roberts, 1987), but it is from the later medieval period that the evidence is more abundant. Pulmonary tuberculosis, or consumption, is a crowd disease, and its increase at this time may be associated with urbanization. It is therefore not merely the number of new town formations in the late Middle Ages which is important for the spread

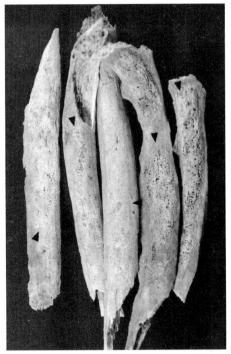

7.9 New bone formation on the visceral surfaces of several ribs (Roman Cirencester, England)

of the disease; the density of population within the towns is critical. In support of this Allison *et al.* (1981) noted that the prevalence of tuberculosis in Peruvian mummies increased with the increasing development of urban centres.

In considering New World evidence, Morse (1961) concluded that tuberculosis was probably non-existent in the American Indian population before the expedition of Columbus. However, irrefutable evidence of pre-Columbian human tuberculosis has been produced (Lichtor and Lichtor, 1957; El-Najjar, 1979; Perzigian and Widmer, 1979; Allison *et al.*, 1981; Buikstra and Cook, 1981; Merbs, 1992), mainly on the diagnosis of Pott's disease. The earliest case so far is dated to 800 BC from Mesoamerica. It is probably significant that most of these pre-Columbian examples are in skeletons from Pueblo, which were centres of relatively high population density. As has been noted, human tuberculosis is a 'population density-dependent' disease. Tuberculosis has been found in buffalo, elk, moose and deer, and perhaps this may have been the source of pre-Columbian human tuberculosis. It is difficult to accept that the disease crossed the Bering land bridge with migrating human groups. This land course disappeared by submersion at the end of the last glaciation and this predates the earliest European tuberculosis by several thousand years.

During succeeding periods the disease has become world-wide and even within living memory has been a scourge and a fear of humans. In the wake of the increasing phenomenon of HIV infection and AIDS, tuberculosis is once again increasing in incidence as a human disease (Grmek, 1989; Brown, 1992; Ryan, 1993). The unfolding story is not yet told. The tuberculous victims of antiquity must have suffered the lingering ill-health, the gnawing and unassuaged bone pain of infective involvement and the extreme emaciation of advanced tuberculosis. No doubt also, the historically later human-type infection of the lungs produced the breathlessness, distressing cough and bloody sputum of pulmonary tuberculosis.

It is not surprising then that in recent times the unfortunate sufferer of tuberculosis was confined to a sanatorium. Rest, fresh air, material welfare and segregation were perhaps the underlying principles of sanatoria before the advent of antibiotics. With a medieval lazar hospital in mind, maybe there has been a mycobacterial legacy even to the twentieth century.

Leprosy

In 1810, Clayton wrote of leprosy that the 'whole distemper was so noisome that it might well pass for the utmost corruption of the human body on this side the grave'. And arguably throughout history few diseases have engendered such fear and provoked such cruel and, at the same time, pious reaction as has leprosy. Much of the medieval attitude to leprosy stems from the supposed biblical references to the disease, references which today are considered largely incorrect. But what of the disease itself? With a world incidence of at least three million patients today, which in tropical Africa is represented by a local incidence as high as 10 per cent, leprosy has the same impact and significance in many parts of the world today as it had in medieval Europe; it has been likened to HIV and AIDS in terms of invoking a similar response from unaffected members of human societies. Leprosy is a chronic infectious disease caused by *Mycobacterium leprae*. Although leprosy is largely a disease of humans, it is not exclusively so; it has been recently identified in the chimpanzee, the Mangabey monkey and the armadillo (Jopling and McDougall, 1988).

The mode of transmission of *Mycobacterium leprae* between people is still uncertain but may be both through skin contact with an infected person, and through exhaled droplets containing bacteria from an individual with a profuse nasal infection (Bryceson and Pfaltzgraaf, 1990). What is certain, however, is that the disease is not inherited and is not transmitted venereally, thus negating prominent medieval thought. After transmission there is an incubation period of some 3–5 years before the presentation of symptoms and physical signs of the disease. The bacterium multiplies slowly, and therefore leprosy is a disease of slow progress; a disease known almost throughout time as the living death. In fact, *'Mundo mortuus sis, sed Deo vivas'* – be thou dead to the world but alive unto God, was the medieval pronouncement to the diagnosed leper. The infection is mainly of peripheral nerves and this, through the motor, sensory and autonomic modalities, is responsible for the majority of skeletal features in the disease and is therefore of profound significance in palaeopathology. The skin, the eyes, bone and the testes may also be involved in the disease process.

Until the sixteenth century, medieval paintings represented leprosy as spots, tumours and pustules distributed over the entire body (Gron, 1973). There can be little doubt that artists of this period recognized the gross deformities of the limbs and face, but it was the early Renaissance artists who first portrayed the limb and facial deformities in leprosy (Hollander, 1913). Notwithstanding this early artistic stricture, there is a sculpture of 1250–1350 from Burton Lazars leprosarium in Leicestershire, England which illustrates the facial features of advanced lepromatous leprosy (Marcombe and Manchester, 1990). A very similar figure is seen on a carving from the high altar of a church in Krakow. A figurine illustrating both the facial and the peripheral limb features of the disease has also been identified (Fig.7.10) in the Abbaye de Cadouin, France (Manchester and Knusel, 1994). It is likely that the sculptor of this most poignant figure had a first-hand and intimate knowledge of a sufferer of

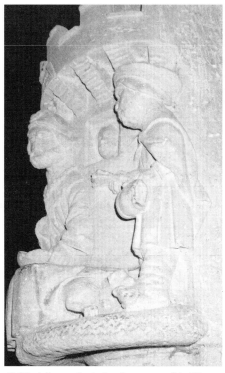

7.10 A figure depicting leprosy and holding a clapper in the Abbaye de Cadouin, France

advanced lepromatous leprosy. Carvings of less certain diagnosis are known from European and Middle Eastern sources (Grmek, 1992).

After the long incubation period, the clinical manifestations of leprosy are variable in severity, bodily distribution and infectivity. The variation is not, however, due to differences in *Mycobacterium leprae*, but is due to differences in immune status of each infected individual (Ridley and Jopling, 1966). At one extreme the infected person exhibits low resistance, the disease is highly infective, and the physical signs involve multiple limbs, face and soft-tissue organs. This pole of the leprosy spectrum is termed lepromatous leprosy. At the other extreme of the spectrum, the manifestation of tuberculoid leprosy is relatively less infective, and the pathological lesions are of one or perhaps two limbs, with less severe soft-tissue reactions.

Involvement of the peripheral nerves results in their loss of function. There is consequent paralysis of muscle groups in the upper and lower limbs and resulting deformity (Fig. 7.11). There is also loss of sensation, particularly of the hands and feet. The skin anaesthesia permits insensitive damage to the tissues, ulceration and secondary infection. The bone changes in the hands and in the feet (Fig. 7.12) and lower legs are the direct result of the secondary infection and the deformity, and consist of inflammatory changes in the bones and joints (Møller-Christensen, 1961;

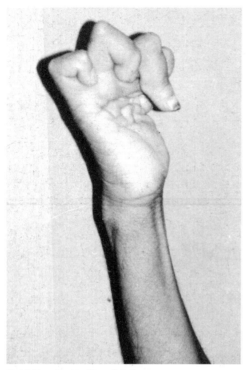

7.11 Paralysis of hand in leprosy

Andersen *et al.*, 1994), joint fixation and deformity, and actual bone absorption, particularly of the toes and fingers (Andersen *et al.*, 1992). Direct infection of the soft tissues around the nose and mouth by *Mycobacterium leprae* results in the characteristic changes in the bones of the face (Møller-Christensen, 1978a; Andersen and Manchester, 1992; Fig. 7.13). The face becomes nodular, the bridge of the nose collapses and is associated with a persistent nasal discharge, the eyes become infected and, in the extreme, blindness supervenes. Invasion of the larynx produces the hoarse, coarse voice characteristic of advanced leprosy.

No wonder that the chronically disfigured and possibly blind man or woman with deformity or loss of fingers and loss of toes provoked such reaction and fear. The diagnosis and misdiagnosis of the disease in antiquity has been, and still is, a subject of debate. The extent to which the non-leprous diseases of the nervous system, and the non-leprous diseases of the skin and eyes, were attributed to the biblical scourge is questionable. Elucidation of the problem comes from the evidence of documents and, more particularly, from the evidence of osteoarchaeology. Some 68 per cent of the skeletons from the medieval leprosarium at Naestved, Denmark, exhibited the changes of leprosy (Møller-Christensen, 1978a).

It is fortunate indeed from a historical viewpoint that leprosy leads to characteristic bone changes and that these changes can be recognized from skeletons of long ago. These changes of the skeleton have been studied, quantified and described by Møller-Christensen during his monumental programme of excavation and research of medieval Danish leper cemeteries (Møller-Christensen, 1953). Subsequent work has further refined the diagnostic criteria and examined the specific pathological processes that lead to the bone changes so familiar to the palaeopathologist (Andersen, 1969; Andersen and Manchester, 1987, 1988). Many of the bone changes of the hands, feet and lower legs have been recognized for many years.

The changes and clinical manifestations of leprosy were present in antiquity just as today, and there is no reason to suppose that the disease has changed its features throughout history. The sufferings of the lepromatous leprous individuals in a twentieth-century African or Indian leprous community are more

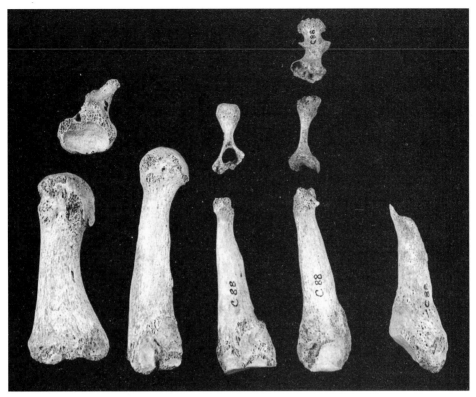

7.12 Bone changes of metatarsals in leprosy (medieval Chichester, England)

or less those of the medieval 'lipper-folk'; but the social reaction and medical treatment have changed. What a piteous spectacle on the medieval scene: poor ostracized men, women or children, of ugly countenance, deformed by loss of members and smelling of the discharging ulcers, who were forced to give notice of their presence with a wooden clapper and then forced to beg with hoarse voice for their material needs. The pattern of social abhorrence and the persistent reaction to leprosy (Jopling, 1991) is unique among diseases in its intensity, inventiveness and ubiquity.

And yet, leprosy appears to have been a late arrival in the history of bacterial disease. Pending the discovery of early skeletons, the earliest history of leprosy relies upon literary sources. The earliest reference to leprosy in humans is in the Sushruta Samhita, an Indian document from the period around 600 BC. The description of loss of sensation, falling off of the fingers, deformity and ulceration of the limbs, and sinking of the nose, are almost diagnostic of advanced lepromatous leprosy (Dharmendra, 1947). A similar description is also identified in a Chinese bamboo book of the third century BC (Skinsnes, 1980; Skinsnes and Chang, 1985). Thus, lepromatous leprosy was established in India and the Far East at an early period, and the clear and accurate contemporary description implies that the authors possessed an acute clinical acumen. It is quite possible

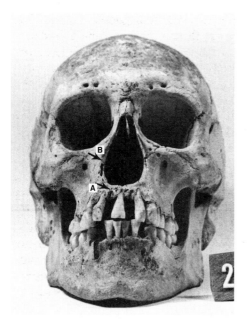

7.13 Facies leprosa: A alveolar bone resorption of maxilla and loss of teeth; B remodelling of nasal aperture (medieval Naestved, Denmark)

that the disease may have had a significant prevalence in those parts of the world at that time.

From whence the bacterium came to infect humans remains unknown. However, it has been found that bacteria similar to mycobacteria can survive on very simple hydrocarbon chemicals which are found in fossil fuels on the ground surface (Chakrabarty and Dastidar, 1989). Could it be therefore that this source resulted in the implantation of potentially pathogenic bacteria into broken human skin, thus establishing disease? Further west, Dols (1979) considers that there is no persuasive evidence that leprosy occurred in ancient Egypt, Mesopotamia or Persia before the time of Alexandra the Great. The literary and osteological evidence for the Mediterranean and European areas is of a later period.

Largely based upon this, the evidence currently available, it has been suggested that leprosy was brought to the Mediterranean from the Indo-Gangetic basin by the returning armies of Alexander the Great (356–323 BC). Its earlier existence in the Far East is, as yet, without corporeal evidence. The Alexandrian Indian campaign was in the years 327–326 BC and, during this expedition, the soldiers or the camp followers may have contracted leprosy. The movement of people, either in 'trade', military or religious expedition, is an efficient vehicle of disease transference. It may be of significance therefore that the earliest corporeal evidence of leprosy known at present is from the Dakhleh Oasis in Egypt (Dzierzykray-Rogalski, 1980). The four skulls showing features of leprosy are of the Ptolemaic period and are dated to the second century BC, a relatively short time after the Alexandrian campaign. It is of interest also that the skulls are of 'European' type and not the Negroid type typical of that area. Dzierzykray-Rogalski suggests that these lepers were members of a high stratum of society who, because of their disease, may have been segregated from the more urban centres of the Empire. If this supposition is correct then, bearing in mind the possible time taken to develop such socio-medical attitudes, leprosy in the Ptolemaic Empire may have been a recognized disease for many years. This is consistent with its entry into the Mediterranean area with the Alexandrian army.

Following this, corporeal evidence of the disease is not recognized until the Egyptian coptic mummies of the fourth to seventh centuries AD from El Bigha near Aswan (Møller-Christensen and Hughes, 1966). The earliest evidence of leprosy in western Europe is of the fourth century AD. A diagnosis of leprosy has been made from the legs and feet of a Romano-British skeleton from Poundbury (Reader, 1974); a skeleton of similar date with unequivocal signs of leprosy has been identified in Scandinavia (Arcini, 1990). Since the western European evidence post-dates the Roman expansion into Europe, it is possible that the disease was transported from the Mediterranean by the Roman Imperial campaigns into northern Europe. The Roman combatant soldier is of course very unlikely to have had leprosy, but camp followers, the group of 'hangers-on' who have accompanied armies since time immemorial, may well have been leprous. The mercantile routes were also, no doubt, a ready road for dissemination of disease. Although less infectious, less mutilating and less obvious than lepromatous leprosy, the tuberculoid and borderline forms, if they existed, should not be forgotten in the transmission of leprosy at this time. From succeeding centuries the evidence of leprosy in Britain becomes more abundant (Lee and Magilton, 1989; Manchester, 1992). Elsewhere in continental Europe Blondiaux (1989) has identified leprous skeletons of a similar early date. A single leprous skeleton dated to about AD 500 has been recorded from France (Møller-Christensen, 1967), and Pálfi (1991) has diagnosed leprosy in a skeleton dated to the tenth century from Hungary.

Much reliance for the early history of the disease in the Near East has, until recently, been placed on the biblical references to leprosy. There are no less than sixteen separate references to leprosy from both Old and New Testaments. However, it has been demonstrated by several researchers (Andersen, 1969; Hulse, 1972, 1976) that biblical references to the disease are probably false and due to a mistranslation of the word *tsara'ath* in the Hebrew version. What is apparent is that the word *tsara'ath* does not denote any specific disease but rather describes the state of ritual uncleanliness. Such a description implies that the individual was not fit to enter a Holy place. It has nothing to do with the infection that we now call leprosy. Because it is now known that leprosy was present in the Near East by the second century BC, discussions on New Testament leprosy are probably irrelevant. The disease was probably known throughout the eastern Mediterranean area at that time. Indeed, the earliest skeletal material diagnostic of leprosy in the Holy Land is from monastic ossuaries of the fifth century in the Judean Desert (Zias, 1985). Regrettably the biblical association remains with the name Lazar, a name suggestive of leper and leper hospital. From the meagre clinical description (Luke 16: xx) it is not possible to state whether Lazarus the beggar was a leper or not. He certainly did not suffer from *tsara'ath* because he was not segregated from society. Further confused medieval thinking has linked the name of this Lazarus with Mary and Martha. Many of England's leprosy hospitals have been dedicated to these three, and, as late as the nineteenth century, the name Maudlin, the abbreviated and conjoined Mary and Martha, had historical associations with leprosy (Richards, 1977). It is perhaps tragic that much of the prejudice against lepers throughout history has been due to an error of translation. Leprosy in the literature of the Graeco-Roman period is referred to by the terms 'elephas' and 'elephantiasis', and in the medieval period by the term 'lepra'. Investigating the written sources of antiquity for the early history of leprosy is clearly very difficult. The attribution of the loosely applied names of the past to the specific disease recognized today is a major pitfall in the investigation of diseases in antiquity.

The spread of leprosy throughout Europe in the medieval period was probably due to expanding trade, the opening of mercantile routes and the increasing movement of people. The developing medieval period saw a gradual increase in leprosy. The osteoarchaeological record becomes more abundant (Manchester and Roberts, 1987) and by the twelfth and thirteenth centuries legal and socio-medical measures aimed at the control of the disease had become established (Roberts, 1986a). The situation in North America is somewhat different in that the evidence for early leprosy is non-existent. This is perhaps expected since by the fifteenth century and the Columbus expedition to America, leprosy in Europe was declining and it is very unlikely that a lepromatous leper would have joined the expedition. Recent excavations in Guam of graves predating European contact with North America, have revealed skeletons with features characteristic of lepromatous leprosy (Trembly, personal communication 1993). Almost certainly, the route of arrival for the disease in Guam was from the Asian mainland. The isolation of North America until long after this period, at least according to currently available evidence, remains a mystery.

The decline and elimination of leprosy in northern Europe illustrates the complex and interrelated bacteriological, social and environmental factors implicated in infectious disease change. These factors differ from country to country and even within individual countries themselves, which may explain the survival of leprosy in one community and its simultaneous disappearance from another. The persistence of the leprosy hospital may not be a true guide to the persistence of leprosy within a society. There is no doubt that by the late medieval period in England the leper was considerably more rare than his or her supposed place of refuge. The leprosy hospital, like the sanatorium in a later period of history, maintained its name and dedication but changed its function. It is well known that by the mid-twentieth century many sanatoria contained few, if any, tuberculous patients but instead accepted patients with other pulmonary diseases. So it may have been with leprosy hospitals in the late medieval period. To all intents and purposes, leprosy was a non-existent disease in England by the sixteenth century, and in the fifteenth century was a rarity (Richards, 1977).

Similar changes took place in southern Scandinavia, and yet in northern Scandinavia and in Iceland, leprosy persisted even until the nineteenth century. What identifiable factors operated in northern Scandinavia in the nineteenth century and in mid- and southern Europe in the late medieval period? It is appropriate to narrow the horizon and consider England alone as representative, because the history of the disease, its hospitals and general population movements are fairly well known. In spite of the vigour with which it was often enforced, segregation of lepers possibly contributed little to the decline of the disease. Leprosy is a highly infectious disease, but the ability of the bacterium to produce clinical disease in patients is poor in comparison with other infectious diseases, and there are, in fact, recorded instances of healthy individuals taking residence in leper hospitals and remaining clinically free of the disease themselves for many years. This illustrates the variation in individual susceptibility to infection, a phenomenon common to most infectious diseases. Effective medical treatment of leprosy in the medieval period was non-existent. Nevertheless, leprosy declined from its fearsome prevalence in the twelfth and thirteenth centuries to its virtual absence in the sixteenth century.

What is apparent during the period of decline of leprosy in the later medieval period in England, is the concurrent increase in tuberculosis. To some extent the evidence for this increase at this time is assumed and is a projected expectation back in time from the known very high prevalence in the urban centres of the seventeenth century. The reaction of the body at microscopic level to *Mycobacterium tuberculosis* and to *Mycobacterium leprae* is essentially the same (Lurie, 1955). It is also noted that there is a degree of cross-immunity induced by these two bacteria. It is found, for example, in modern investigations that BCG vaccine, which is normally used for protection against tuberculosis, does offer some protection against leprosy (Clark *et al.*, 1987; Jopling and McDougall, 1988). It was suggested by Grmek (1983) that there is an evolutionary chain of mycobacterial development from the non-pathogenic through and including the human pathogens. In this chain *Mycobacterium tuberculosis* is regarded as an earlier entity than *Mycobacterium leprae*. If this phase of bacterial evolution has resulted in a decrease in bacterial virulence (and the relatively low pathogenicity of *Mycobacterium leprae*, and the variable human susceptibility may suggest this) then due to biological competition, tuberculosis will take precedence over leprosy. Exposure to tuberculosis, regardless of whether it results in overt disease or rapid self-conquest of infection, may therefore induce a degree of immunity to leprosy, and will therefore reduce the chances of contracting leprosy (Manchester, 1991).

This is clearly of only passing interest to the individual with relentlessly advancing tuberculosis. However, the human-type tuberculosis has its primary focus of infection in the lungs and it is a common response today (and, presumably, in antiquity also) that this process becomes arrested early without advancement of the disease. Henceforth the individual is immune to tuberculosis and, by the above reasoning, in part to leprosy also. Therefore an increasing community exposure to tuberculosis may result in a decreasing community incidence of leprosy. Clearly, those individuals dying with tuberculosis will not prevent leprosy gaining or maintaining a foothold in a community; but the background of people immune by exposure to tuberculosis will fulfil this role. Exposure to tuberculosis is likely to be more widespread through human-type bacilli, and a prerequisite for this is close human-to-human contact. This is achieved by urbanization. The revival of urban living in Europe gathered momentum from the tenth century and the number of new town foundations reached a peak in the late thirteenth century (Pounds, 1974). The early fourteenth century onwards witnessed a falling off in the number of new foundations. What should be significant, however, is not merely the number of urban centres developing within a territory, centres defined by social organization rather than number of inhabitants, but the actual population size and density within these centres. At the end of the thirteenth century, the period of maximum demographic growth, very few urban centres had populations in excess of 50,000 and these were mostly in Italy. Perhaps no more than 15 or 20 towns had populations greater than 25,000, and again most of these were in Italy. The number of towns containing smaller populations is greater, with the majority containing 2,000–10,000 inhabitants (Pounds, 1974). As to England, in 1199 Peter of Blois reported that London had a population of 40,000, a figure incorrect for that period but possibly correct for the mid-fourteenth century (Green, 1971). The development of urban centres was somewhat later in northern Scandinavia, and it is observed that the decline of leprosy there was also later than in England.

The osteoarchaeological record may be supportive of this hypothesis. Leprosy is attested in several hundred skeletons in Europe as a whole (Møller-Christensen, 1967). Tuberculosis is not uncommon in both the skeletal and the literary record. And yet the presence of both tuberculosis and leprous lesions in the same skeleton is rare. A skeleton with evidence of both has been described from the medieval cemetery at Naestved in Denmark (Weiss and Møller-Christensen, 1971a). The tuberculous changes are suggestive of human-type infection of the lungs, but spinal involvement is also present. The rarity of this combination of diseases is support for the mutually exclusive nature of leprosy and tuberculosis, and, by inference, for the above hypothesis. And yet in modern groups, pulmonary tuberculosis was a major cause of death in leprosy hospitals. Although tuberculosis frequently occurs in leprous patients, leprosy rarely develops in tuberculous patients (Jopling, 1982). It seems that although tuberculosis confers some immunity to the development of leprosy, the converse does not apply.

Whatever the manifold reasons for the decline of leprosy, Europe is now largely spared this most emotive and mutilating of the mycobacterial diseases. The scourge is now a problem of the tropical and semitropical areas of the world. When prejudice, fear and geographic and economic barriers have been overcome, leprosy may also disappear from these zones and become a disease of purely antiquarian interest.

Treponemal disease

For many years the human diseases caused by bacteria of the genus *Treponema* have been the subject of controversy. These diseases are pinta, yaws, endemic syphilis and venereal syphilis. The controversy centres on whether these are different disease entities caused by different species of bacteria within the genus, or whether they are merely different clinical manifestations of infection by one species, *Treponema pallidum*. If they are truly separate diseases, then collectively they may be referred to as the treponematoses. If they are but different clinical manifestations, then the disease entity is the treponematosis. Upon this distinction depends the most emotive controversy, regarding the evolution and history of syphilis.

Although to many this may seem an argument of bacteriological nicety, this controversy is of more worldly significance. No finger of rectitude is pointed at pinta, yaws and endemic syphilis, but in the past, and even today, certain moral judgements surround the problem of venereal syphilis. Much time and thought has been devoted to the question of global venereal syphilis and its New World or its Old World origin.

Before discussing the evolution and spread of the treponemal diseases, it is appropriate to consider *Treponema* and its identity. Pinta, yaws and syphilis (both endemic and venereal) have been customarily attributed to the bacterial species *Treponema carateum*, *Treponema pertenue* and *Treponema pallidum*, respectively, and it is the specificity that is under scrutiny. These three 'species' are indistinguishable in appearance and physical laboratory characteristics (Dooley and Binford, 1976). Certain immunological changes in the blood of infected individuals are indistinguishable in the three bacterial infections. These facts, together with some epidemiological aspects of the diseases themselves, have led to the conclusion that there is only one species of *Treponema* involved in these infections, and that has been labelled *Treponema pallidum* (Hudson, 1958). Counter arguments based on the different clinical features and on the different geographic distribution of the individual diseases have led to the conclusion that the bacteria are, in fact, separate species (Hackett, 1963). The problem is not solved and no doubt awaits further refinements of bacteriological techniques.

However, if the laboratory questions are as yet unanswered, the clinical effects of infection have been known for many years. The basic pathological changes, both gross and microscopic, of the infectious diseases of pinta, yaws, endemic syphilis and venereal syphilis are identical. Differences between them are purely quantitative and of degree, and are not qualitative. There is, however, valid reason for regarding pinta as a somewhat different problem, despite the identical reaction of inflammation. In this disease the pathological change is of the skin only, unlike the other diseases. It is therefore not manifest in skeletal material. Also, it has not been found possible to inoculate animals with this infection under experimental conditions, as is possible with the other infections of the group. The clinical severity in terms of morbidity and mortality does seem to progress from pinta, the least significant, through yaws, endemic syphilis, to venereal syphilis, at which point, for the present anyway, the story stops. But evolution, if this is what is in evidence, is not a finite phenomenon and there is no reason to suppose that an end point has been reached in the treponemal diseases any more than in the other infections.

Yaws, endemic syphilis and venereal syphilis are all associated with inflammatory changes in most tissues from the body surface to the bones. Venereal syphilis, being the most severe, is also characterized by affection of the arterial circulation and the nervous system. All are purely human diseases. All are transmissible from infected person to non-infected person without the intervention of an intermediate animal host. Only venereal syphilis is transmissible from infected mother to unborn child. All are characterized by recognizable clinical stages of development. The early stage is at the site of entry of the bacteria and is a relatively mild inflammatory lesion. A later stage marks the generalized spread of bacteria within the body and is characterized by skin and soft-tissue changes. In the later stage there is inflammatory change in the bones, which is mainly of a destructive nature but which also demonstrates considerable regeneration and repair. It is with the evidence of this stage that the palaeopathologist is concerned. It is from this stage alone that the corporeal evidence for the antiquity of treponemal disease comes. A final stage of venereal syphilis is the involvement of the heart, arteries, brain and spinal cord.

It must be remembered that, albeit uncommonly, an individual can overcome their disease in an early stage and recover. Thereafter they will remain immune to further attacks of this disease. Because infection by one of the group will confer immunity to the other diseases, that is, there is cross-immunity, a recovered individual will thereafter be immune also to the other treponemal diseases. This is possibly of significance for the evolution of endemic and venereal syphilis.

As already stated, the diseases differ quantitatively and in the prevalence of bone involvement (Rothschild and Heathcote, 1993; Hershkovitz et al., 1994; Rothschild and Rothschild, 1994). Pinta need not, of course, be considered further in the present context. The bone changes of yaws, endemic syphilis and venereal syphilis are of osteomyelitis, induced in part by an inflammatory reaction specific to *Treponema* (Canci et al., 1994). This reaction, which results in gross bone destruction, is called a gumma. However, unlike some of the cases of non-specific osteomyelitis discussed earlier, the osteomyelitis of the treponemal diseases is accompanied by extensive bone regeneration and exhibits specific microscopic characteristics (Schultz, 1994). In consequence, in the later stages of the bone infection, the particular bone assumes a much altered shape. As might be expected, the frequency of bone involvement in these diseases increases from about 3–5 per cent of all cases of yaws to 10–12 per cent of all cases of venereal syphilis, with endemic syphilis lying between the two. In yaws the tibia is the most commonly involved bone (Dooley and Binford, 1976), and only to a lesser extent are the other bones of the skeleton involved. The skull is infrequently involved but, when it is, the destruction is generally more severe than in syphilis, particularly in the oral and nasal areas (Manchester, 1994). The usual result is a few irregular crater depressions of the skull surface. Occasionally the destructive element may be extensive. This may result in the condition of gangosa in which the whole nasal area and upper jaw may be destroyed and associated with extensive destruction of the soft tissues of the face, a severe and mutilating stage even surpassing the mutilations of leprosy. More common, however, is the tibial osteomyelitis which, due to the deposition of new bone, gives rise to the sabre shin, so called because of its shape.

As with yaws, skull involvement in endemic syphilis is uncommon, but may result in extensive destruction of the nasal area and upper jaw. Also in common with yaws, the tibia is the most commonly affected bone, resulting in the sabre shape (Anderson et al., 1986; Hershkovitz et al., 1994). The difference between these two diseases, yaws and endemic syphilis, lies in the earlier stages of each disease and in their individual geographic environment. Both diseases are common and endemic in hot climates, but yaws has a predilection for the humid tropics whereas endemic syphilis is prevalent in the arid zones lying north and south of the yaws territory (Froment, 1994). In fact, to avoid confusion of terms in syphilis, endemic syphilis has been renamed treponarid (Hackett, 1963) but the new term has not yet come into universal usage.

Pinta is a disease usually acquired during the third decade, whereas yaws and endemic syphilis are infections primarily of children, but of course children become adults and the lesions persist.

The emotive discussions on treponemal diseases, often with undertones of morality, largely surround venereal syphilis. The names given to the disease perhaps betray the interest in the condition and suggest an element of blame in its origin. Mal de Naples, Arboyne pimple, Scottish sibbens, Swedish saltfluss, Morbus gallicus and Spanish pox are but a few. In view of the arguments regarding its New World or its Old World origin, it is surprising that a name implicating North America does not seem to have been used.

For all the similarities that yaws and endemic syphilis possess, venereal syphilis displays several differences. The mode of transmission from person to person is perhaps the most obvious difference; yaws, endemic syphilis and also pinta are transmitted by bodily contact which is not of the intimacy of sexual intercourse. They are, as mentioned, diseases with an onset in childhood. Venereal syphilis is acquired in adulthood through the act of sexual intercourse with a person infected with *Treponema pallidum*. Pathologically the most striking and significant difference is in the severe, incapacitating and frequently fatal circulatory and central nervous system involvement of venereal syphilis, features not manifest in pinta, yaws or endemic syphilis. The most advanced stage of venereal syphilis has given rise to the apt term general paralysis of the insane. The affected individual with stumbling faltering gait, given to bouts of irrational madness, has good reason to regret his or her previous indiscretion. Relief from worldly suffering may come dramatically from the rupture of a grossly dilated major artery and the consequent catastrophic haemorrhage. It is noteworthy, however, that only 10–12 per cent or so of venereal syphilitic individuals possess bone changes. Since the only truly reliable evidence of syphilis in antiquity is derived from osteoarchaeological study, it is quite probable that the prevalence of venereal syphilis in the distant past may be underestimated by as much as 90 per cent. This may in some measure explain the apparent rarity of the disease in past society. Like yaws and endemic syphilis, the tibia is the long bone most frequently affected in venereal syphilis (Clairet and Dagorn, 1994), presenting as a deformed osteomyelitic bone, but multiple bone involvement throughout the skeleton is frequently noted. Venereal syphilis may also result in destructive change of joints, characteristically the knee. The joint itself may be the seat of infection or, at a later stage of the disease, may become damaged by the loss of sensation due to nervous system involvement. This so-called Charcot joint adds further to the unstable gait of the relentlessly advancing syphilitic disease. In contrast to the other two diseases however, the skull is commonly affected in venereal syphilis and it is upon this change that a palaeopathological diagnosis is mainly reached. The plate bones of the cranial vault exhibit a characteristic 'worm-eaten' appearance that has been given the name caries sicca (Fig. 7.14). Most commonly the parietal and frontal bones of the vault are affected, the pathological process being one of gross destruction and irregular repair. The inflammation commences within the internal substance of the skull bones themselves and gradually spreads both outwards and inwards. Eventually perforation of the skull may result (Hackett, 1981). Although changes do occur at the nasal area and palate (Fig. 7.15), these are not so marked as in yaws and endemic syphilis.

There is yet another difference that adds a further dimension to the

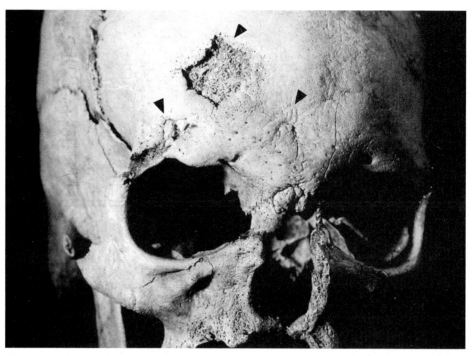

7.14 Involvement of skull surface in caries sicca

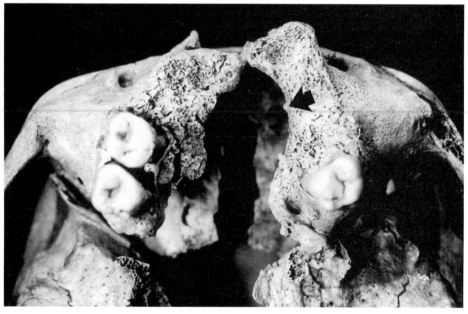

7.15 Palatal destructive lesions of Fig. 7.14

treponemal diseases. This is the ability of the *Treponema pallidum* of venereal syphilis to pass from an infected mother across the placenta to an unborn child. This unwelcome infection of a totally innocent victim gives rise to congenital syphilis. It may suggest a difference between the species of *Treponema*, but the absence of congenital infection in endemic syphilis is rather puzzling, except of course that this latter is largely a disease of the young who are not as yet involved in reproduction. It is probable that transplacental passage of the bacterium occurs in pregnancy during the secondary stage of venereal syphilis, during which phase there is haematogenous spread of *Treponema*. It is considered (Grmek, 1994) that pregnancy will not occur during this secondary stage in endemic syphilis because of the young age of the infected female. The clinical features of congenital syphilis are in some respects similar to those of acquired venereal syphilis. The osteomyelitis of the tibia produces the sabre shin so characteristic of the treponemal infections, the multiple bone involvement (Panuel, 1994) and the notched, so-called Hutchinson's, teeth and mulberry molars are the cardinal features of this disease. The rarity of congenital syphilis in palaeopathological contexts is largely due to the fact that the disease carries a 50 per cent mortality in the very young. The skeleton of a newborn case of congenital syphilis recovered from an archaeological excavation will rarely, if ever, be recognized for what it is. As always, it is seen that palaeopathological diagnosis is so dependent upon age at death, preservation and recognition.

For many years the search for the origin and evolution of the treponemal diseases centred on venereal syphilis and its relation to the trans-Atlantic expeditions of Christopher Columbus (Baker and Armelagos, 1988). In general, Europeans chose to relate the European onset of the disease to the return of the Columbus expedition, which, it was said, infected Europe with the treponemes from America. The Americans, in their turn, chose to regard the disease as of Old World, but not necessarily European, origin. Although the argument has not ended, and some still see the answer to the treponemal question around 1493 (Møller-Christensen, 1969b, 1978b), it is probable that the recent, but pre-antibiotic, global distribution of pinta, yaws, endemic syphilis and venereal syphilis holds the key to the origin of these most elusive diseases of antiquity (Hudson, 1968).

Figure 7.16 indicates the world-wide distribution of the treponemal diseases at about 1900, that is, before effective antibiotic therapy. It is noted that pinta occupies the area of Central America only; yaws, the belt around the equator in many countries; and endemic syphilis, in the arid regions north and south of the yaws territory. Venereal syphilis is widespread, and to some extent without geographic frontiers, but with a predilection for the crowded urban centres of civilization. It is considered (Hackett, 1963) that pinta was the primitive human precursor and, at about 15,000 BC, was widespread following the migrations of people out of Central Africa. It was carried to the Americas across the Bering land bridge and, for some reason not understood at present, there it remained, even after its disappearance elsewhere. Thus, a Central African cradle is accepted, as is the primeval status of pinta. Contrary to this opinion of the primogeniture of *Treponema carateum*, Grmek (1994) notes that a species that is isolated in a

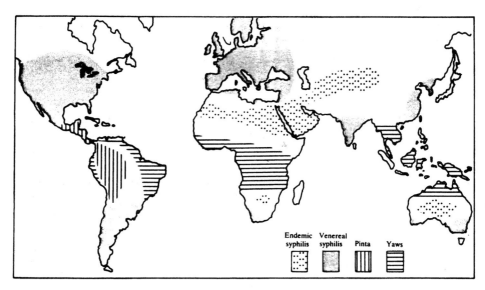

7.16 Distribution of the treponematoses AD 1900 (after Hackett, 1963)

territory at the edge of the geographic area in which its group has expanded should not be considered primitive. This is precisely the case with pinta in the modern world, isolated as it is to Mesoamerica. On this basis, Grmek considers that yaws, not pinta, is the most ancient clinical manifestation of treponemal infection in humans. Thereafter opinions vary. Some (Hudson, 1958, 1965) regard pinta, yaws, endemic syphilis and venereal syphilis as different clinical manifestations of but one disease, treponematosis.

The proposition holds that the migration of people carried the treponeme to different climatic areas and that this climatic variation resulted in the apparently different diseases. The change was not, however, of the bacterium but rather of people's social adaptation to their new environment. The absence of clothes in the humid tropics allowed the easy transference by skin-to-skin contact in yaws. The more huddled, closely knit villages of the arid Near East encouraged the treponeme to become endemic, particularly in the increased child population. Such a change is due to many factors, not least an increased population size unit, a more settled existence and, as a cause or a consequence, the more year-round assured food supply. With increased urbanization of the temperate zones, the relaxation of sexual attitudes, increased climatic necessity for clothes and increased element of unsettled and maritally unattached individuals, the treponeme was encouraged to find new routes of transmission. In such circumstances transmission by the intimacy of sexual intercourse replaced the more casual skin contact of yaws and endemic syphilis. Venereal syphilis entered the scene and, like many infections, its spread was facilitated by urbanization, prostitution and military and religious pilgrimage (Hudson, 1963). Prostitution, the familiar reservoir of venereal infection, has no place in village society.

It has been found that there is a back and forth transition from one treponemal disease to another even within a single group of people on changing from one environment to another. This support for Hudson's theory has led to his statement that every social group has the kind of treponematosis that is appropriate to its geographical and climatic home and its stage of cultural development (Hudson, 1965). It is also noted that there can be differing presentations within separate peoples living in the same geographic environment. For example, in the yaws regions, groups such as Europeans with higher standards of living rarely develop yaws but do develop venereal syphilis (Cockburn, 1961). The relationship between geographic area, climatic environment and treponemal infection is therefore by no means straightforward.

The second major theory of treponemal evolution regards the causative bacteria of pinta, yaws and syphilis as separate species of the genus *Treponema* (Hackett, 1963; Brothwell, 1970) and ascribes their origin to the mutation of the primeval *Treponema carateum* under the influence of climatic variation. Mutation is a phenomenon that must be common in the rapidly multiplying world of bacteria. By the Darwinian process of natural selection, certain mutants may be better adapted to the new climate. Their reproduction at the expense of the parent species will thus ensure the new clinical presentation of disease. The two theories, which, in practice, are not so widely different, centre around the taxonomy of *Treponema*.

Notwithstanding these theories, there remains to be explained the startling, almost meteoric, rise to importance of venereal syphilis in sixteenth-century Europe. Lending support to the Columbian theory, documentary records attest the near-epidemic status of the disease around 1500. Clearly, a decade or so after the return of Columbus' force, be it syphilitic or not, is insufficient time to unleash a European pandemic. This is not an epidemiological reality with a chronic disease such as syphilis. It is possible, however, that Columbus brought back from the Americas a more virulent strain of *Treponema pallidum* and that this was responsible for converting a long-standing and comparatively mild disease in Europe into one of fulminating character. It has been further proposed (Hackett, 1967) that venereal syphilis in Europe prior to the Columbian expeditions was not identified specifically from several other diseases, including leprosy. Possible support for this is noted in the medieval belief in the venereal mode of transmission of leprosy. However, skeletal evidence from medieval leprosy cemeteries does not support this proposition.

Holcomb (1940), in discussing the possible medieval diagnostic confusion of leprosy, cites syphilis as one of the confusing diseases. He refers to the writings of observers as early as the fourteenth and fifteenth centuries, among them being Paracelsus and Guy de Chauliac. These workers refer to diseases that may now be interpreted as venereal syphilis. There is, however, no general agreement on these interpretations, which rely so much on the observations, acumen and accuracy of recording of the early physicians.

Doubtless, discussions of these theories will continue for many years, but what of the skeletal evidence? Clearly, palaeopathological evidence of pinta is not found. In order to place in true perspective the corporeal evidence of treponemal infection from antiquity, it must be restated that less than 15 per cent of infected individuals display bone changes of their infection. Taking into account such aspects as the often-assumed earlier age at death in antiquity, it is likely that in studying the skeletal evidence from the past, one is seeing merely the tip of the iceberg. The earliest evidence of yaws comes from the Mariana Islands and is dated to about AD 850 (Stewart and Spoehr, 1967). The diagnosis has been made on the classic cranial and long-bone features of the disease. Evidence of yaws from later periods has come from pre-European-contact Australia, pre-contact Tonga, Easter Island, Borneo and Puerto Rico (Steinbock, 1976), and Guam (Rothschild and Heathcote, 1993).

The separation of venereal from endemic syphilis in early skeletal specimens depends upon the geographic origin of the specimen just as much as the bone lesions. An example of endemic syphilis showing skull and long-bone changes in an Australian Aboriginal skeleton of pre-European-contact date has been described (Sandison, 1980b). A further case has been described in a skull from Tasmania, and it is suggested that the disease accompanied the original inhabitants on their migration from Australia into Tasmania some 10,000 years ago (Hackett, 1974). A European example has also been noted from this period (Anderson et al., 1986).

For reasons already discussed, which were perhaps not always scientifically motivated, concentration of thought has been on venereal syphilis almost at the expense of the other treponemal diseases.

The early evidence of syphilis in the Old World is sparse indeed. Examples from Siberia dated as early as 1000 BC have been diagnosed as possible syphilis (Steinbock, 1976). An extensive examination of several thousand early Egyptian and European skeletons has failed to reveal evidence of syphilis prior to AD 1500 (Møller-Christensen, 1969b). A single female skull with typical caries sicca has been discovered in the burial ground of Spitalfields, London, and dated prior to 1537 (Morant, 1931). Unfortunately the terminus post quem is 1197 and further dating precision cannot be made. Evidence of the early presence of syphilis in England has also come from the cemetery of St Helen-on-the-Walls, York. A skull from this cemetery displays caries sicca. The burials are mainly dated to the fifteenth and sixteenth centuries (Dawes and Magilton, 1980) and this particular skull has been radiocarbon dated to before AD 1492. With increased cemetery excavations, skeletal examination using improved diagnostic techniques and dating precision, further examples of pre-Columbian treponemal disease have been identified in Europe (Stirland, 1991a, 1994; Power, 1992; Gladykowska-Rzeczycka, 1994; Henneberg and Henneberg, 1994; Roberts, 1994). A diagnosis of congenital syphilis and thus venereal syphilis has been proposed for fetal remains from Hyères, France (Pálfi et al., 1992).

Evidence of early treponemal disease in the Old World may be inferred from the documentary records of treatment, but this is, of course, circumstantial evidence only. It appears that in the twelfth and thirteenth centuries, the Crusading forces in the Levant were using 'Saracen ointment' to treat a disease that they diagnosed as leprosy. This ointment contained mercury and, for whatever disease it was efficacious, it was certainly useless in the treatment of leprosy. For many years, mercurial compounds were used in the treatment of syphilis. The suggestion is therefore that the Crusaders were using their mercurial ointments to treat syphilis. Such evidence is tentative when compared to the irrefutable evidence of palaeopathology.

In contrast to the sparse evidence from the Old World prior to AD 1500, North and Central America afford indisputable evidence of pre-Columbian syphilis. Cases of the disease have been diagnosed from Pecos Pueblo, New Mexico; from Arizona; from Alabama; from Ohio (El-Najjar, 1979) and North Carolina (Reichs, 1989). Skeletal evidence of the cardiovascular sequelae of late-stage venereal syphilis is rare indeed. From the northern plains of North America, a single specimen exhibiting erosion of the posterior surface of the manubrium and the anterior surfaces of the second and third thoracic vertebrae is indicative of an aneurysm of the aorta, an arterial dilatation probably responsible for death of the individual (Walker, 1983). The skeleton of an American Indian child dated by association to before AD 1400 has the skull and long-bone features of congenital syphilis, thus supporting the venereal origin of the disease.

Ideas concerning the bacteriology and the history of the treponemal diseases will no doubt be modified from time to time. With increasing archaeological excavation and with firmly established diagnostic criteria, the evidence for early treponemal disease will accumulate. The evolutionary models already discussed, based in part on theory and in part on the observed skeletal evidence, suggest that human infection due to bacteria of the genus treponema existed in both pre-Columbian Europe and pre-Columbian America. Infective diseases are not solely microbiological entities but are a composite reflection of individual immunity, and social, environmental and biological interaction.

Parasitic infection

In many parts of the world today, particularly those bordering the tropics, infection by the larger parasites is a cause of considerable morbidity. By and large it is the endoparasites, which live within the host's body, which tend to give rise to chronic disease and are therefore responsible, in part, for the chronic ill-health that characterizes some of the poorer nations of the world, at least in the recent past. A similar situation must have existed in the more distant past also. Since many of these parasites do not solely attack humans but have animal host stages in their life cycle, a prerequisite for human infection is a close animal-to-human contact. Many parasites have infected humans only since, in the evolutionary process, the latter have become omnivorous, eating meat as well as vegetable foods. Several parasites, either as adults or at some stage in the life cycle, live within the flesh of animals. It is by eating such flesh that humans become infected. This may, in part, explain the food taboos of certain religious groups. For example, the Jewish avoidance of pork may be due to their knowledge in the distant past of infection of pigs by *Taenia solium*, and its transference to humans by the eating of infected pork. This knowledge was obviously not gained by scientific observation but was the result of years of conscious experience. Parasitic infection of people is likely to have become more widespread with animal domestication, and its increase may therefore have run parallel with tuberculosis.

Unfortunately in palaeopathological terms, the evidence for these parasitic infections is sparse, but techniques of investigation are improving. The range of parasitic infections in antiquity is becoming known (Sandison, 1981). The parasites themselves are, like our own flesh and blood, soft tissues. Just like our own soft tissues, these parasites putrefy and disappear after burial of the host. Occasionally, however, parasitic remains are discovered in mummified human remains. Perhaps the earliest observation of this kind was made by Ruffer (1910). He found eggs of the parasite *Schistosoma haematobium* in the kidneys of two mummies of XX Dynasty date. This condition, known at one time as bilharziasis, induces bleeding into the urinary tract and, even today, is a source of considerable morbidity in parts of Africa and the Mediterranean. In more recent mummy investigations, evidence of many more parasites has been found.

Unfortunately, the osteoarchaeological evidence of parasitic infection consists of very few examples. A worm of the genus *Echinococcus* lives in the intestines of dogs and foxes. The parasite eggs are passed in the faeces of these animals and if, due to food or water contamination, they are ingested by humans the eggs enter the life-cycle phases of the worm. They develop into multiple cystic structures called hydatid cysts which inhabit various organs of the body, principally the liver and, to a lesser extent, the lungs. By good fortune, at least for the palaeopathologist if not for the affected individual, these cysts calcified in a medieval Danish woman and were discovered on excavation (Fig. 7.17). Seventy-two identified cysts and many fragments of similar cysts were found in the area of the abdominal cavity (Weiss and Møller-Christensen, 1971b). A solitary cyst measuring 47 × 35 mm was found in the chest cavity of a Romano-British woman. This hydatid cyst was presumably in the lung (Wells, 1976). A solitary egg-shaped lesion was found in the area of the abdomen of a skeleton from medieval Winchester. The lesion was shown on radiography to have a smooth inner lining characteristic of a calcified hydatid cyst (Price, 1975).

People have for a long time lived in fairly close association with dogs. Animals may have been used for hunting or may, as in recent times, have been kept as pets and companions. The potential for this parasitic transfer from dog to human has been ever present. The squalid and unhygienic lifestyle of the medieval town possibly increased human population prevalence. It is then surprising that more evidence of such cysts is not forthcoming. These cysts are, however, thin walled and fragile and may not have survived their environment of deposition over several hundred years of burial. Their presence should nevertheless be looked for during the archaeological excavation of human skeletal remains.

Knowledge of the endoparasitic infections of humans in antiquity is becoming more extensive, arising from a perhaps unexpected source. The excavation of settlement sites is producing material from latrines and rubbish pits, and certain environments will preserve evidence. Examination of this material is revealing the presence of parasitic eggs which were presumably passed in the faeces of humans and animals of antiquity (Reinhard, 1990; Reinhard *et al.*, 1992). Fortunately the eggs of these worms of the distant past have specific and characteristic forms.

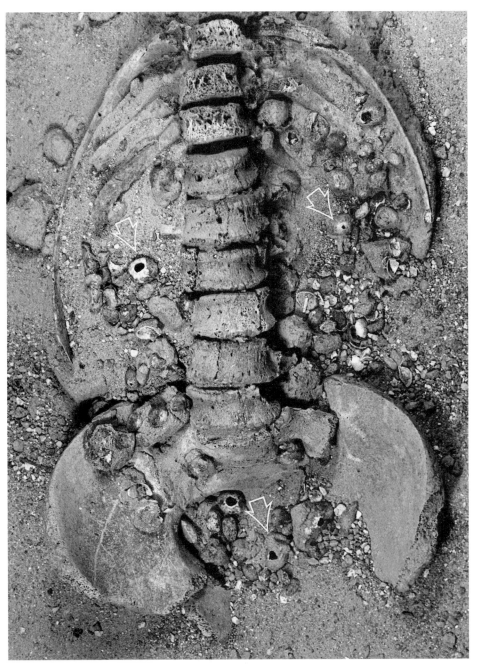

7.17 Calcified cysts in the abdominal cavity of a female burial, medieval Denmark (some arrowed)

Microscopic examination of latrine deposits not only confirms the infection of earlier people but allows a specific diagnosis to be made. Eggs of *Trichuris trichiura* (whipworm) and *Ascaris lumbricoides* (roundworm) have been found in the medieval cesspits of York, England (Jones, 1985). With such knowledge, the clinical symptoms and consequences of infection can be deduced. Abdominal discomfort, diarrhoea and constant blood loss associated with tape worm infection must have accounted for much morbidity in past populations. Maybe the chronic iron deficiency anaemia causing cribra orbitalia and porotic hyperostosis, to be considered in the next chapter, is in part due to such infection. These microscopic findings of environmental archaeology are reliable but circumstantial evidence of parasitic infection of humans.

Of much wider distribution and of much less clinical significance are the infestations of humans by ectoparasites. These organisms do not enter the body but live on the skin surface and hair. For survival they suck the blood of the host. Ectoparasites such as the flea, head and body lice, and ticks usually cause no more serious problem than a rash and the social embarrassment of itching. Occasionally, however, these arthropods may be the vectors of serious disease. Harbouring smaller organisms, notably the different species of *Rickettsia*, within their intestinal tract, the human ectoparasites may transfer these agents of disease directly to the bloodstream of humans. The infectious disease of typhus is a serious, sometimes fatal, sequel to life in insanitary conditions. Also known as camp fever, typhus was well known to campaigning troops in recent wars. No doubt it was common too in earlier times, particularly among the besieged and the besiegers in prolonged medieval warfare. But there is no skeletal or mummified evidence of this acute infectious disease. There are, however, preserved ectoparasites in mummified remains. Of a small series of North American Indian mummies examined, 44 per cent had head lice (El-Najjar and Mulinski, 1980). The eggs of head lice are also common findings in the mummies of Peru (Vreeland and Cockburn, 1980). In addition, Zias and Mumcuoglu (1991) found head lice preserved in hair combs in Israel.

Although the palaeopathological evidence of ectoparasites is scant, when found their prevalence in a burial group is high. It is deduced therefore that ectoparasitic infection was commonplace in antiquity. Presumably, the diseases such as typhus, dependent upon their parasitism, were also common. It is unfortunate that knowledge concerning the range and prevalence of parasitic infection in the distant past is incomplete because of the limited nature of preservation. Such evidence as there is suggests that the problem was as widespread and varied, if not more so, as it is today. The improvements in food care, hygiene and animal husbandry during the passage of time have, by and large, restricted the problems today to the less developed areas of the world.

CHAPTER 8

Metabolic and Endocrine Disease

If anyone anything lacks. . .

(W.S. Gilbert 1836–1911)

INTRODUCTION

Unfortunately, classification in clinical medicine is not all-embracing. There exist diseases of palaeopathological significance which do not lend themselves to the foregoing classes used in the present volume. These diseases may loosely be considered as the abnormalities of deficiency or excess, not only of dietary constituents, but also of hormones, those chemicals manufactured by the endocrine glands of the body for the maintenance of its health.

Past societies are often assumed to have trodden that fine knife-edge between subsistence and starvation. As has been noted in connection with population expansion, the improved techniques of hunting and refinement of agricultural methods shifted some groups away from starvation, albeit temporarily, even if there was a greater risk of dietary deficiencies through reliance on a less varied and poorer-quality diet (Cohen and Armelagos, 1984). Starvation is still a familiar sight today in the less developed areas of the world, particularly where the rainfall level is critical. No doubt in the past an increasing community size still stretched the food resource. It is not just the total lack of food, the overall starvation problem, which is of relevance. A lack of quality, particularly in respect of the essential vitamins and chemical trace elements, is just as important. Evidence of chronic food shortage, by living on the wrong side of the 'knife-edge', may be deduced from the study of skeletal and dental remains. Many factors may be involved in the production of such skeletal and dental abnormalities, and a direct causal relationship with poor diet cannot be inferred as it is likely that multifactorial causes may be implicated.

The metabolic diseases can also be described as 'indicators of stress', a term used increasingly in the anthropological literature over the past 20 years. The abnormalities observed in skeletal and dental remains represent the individual's adaptive response to stressors working on the body during his or her growing years. That response will be determined by a number of factors, e.g. the individual's immune status and genetic predisposition. What is clear is that a skeleton with no indicators of stress may either suggest a healthy person or it may represent somebody who never recovered from the insults to the body, i.e. they were continually stressed. Selye (1950) suggests that stress is a non-specific response to stimuli, i.e. the body can be stressed by multiple stressors but it displays a very characteristic form and composition when it adapts. Factors in a person's environment may buffer the impact of stress but others may enhance it, and some populations may overcome some stressors but some may not. Although seen as physiological stress, some authors have considered stress as being instrumental in predisposing to disease (Bush, 1991). It is known, for example, that emotional stress can lead to the formation of enamel hypoplastic lines on the teeth (see Chapter 4), and Harris lines of arrested growth in the long bones (see later). Although it may be possible to identify factors in a population's environment, culture or biology that may cause physiological stress, it is virtually impossible to read into their psychology. Goodman et al. (1988) provide a useful summary of the recognized stress indicators shown in prehistoric, historic and contemporary populations. A number of these indicators have already been discussed, and two are particularly relevant here. Mortality rates provide an indication of how healthy and adaptive (or not) a population was by their age at death profile, always assuming that their ages have been determined accurately (see Chapter 2). High infant mortality, for example, suggests that an acute disease may have precipitated deaths in this age group. In addition, integrating mortality data with identified stressors may highlight earlier death in individuals who were stressed (Huss-Ashmore et al., 1982). Also, final attained stature, when compared to that expected of the group, may differ; decreased stature may indicate poor nutrition during growth. For the purposes of this chapter those 'indicators' that show a clear relationship with nutritional inadequacy will be considered; these are anaemia, osteoporosis and Harris lines, plus the specific vitamin deficiencies of scurvy and rickets. Dental enamel defects and periostitis are discussed in Chapters 4 and 7, respectively.

EVIDENCE FOR DIET

Evidence for the type of diet enjoyed by early people may come from the detailed chemical analysis of bone and teeth. The level of trace elements in these tissues has been used as an indicator for dietary status in earlier societies (Price, 1989; Burton and Price, 1992). Burton and Price (ibid.) examined barium/strontium ratios to compare human bones from inland archaeological sites without access to marine resources, from coastal sites where marine foods dominated the diet and from coastal sites where agricultural resources were the mainstay of subsistence. Low barium/strontium ratios characterize marine resources; this should be reflected by these ratios in humans who have consumed such resources. A successful distinction was made between the populations showing large differences in consumption of marine resources, although several problems were highlighted in the analysis, not least diagenetic alteration of those elements.

Plants and terrestrial vertebrates metabolize strontium and calcium differently. The ratio of these two elements is therefore different in these two major life forms. In consequence, people consuming a diet rich in meat have a different strontium:calcium ratio in their bones from those with a more vegetarian diet. Such trace element analysis has been used not only for palaeodietary research, but also to investigate social ranking within cemetery groups. It is suggested that dietary type, either vegetarian or containing more meat, may reflect different ranks within a hierarchical society (Schoeninger, 1979).

The analysis of trace elements does, indeed, have its problems, particularly because of the influence of burial on the skeleton and uptake of elements from surrounding soil, the very elements being analysed as dietary indicators. Price (1989: 251) suggested methods for discovering and controlling for the effects of diagenesis, which he stressed must be developed. In addition, some elements seem to be more useful than others, but often their relationship to diet is unclear. Strontium, zinc, barium and sodium were elements considered the most useful and promising (Price, ibid.). The diagenesis problem (Hanson and Buikstra, 1988) has been addressed by some researchers (Pate and Hutton, 1988; Lambert et al., 1989; Price et al., 1992), and consideration of the part of the bone being analysed with respect to the results obtained have been investigated (Grupe, 1988a). Grupe found that the outer compact bone is less susceptible to diagenesis and that trabecular bone was giving less reliable data. Clearly, more work is necessary to eliminate the problems inherent in trace element analysis and palaeodietary studies.

Further evidence of dietary type may come from an analysis of the proportions of carbon isotopes present in human bone (Schwarz and Schoeninger, 1991; Katzenberg, 1992). Analysis of stable isotopes in bone collagen has concentrated on answering questions about the introduction of maize into parts of North America, the reliance on animal versus vegetable protein, and the consumption of marine or terrestrial foods (Katzenberg, ibid.: 105). Work in the UK has examined stable carbon and nitrogen isotope ratios of bone from prehistoric Scotland (Antoine et al., 1988); although a marine-based diet was expected for these island groups, a mixed marine–terrestrial diet was inferred from the results. Simultaneous trace element analysis of this material gave confusing results due to post-mortem deposition of elements in the bone. The problems of diagenesis do not seem to be as acute in isotopic analysis; if collagen is preserved then 'carbon isotope ratios are reliable' (Price, 1989: 251).

The data produced by these methods used to analyse the chemistry of dental and skeletal material can potentially indicate the type of diet an individual was eating; when compared to the palaeopathological record it may shed some light on dietary status and its effect on health.

ANAEMIA

The study of the skeletal changes of anaemia have attracted a great deal of attention in the twentieth century and these data have been applied to questions such as: what happened to a population's health when they started to practise agriculture, and was it more unhealthy to live in an urbanized or a rural community? There are a number of anaemias of different aetiology but this section will deal mainly with the most common form of anaemia, that caused by iron deficiency. Even today much of the world's population has been estimated to be iron deficient (Kent, 1992: 2).

Anaemia can be defined as a reduction in concentration of haemoglobin and/or red blood cells below normal (Wintrobe, 1974). Iron is needed for the development of haemoglobin in newly formed red blood cells in bone marrow, but in anaemia a person's red blood cells become pale and small, and they have a much shorter life span, up to half the normal life of 120 days. Iron is usually stored in the liver and the spleen when old blood cells are broken down. Around 90 per cent of the iron in old red blood cells is needed to form new cells and, as iron deficiency develops, these stores are depleted while the body attempts to absorb increased amounts of iron. Apart from being needed for haemoglobin formation in red blood cells, and hence transfer of oxygen to the body cells, iron is also necessary for transmission of nerve impulses for collagen (protein) synthesis, and contributes to the strength of the immune system.

Iron is found in high quantities in red meat, legumes and shellfish, for example, and is absorbed via the intestines. Iron from plants is harder to absorb, and compounds called phytates in staple cereal crops, such as maize, inhibit iron absorption (whereas vitamin C aids absorption). Cereals are themselves poor sources of iron (Stuart-Macadam, 1992), and it is notable that iron is added today to most of the cereals we eat at breakfast. Thus, the transition from a hunter-gathering to an agriculturally based economy relying on these crops for an adequate varied diet, may have led to iron deficiency in the past. The picture is not that clear cut, however, because many factors can predispose to the development of anaemia (Kent, 1987). In fact Walker (1986) quite categorically states that his study of 400 crania from a Californian fish-dependent group of people living in the prehistoric and historic periods, revealed that this iron-rich diet did not prevent the occurrence of anaemia. However, some fish do have a low iron content, e.g. white fish has 0.5 mg/100 g compared to 7.0 mg/100 g in kidney and liver and 1.9 mg/100 g in beef (HMSO, 1985). These results, of course, support the suggestion that diet is only one of the causes of the bone changes of anaemia.

Apart from an iron-deficient diet, excessive blood loss through injury, chronic disease such as cancer and parasitic infection of the gut probably had a large part to play in the past. It is known from the survival of parasites in archaeological deposits that humans were subject to gut infections (Reinhard, 1988); their prevalence, both geographically and through time is, however, unknown. Last, but certainly not least, is the impact of infection on a population; most nutritional deficiencies are aggravated by infection, and work on the medieval skeletons from a Danish leprosy hospital at Naestved indicated that two-thirds of the group with bone changes of leprosy had skeletal indications of anaemia. At that time Møller-Christensen (1953) believed the lesions in the orbits to be the result of leprosy. Carlson et al. (1974) consider the role parasitic infection had in influencing the occurrence of cribra orbitalia in skeletons from prehistoric Nubia, and Stuart-

Macadam (1992) summarizes the evidence for infectious disease as a major aetiological factor in the development of iron-deficiency anaemia. It is believed that the process of infection leads the body to withhold iron from the pathogens, which need it to survive and reproduce in the body; this makes the body iron deficient. If this theory holds true, then changes in settlement pattern and increasing population density with the transition to agriculture would have led to an increase in infectious diseases; the study of infectious disease in some populations seems to support this theory (Cohen and Armelagos, 1984), although others do not. There are studies (e.g. Møller-Christensen, 1953; Mensforth *et al.*, 1978) where porotic hyperostosis and infection were observed in the same skeleton. If iron-deficiency anaemia is induced by the body as a response to infection, both porotic hyperostosis and infection should not occur together. However, a multitude of factors acts on an individual at different times during his or her life. Therefore, infection and anaemia could reflect different aetiological factors. As Stuart-Macadam (1992: 159–60) suggests, these causes could be a function of many factors such as climate, geography, hygiene, diet, time period and economy.

Fatigue, pallor, shortness of breath and palpitations characterize the disease, with more severe forms creating gastrointestinal disturbances and abnormalities in the skeleton. The bone changes probably only occur in childhood (Stuart-Macadam, 1985), although adults do display the lesions. On the basis of studies of radiographs of patients with anaemia, specific criteria for identification of this disease in archaeological groups have been identified (Stuart-Macadam, 1987). Although anaemia occurs in all areas of the world in the past and today, the bone changes vary in extent and severity. Thinning of the outer table of the skull, due to vertically orientated trabeculae in the diploë causing pressure on the table (the 'hair-on-end' appearance radiographically), and thickening of the diploë between the two skull tables are two of the main criteria highlighted (Figs 8.1 and 8.2). These changes are the result of the body's attempt to produce more red blood cells in the marrow to compensate for lack of iron. Apart from the (external) skull lesions, particularly seen on the parietal and occipital bones, the orbital roofs are affected (Fig. 8.3) in the form of 'holes' in the bone surface (cribra orbitalia). The skeletal changes appear to come in two forms: the orbital lesions alone, and both orbital and vault lesions together – the bones are often symmetrically affected and vault lesions do not tend to occur without the orbits being involved. It has been suggested that the vault lesions indicate a more severe form of the anaemia (Stuart-Macadam, 1989a) but that, because of the similarity of orbital and vault lesions radiographically, both are caused by the same aetiological factor. What is clear is that in archaeological populations in Britain the vault lesions are rarely seen, with cribra orbitalia being much more common. In fact, an increase in porosity of the vault surface is often observed (Fig 8.4), sometimes with no attendant cribra orbitalia.

In a study by Stuart-Macadam (1991) of 752 individuals from a Romano-British site at Poundbury, Dorset in England, 230 had bone changes supporting a diagnosis of anaemia. One hundred and seventy-three (75 per cent) had orbital lesions only, seven (3 per cent) had vault lesions only and 50 (22 per cent) had

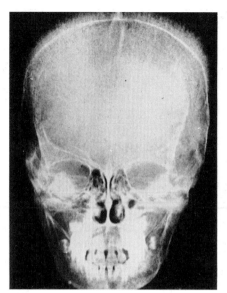
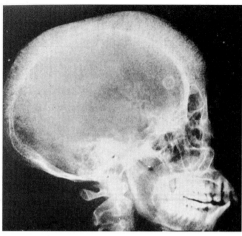

8.1 Radiograph of hair-on-end appearance in porotic hyperostosis of anaemia

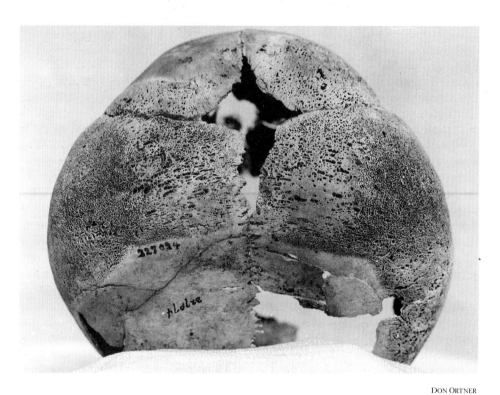

8.2 Cranial vault lesions in anaemia: NMNH 327074, 1–2 year old individual, Pueblo Bonito, New Mexico

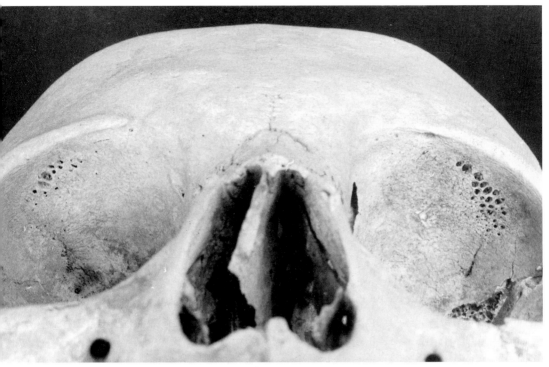

8.3 Cribra orbitalia in both orbits (medieval France)

both. Juveniles had a significantly high prevalence of both orbital and vault lesions, and the lesions were more severe. A similar picture was seen in the analysis of a medieval Christian population from Upper Nubia derived from two cemeteries (Mittler and Van Gerven, 1994); active lesions of anaemia were only observed in the young (up to the age of 12 years) and the frequency of lesions decreased after this time. The presence of these active lesions obviously indicates that the individual had not yet adapted to the disease at the time of death, i.e. the bones are unhealed; in fact studies do show that there is an increased mortality in individuals with cribra orbitalia (Huss-Ashmore *et al.*, 1982). Novel methods of diagnosing anaemia by measuring the iron content of the bone and other organic material in skeletons with and without bone changes of anaemia have indicated a correlation between lower iron levels and anaemia (Fornaciari *et al.*, 1981; Sandford *et al.*, 1983).

Although iron deficiency anaemia is the most commonly observed anaemia today (and probably in the past), two genetic anaemias characterized by abnormal haemoglobin should also be discussed. Both these anaemias produce bone changes in areas of the skeleton other than the skull but, essentially, the skull changes are the same for all the anaemias. Thalassaemia is a genetically determined disorder caused by a problem of haemoglobin synthesis (Steinbock, 1976). Pale cells with low haemoglobin content are produced but are rapidly

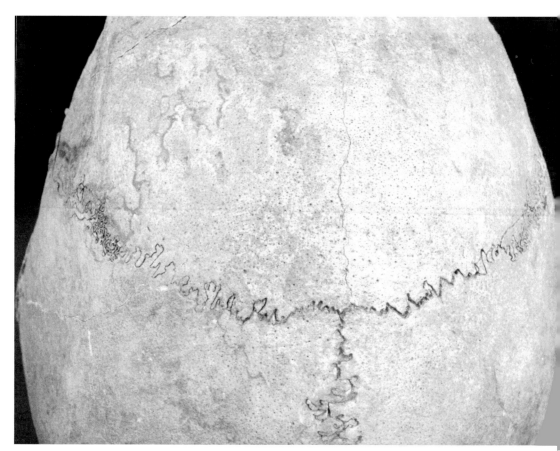

8.4 Increased porosity on frontal and parietal bones (British)

destroyed. A high frequency of the disorder is seen around the Mediterranean, in the Middle East and the Far East. Bone abnormalities in the paranasal sinuses, mastoids and facial bones are seen in addition to the vault and orbital lesions already described. The metacarpals and metatarsals enlarge with thinning of their cortices, and generalized osteoporosis of the spine develops.

The other type of genetic anaemia is sickle-cell anaemia, where abnormal elongation of red blood cells occurs. Two reactions are precipitated in the skeleton: first, bone changes in the skull, vertebrae, pelvis, hand and foot bones occur due to marrow overactivity and enlargement as the body tries to produce more red blood cells; and, secondly, necrosis (death) of bone due to blockage of the blood vessels by these abnormal cells (Steinbock, 1976) develops. Apart from the macroscopic and radiographic features of sickle-cell anaemia, microscopy has also been used for diagnosis. Maat and Baig (1991) identified fossilized sickle cells using scanning electron microscopy in bone from a 2,000-year-old skeleton which supported the macroscopic bone lesions of anaemia; without this information, the diagnosis of the type of anaemia would not have been possible. Today, West, Central and East African populations have high rates of sickle-cell anaemia.

It has been noted that people with sickle-cell anaemia and thalassaemia have a resistance to malaria because the infection cannot develop fast enough between formation and death of red blood cells during their short life span (Steinbock, 1976: 234). Very few cases of sickle-cell anaemia and thalassaemia have been identified in the archaeological record, perhaps because the cranial changes are so similar for all the anaemias. What is clear, however, is the need to consider the geographic context of skeletal material, which may help with the diagnosis of the genetic anaemias in the future.

VITAMIN C AND D DEFICIENCIES

Deficiencies of particular vitamins also produce more specific skeletal changes. It might be assumed that in the hunter-gatherer or agriculturalist past, vitamin C deficiency was unlikely to occur. This vitamin is found in fresh fruits and uncooked vegetables, natural produce which probably contributed to the staple diet of many past human groups. With the transition to agriculture the availability of vitamin C from fresh foods may have been reduced, together with losses due to cooking of foods and prolonged storage, both common in settled communities; scurvy, the clinical manifestation of vitamin C deficiency, is known, albeit rarely, from osteoarchaeological remains.

This vitamin is necessary for the bodily combat of infection, for the absorption of iron and it is essential for the normal formation of the body tissues (especially collagen). In addition to reducing the resistance to infection, vitamin C deficiency predisposes to bleeding into the skin and beneath the periosteum (membrane surrounding the bones). Apart from faulty formation of the periosteum and the ligaments holding the teeth in the sockets, the cement substance in the blood vessels is defective and predisposes the individual to haemorrhage into the soft tissues, bones (especially the jaws) and joints. The result is the formation of new bone on the skeleton as a response to bleeding. Most commonly the gums swell and bleed, and this leads to the development of periodontal disease (see Chapter 4).

Skeletally the evidence for scurvy consists of new bone formation, potentially anywhere on the skeleton. Recent work (Ortner, 1984; Roberts, 1987) suggests that the new bone may be localized in the jaws, in the orbits and along the lines of the temporalis muscle (important for chewing). The change in the orbits is characteristically new bone formation, not to be confused with the lesions of anaemia (Fig. 8.5).

Perhaps prolonged winters in an inhospitable northern climate in Europe, for example, and the consequent absence of fresh produce for many months would create this scurvy of antiquity. It is proposed that scurvy as a disease would have been more common in settled agricultural communities where gathering of fresh fruit would have been limited and consumption of staple crops would have reduced vitamin C intake. Reliance on staple crops such as maize, containing little vitamin C, would also have predisposed people to scurvy. Certainly, the long sea voyages of later centuries were a noted cause of the disease and, as is well known,

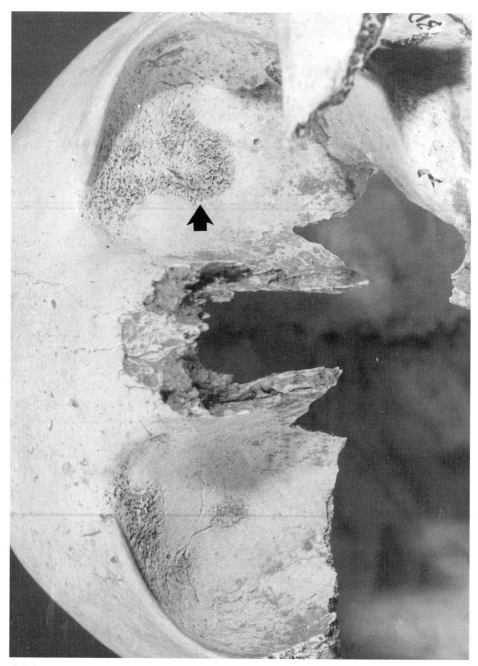

8.5 Orbital new bone formation representing scurvy (1st century BC, Beckford, Worcestershire, England)

provided observations that were used for the early recognition and treatment of scurvy. Other predisposing factors are premature or twin births, infection and feeding with prepared infant foods (Stuart-Macadam, 1989b: 202); this latter cause may not be relevant if one assumes that in most societies in the past children were breast-fed.

For all this, however, scurvy is a palaeopathological rarity, probably due to non-recognition or misdiagnosis in the palaeopathological record. Evidence in palaeopathology consists of the identification of the bony reaction to haemorrhage; in addition, periodontal disease, ante-mortem tooth loss, haemorrhage into the joints and radiopaque lines on radiographs of long bones are also highlighted as potential scurvy indicators. Ortner (1984) highlights the orbital roofs as being one of the areas to examine for haemorrhage and new bone formation. Ortner (1984) and Roberts (1987) describe two of the few convincing cases in the archaeological record. The former is of an 8-year-old child from Alaska with reactive bone change in the orbits and jaws, extending to the anterior portions of the temporal bones, all suggestive of mechanical chewing stress and haemorrhage. Similar changes were observed in a 3–4-year-old child from a cemetery in Britain dated to between 100 BC and AD 43. A final example comes from The Netherlands (Maat, 1982), where historical evidence for scurvy was considered in the examination of fifty whalers' skeletons buried between AD 1642 and the end of the eighteenth century on an island called Zeeusche Uytkyck. Thirty-nine of the fifty skeletons had evidence of scurvy, including bleeding into the joints and gums. The rarity of scurvy in the archaeological record may be the result of the availability of adequate sources of vitamin C in the past. It is, however, likely that cases are not being recognized or are being misdiagnosed, especially if the orbital lesions are being mistaken for the changes of anaemia. The widespread new bone formation in this deficiency disease may also be a complicating factor, considering the number of disease processes that can initiate this patterning of skeletal abnormalities.

Vitamin D deficiency can also produce chronic abnormalities in the skeleton. This vitamin is necessary for absorption of calcium and phosphorus and the mineralization of osteoid (the organic matrix of bone) and cartilage, and its deficiency leads to a 'softening' of the bones. If this chronic deficiency occurs during the growing period, the disease is called rickets. The weight-bearing bones of the legs become bent and deformed when walking commences (Fig. 8.6); there is no reason not to suspect that the arm bones may also deform when crawling commences. Other bones of the body also deform under the influence of muscular contraction. The ends of the growing long bones expand and, in appearance, resemble the widened end of a trumpet; this reflects excessive unmineralized cartilage causing increase in length and width in the growth plates of the bones. In addition, the costochondral areas of the ribs become nodular prominences (rachitic rosary), the pelvis is retarded in growth, dental development and health may be affected and the skull tables may be thinned, usually in the area subject to pressure when the infant is resting (Steinbock, 1976: 266). The squat, bow-legged little figure is not so familiar in England today as he or she was 100 years ago. The woman in labour unable to give birth because of the obstruction of a deformed

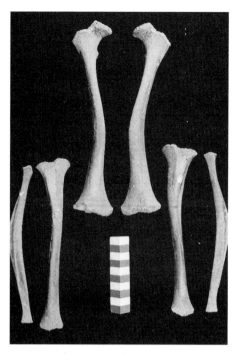

DON ORTNER

8.6 Rickets in long bones: FABC B–37, 8-year-old male, First African Baptist Church, AD 1823–1841, Philadelphia, USA

pelvis was a recognized hazard of past obstetric practice. The child fortunate enough to have been born and to have survived the precarious neonatal period was pushed further on their ricketty road by the inadequacy of their mother's milk. A chronically underfed woman would produce the calcium-deficient milk so imperilling her infant's well-being and reducing her already low health status.

The ingestion of vitamin D from, for example, fish oil and animal fat is not the only source of the vitamin. The human skin is able to effect a chemical change so producing vitamin D from a chemical precursor; 90 per cent of the body's vitamin D requirement is produced in the skin. This change is, however, dependent upon ultraviolet light. In the past the only source of this was sunshine. Clearly, the children of antiquity, spending their days outside, were unlikely to develop rickets, even during the northern winter months. Urbanization and the later industrial revolution in the cities were the sources of such a danger; vitamin D deficiency has been termed a disease of civilization. The huddled, overhanging houses of the city would black out any sunlight that managed to penetrate the barrier of industrial smoke. The poor, often underfed children were compelled to work the daylight hours in the noise, danger and shelter of the factory. In such circumstances rickets was prevalent. In fact, Hess (1929) noted that the prevalence of rickets coincided almost exactly with a deficiency of sunlight. Fildes (1986) noted that rickets was a common disease in England in the seventeenth and eighteenth centuries ('the English disease') and Madonna and Child paintings produced in The Netherlands of the fifteenth and sixteenth centuries show characteristic deformities in the form of bowed legs and deformed chests. It was described in seventeenth–century England as a new disease, which does support the lack of evidence before that time in the British archaeological record. Massage and splinting of affected limbs, and special boots and long coats to hide deformities were advocated (Fildes, ibid.: 128), while the livers of birds and fish, and later (post-1780s) cod liver oil, were dietary recommendations; of course, cod liver oil is high in vitamin D but it should be remembered that 90 per cent of this vitamin is formed by the action of sunlight on the skin. It seems that this was not understood until very much later.

The osteoarchaeological evidence of rickets is not plentiful, particularly in the more distant past. Evidence of the disease has been found in Neolithic skeletons from Denmark and Norway (Sigerist, 1951) and more plentiful evidence comes from Hungary during the Roman period (Wells, 1964a). The rarity of this disease in antiquity is attested by Gejvall, who records (1960) that in his extensive examination of human remains, only two cases were identified. Møller-Christensen's study of 800 medieval skeletons from the Æbelholt Monastery in Denmark revealed only nine cases of rickets (Møller-Christensen, 1958). A classic example of rickets has been highlighted in a 7-year-old child from the medieval cemetery of St Helen-on-the-Walls, York, England (Dawes and Magilton, 1980). A recently reported case from Ireland (Power and O'Sullivan, 1992) illustrates well the bending deformities of the lower legs; associated with these deformities was short stature, developmental defects of the teeth and retention of three deciduous teeth. Perhaps the examination of the later burial grounds of the Industrial Revolution period would even the balance on the palaeopathology of rickets, but at present this disease of civilization appears to have been a rarity in past populations. It may be that much of the evidence for rickets is lost, since, if deformities were fairly mild in childhood, remodelling in adulthood may have obscured them from identification (and some adult bones do show abnormal bending deformities of a minor degree). However, recent work on a later (post-medieval) population of Spitalfields, London, dated to the eighteenth/nineteenth centuries AD (Molleson and Cox, 1993), showed that at least twenty children and fifteen adults had rickets. Feeding with prepared infant foods, swaddling and keeping infants housebound for the first year of life may all be factors contributing to the prevalence of rickets in this population.

Osteomalacia is the adult counterpart of childhood rickets. Softening of the bones occurs as a result of dietary calcium deficiency, or as a result of abnormal loss of calcium from the body in kidney or intestinal disease. The loss associated with prolonged suckling of infants has already been mentioned, but multiple pregnancies in rapid succession will also deplete calcium stores (Steinbock, 1976: 272). The result of this bone demineralization in adults is not bending of the bone characteristic of rickets, but rather the collapse and deformity of the vertebrae under weight-bearing stress and the deformity of the pelvis, which is of such catastrophic obstetric significance. Bending deformities in the long bones are rare unless it is a severe case, and flaring of the ends of the bones is not present, due to closure of the growth plates. The frequency of minor degrees of vertebral collapse in skeletal remains suggests that osteomalacia may have been a common feature of earlier people, but diagnostic precision rests upon the characteristic radiographic or microscopic findings in these early skeletons, as there are many causes of vertebral collapse, such as tuberculosis and osteoporosis.

HARRIS LINES OF ARRESTED GROWTH

A less-specific condition (in terms of aetiology) seen in skeletal material is Harris lines of arrested growth. They are seen as dense, opaque transverse lines, particularly on the radiographs of long bones; the tibia, femur and radius tend to

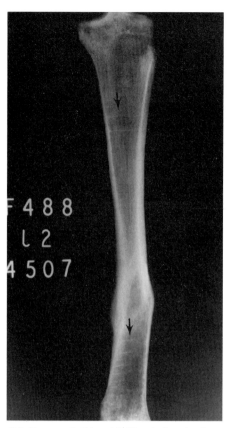

8.7 Fractured tibia with Harris lines in the proximal and distal ends (4th century AD, Baldock, Hertfordshire, England)

be the most often affected bones (Fig. 8.7). These lines represent periods of stress when the bone growth in length has been arrested. Nutritional deficiencies or childhood disease, since these lines can only occur when the bones are growing, have been implicated as causes, based on experiments on animals and observations on humans (Harris, 1931). For a line to occur in a bone, the individual has to have recovered from the stress episode, i.e. a person continually malnourished and diseased will not display Harris lines; they are, in effect, 'recovery lines'. These lines mark the ends of the bone when the growth arrest occurred so, in theory, calculation of the age at formation should be possible (Hunt and Hatch, 1981; Hummert and Van Gerven, 1985). Based on modern growth rates, it has to be assumed that growth occurred at the same rate in the past – not an easy assumption to make. However, the study of the age distribution of Harris lines in a population will provide more information on the major stress periods in an individual's life, e.g. weaning or childhood disease (see Goodman and Clarke, 1981 for an example). One of the major problems in analysis is that as the individual ages the lines can become invisible, i.e. remodelled away, because of continual bone turnover.

The mechanism behind line formation starts with arrest of cartilage proliferation at the growth plate; the thin layer of cartilage cells below the plate are replaced by osteoblasts which form a thin layer of bone (Steinbock, 1976: 46). When the stress has been overcome, the osteoblasts recover immediately and begin laying down bone, visible on a radiograph as a transverse line. Since Harris lines are formed in the growing years, the study of subadult individuals would seem to provide the most reliable prevalence rates, but most researchers have analysed skeletons over the full age range. However, if the adults are not considered (due to the vagaries of Harris line survival in the bone), differences between the sexes cannot be studied (Martin *et al.*, 1985). The recording of Harris lines has its problems too. It appears to be generally accepted that if a line extends 50 per cent or more across the bone shaft it should be recorded; but if a line was being resorbed at the time of the person's death, it may not extend that far across the bone, so should it be counted? Interobserver error has also been noted as a problem in the recording of Harris lines (Macchiarelli *et al.*, 1994). Results of tests showed a substantial interobserver disagreement of Harris line estimates when recording them on radiographs and bone sections. If standardization of recording is not practised, and interobserver error not accounted for between researchers, results cannot be reliably compared.

The association of Harris lines with other indicators of stress has been examined on skeletal groups (e.g. Clarke, 1982) with inconclusive results, suggesting that the aetiology of these particular 'indicators of stress' is complex, and that the same cause cannot be implicated for all stressors. Furthermore, many studies of hunter-gathering and farming populations in the past have noted the decrease in number of lines with the transition to agriculture (Cohen and Armelagos, 1984). Although it provides an indication of particularly problematic periods in terms of health during a person's growth, the study of Harris lines has many problems.

OSTEOPOROSIS

Osteoporosis is, today, accepted as the most common of the skeletal metabolic diseases; it is also seen in other animals (Sumner *et al.*, 1989). The osteoporoses are 'a heterogeneous set of disorders characterised by a reduction in total bone volume caused by thinning of the cortical walls of the long bones . . . thinning and loss of trabeculae, and increased porosity, principally of cancellous bone' (Burr and Martin, 1989: 197–8). Relatively little is known of its frequency in the past, due to problems in diagnosis. There is no reason to suspect that frequency rates were any less than today. However, because of increased longevity and an increasing incidence of the disease with age, its prominence is a subject for media attention.

Age is the most common correlate of osteoporosis (Woolf and St John Dixon, 1988), but a multitude of disease processes include osteoporosis as one of their many clinical features, e.g. rheumatoid arthritis. Osteoporosis does not seem to select for any particular ethnic group or social class, although studies have shown Black groups to have a higher bone mass than White groups (Nelson *et al.*, 1991) and, therefore, more bone has to be lost before osteoporosis is visible in the former group. Although ageing is the most common cause of osteoporosis, general factors such as diet, sex, lack of exercise, circulating sex hormones, prolonged lactation and a high number of pregnancies, smoking, caffeine and alcohol all have their part to play. Of course, some of these factors may be more significant for some groups both today and in the past. During their lives, females always have lower bone mass than males, and the difference increases after the menopause when lower levels of oestrogen circulate around the body. Oestrogen is a hormone which, among other functions, prevents excessive destruction of bone by osteoclasts. The age at menopause today has a mean of 50 years (Woolf and St John Dixon, ibid.: 168). Documentary records from classical Greece and Rome (Amundsen and Diers, 1970) suggest that the menopause occurred then around

40 to 50 years of age. This is a factor to bear in mind in the study of past human groups. If, as some researchers suggest, women died in their earlier years, the menopause may not have been significant in the development of osteoporosis. Obviously longevity will vary between groups from different eras and geographic locations.

Diet appears to be another major factor in influencing osteoporosis development. Calcium is the most abundant mineral in the body and it is crucial to the formation of teeth and bones. Disturbances in calcium intake alter the rate of mineralization of new bone matrix formed. A high intake of calcium throughout life is associated with higher bone mass, but the effects of calcium supplementation on osteoporosis development in post-menopausal females varies between studies. Of course, vitamin D is also essential to allow the absorption of calcium (and phosphorus), and a high-protein diet leads to inhibition of calcium absorption and an increase in urinary calcium is seen (Stini, 1990). Calcium depletion may also be caused by factors such as prolonged lactation, frequent pregnancies and reduced access to dairy foods. Furthermore, fluoride may protect against osteoporosis but further studies are needed, and obesity ensures a higher bone mass and prevents osteoporosis (Woolf and St John Dixon, ibid.: 46). Finally, higher bone mass is seen in people who exercise regularly. Mechanical demands on the skeleton actively promote increased bone mass. Of course, starting exercise post-menopausally after never having exercised before would not prevent osteoporosis.

Diet and exercise would be considered (along with age) as relevant factors in osteoporosis development in the past, and quality of diet (Martin *et al.*, 1985, 1987) is an area of study relevant to the consideration of disease in general. Linked with osteoporosis would be an assessment of the frequency of indicators of stress, such as mortality, stature, enamel defects, Harris lines and the cranial changes of anaemia – a complex aetiological web which contributes to our understanding of osteoporosis prevalence.

Calcium is available in high quantities in dairy foods (milk and cheese) and vegetables such as broccoli and spinach (in quantity). Thus it may be expected that osteoporosis should be more prevalent in populations practising hunter-gathering rather than agriculture. Some studies show this not to be the case, where cortical thinning, decrease in bone circumference and slowing of growth occurs in a higher frequency in farming groups (Cohen and Armelagos, 1984). However, not all studies show a consistent picture where the protein content of the diet is concerned; it would be expected that earlier hunting groups would have more ready access to protein from hunted animals (the best balanced protein for humans) – could this high protein diet lead to osteoporosis? In this respect, and considering the reduced intake of protein from animals, agricultural communities would be expected to have less osteoporosis. If, as studies show, osteoporosis had a potentially higher frequency in hunter-gatherers because of reduced access to calcium from dairy products and high protein diets, perhaps the effect of exercise counteracted its occurrence. Consideration of workload or exercise in past groups may also help in the aetiology of osteoporosis. Mobile hunter-gatherers would be more likely to undertake regular exercise, thereby strengthening the skeleton throughout their lives, whereas settled farmers may not be so active. However some, but not all, studies comparing hunter-gatherer and agricultural groups show increased rates of osteoarthritis in the latter groups, possibly indicating increased workload. What is clear is that osteoporosis can be considered multifactorial in aetiology.

Most osteoporosis is diagnosed today when a person sustains a fracture, especially in the most frequently affected areas of the body in this disease; the wrist (Colles fracture of the radius), the hip (fractured neck of femur) (Fig. 8.8) and compression fractures of the vertebral bodies of the spine ('cod fish vertebrae'), leading to kyphotic deformity or 'dowager's hump'. In many respects the skeletal evidence for fractures in the past does highlight a possible underlying osteoporosis. There are a multitude of diagnostic methods available to the modern clinician but, as Pfeiffer and Lazenby (1994: 36) have pointed out, 'The methods of bone mass quantification applied in the clinical arena may not be easily transferable to dry, long-buried bone tissue'; radiography (to look at cortical and trabecular bone density, thickness and porosity), densitometry of X-rays, photon densitometry (bone mass measurement), microradiography (mineral content), computed tomography (bone mineral content and bone mass), the metacarpal index (cortical bone volume), relative stature through time and clinical laboratory investigations (blood calcium, phosphate and alkaline phosphatase). Some of these are available to the palaeopathologist but some are obviously not.

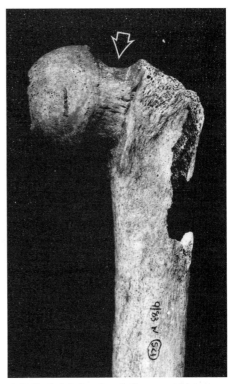

8.8 Healed femoral neck fracture (4th century AD, Gloucester, England)

Radiography is probably the most common non-invasive diagnostic tool used, but suffers from a number of limitations; the most common of these are the effects of burial in the ground on the body and on loss of bone, i.e. post-mortem effects. What a person sees on a radiograph as bone loss may purely be the result of post-mortem damage. Invasive methods, such as examining the microscopic structure of bone (histomorphometry) or assessing actual bone mineral content, have been applied to archaeological populations to assess bone loss (Martin *et al.*, 1985). The use of these methods is very much determined by the preservation of the skeletal material being studied (as for radiography). Recent work has shown the value of scanning electron microscopy (SEM) in assessing osteoporotic

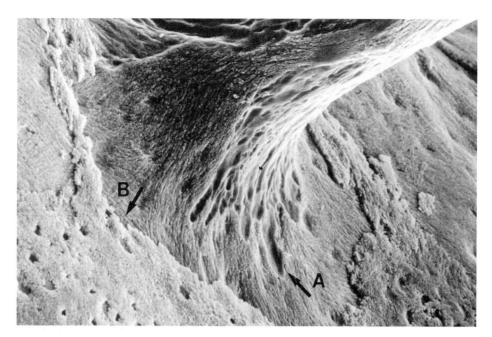

DON ORTNER

8.9 Scanning electron micrograph of rib section from 79-year-old female from the Terry Collection, Smithsonian Institution, showing A: Howship's Lacunae (indicating osteoclastic resorption) and B: new bone formation (indicating osteoblast formation)

changes in bones from archaeological populations (Roberts and Wakely, 1992). SEM records the topographic features of bone, and excessive bone resorption, with reduced formation, may be identified in sections of bone (Fig. 8.9). The presence of healing microfractures in trabeculae of vertebrae suggests that these increase with age and osteoporosis (Vernon-Roberts and Pirie, 1973; Mosekilde, 1990). These can be interpreted as a repair mechanism to preserve the bone integrity. It is suggested that these features could be used to diagnose osteoporosis before any more significant changes in the skeleton occur, such as reduction in mineral density or structural collapse of bone. The study of osteoporosis in archaeological populations has great potential, considering its incidence today.

ENDOCRINE DISEASE

The endocrine diseases are rarely seen in palaeopathological contexts and are therefore not discussed in detail here; the interested reader is referred to Ortner and Putschar (1981). However, they warrant brief consideration in this chapter.

The endocrine system consists of a series of ductless glands whose cells secrete hormones into the blood. Hormones are chemical substances, formed in a body organ or gland, which are carried by the blood to influence growth, function and nutrition elsewhere in the body. Over- and undersecretion of hormones leads to endocrine disease. Although there are several endocrine glands (pituitary, thyroid, parathyroids, adrenals, ovaries, testes and pancreas), only the pituitary and thyroid glands are relevant in palaeopathology, because these glands control skeletal growth (pituitary) and maturation (thyroid). The pituitary gland lies inside the skull and the thyroid gland is situated in the neck.

Hyperpituitarism is characterized by excessive production of growth hormone by the pituitary gland. Gigantism or acromegaly may occur, producing taller than normal individuals. Hyperpituitarism occurring during growth produces gigantism, and in adulthood, acromegaly. In acromegaly bone deposition occurs and leads to enlargement of bones, increase in thickness of the skull vault, enlarged frontal sinuses, spinal osteophytes, prominent tendinous and ligamentous insertions and extreme height. Few convincing cases have been described in palaeopathology. Hypopituitarism, or a deficiency in growth hormone during growth, leads to dwarfism. Tumours, infection or injury to the pituitary gland and genetic factors may be implicated for the abnormality. It is a cause of a large percentage of people with short stature today. Stunted growth, delayed development of the dentition and fusion of the secondary ossification centres, and a short, gracile, proportional skeleton results. Disproportionate dwarfism, e.g. achondroplasia, can be differentiated relatively easily from this condition (see Chapter 3). There are many causes of short, proportional stature, such as chronic infection, but the distribution and character of bony abnormalities seen in pituitary dwarfism should differentiate these conditions in skeletal remains, but not always in artistic representation.

Two probable cases have been described by Ortner and Putschar (1981: 302–3) and Roberts (1988b). In the latter case a proportionately short female adult skeleton, excavated from a fourth-century AD cemetery in Gloucester, England, was diagnosed as having pituitary dwarfism (Fig. 8.10). This was based on delayed fusion of the secondary ossification centres, a gracile skeleton, abnormalities of the dentition and a reduced stature (131.2 cm compared to the mean for females in that cemetery of 153 cm). Interestingly, the only possible cause of this disorder identified on the skeleton was in the form of long standing plaques of new bone on the endocranial surface of the skull, suggesting possible infection.

Hyperthyroidism, or thyrotoxicosis, is characterized by excessive amounts of thyroxine produced by the thyroid gland. Iodine is necessary for the formation of thyroxine, and there appear to be several areas of the world where iodine deficiency exists in groundwater, e.g. Switzerland, parts of the US and England (Bloom, 1975: 202). In fact, 10 per cent of the world population is affected by a deficiency of iodine (Cotran *et al.*, 1989: 1227). Enlargement of the gland (goitre) may result from excessive iodine in the diet, which stimulates overproduction of thyroxine (toxic goitre), but a lack of iodine can also lead to swelling of the gland, yet no hyperactivity (non-toxic goitre), even though there may be an increase in thyroid stimulating hormone (TSH) by the pituitary gland. Increased bone resorption and osteoporosis, with cartilage calcification, characterize the disorder, with fatigue, nervousness, weight loss and palpitations as some of the signs and symptoms. Although there have been many representations of goitre in art, no cases of thyrotoxicosis have been reported palaeopathologically. Hypothyroidism

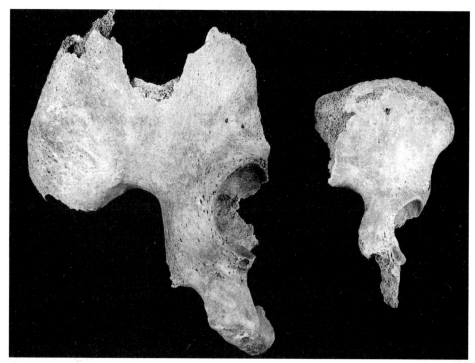

8.10 Innominate bone of pituitary dwarf compared to normal size (4th century AD, Roman Gloucester, England)

(cretinism in the young and myxoedema in adults) involves a thyroxine deficiency. This may be the result of wasting, atrophy or destruction of either the thyroid or pituitary gland, or a deficiency in iodine in local water. Bone changes may consist of delayed maturation of the skeleton, irregular fragmentary ossification centres, prominent cranial sutures and wormian bones, accompanied by generalized osteoporosis (Ortner and Putschar, 1981). The individual (if affected in the growing years) is short but proportionately so. The clinical features of the disease are very much opposite to those of thyrotoxicosis – mental retardation, constipation, lethargy, slow heart rate, decreased sweating and weight gain. Although there are some differences in the skeletal changes compared to pituitary dwarfism, in archaeological populations diagnosis of one of the two conditions may prove difficult. In fact, no cases of hypothyroidism have been reported to date.

Related to the pituitary gland disorders is hyperostosis of the endocranial surface of the frontal bone of the skull; this is believed to occur shortly following pregnancy. Prominent thickening, and formation of nodules, of new bone on the frontal bone in post-menopausal females occurs (Fig. 8.11). These changes are probably the result of altered pituitary gland secretion of hormones (Ortner and Putschar, 1981: 294). In archaeological populations it has been rarely reported (but see Armelagos and Chrisman, 1988).

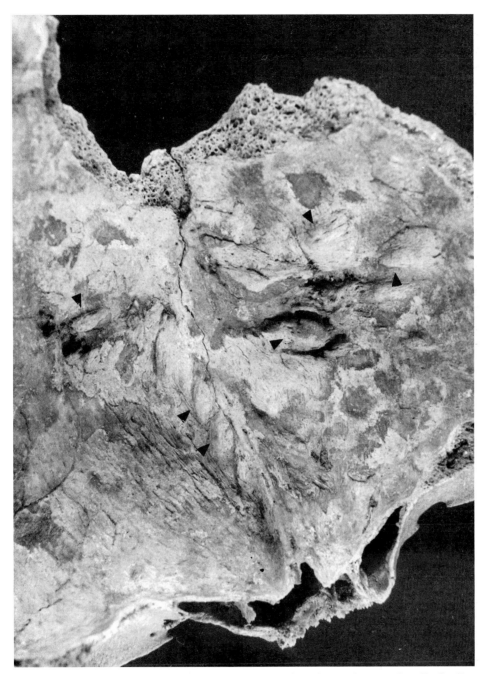

8.11 Hyperostosis frontalis interna (8th–10th century AD, Raunds, Northamptonshire, England)

PAGET'S DISEASE

A final condition to consider in this chapter is Paget's disease, osteitis deformans or 'matrix metabolic madness' (Cotran *et al.*, 1989: 1328). Another rarely reported condition in the palaeopathological literature, it does deserve discussion due to its frequency in modern populations; Caucasians in Europe, North America, Australia and New Zealand are most commonly affected, and frequencies of 10 per cent in males and 15 per cent in females are apparent by the ninth decade of life (Cotran *et al.*, ibid.: 1329). Its specific cause is unknown, but may be the result of a low-grade viral infection with a long incubation period. People with Paget's disease tend to be lethargic and withdrawn, and they have an increased heart rate and blood flow, leading to a very warm skin. Today, it tends to affect persons over 50 years of age. Its prevalence in the past was probably of the same order, but numerically it was probably not as common as today if a reduced longevity is assumed.

The disease is characterized by pain in the affected part and by increasing deformity of the bone due to 'softening'. A localized increased bone turnover rate characterizes the disease, resulting in a 'mosaic' patterning of the bone, both radiologically and histologically; this is the result of woven and fibrous bone

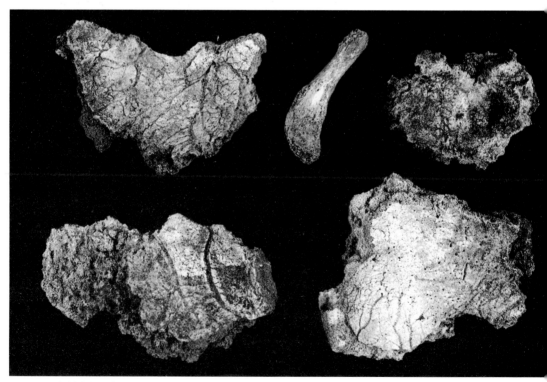

8.12 Skull fragments with impressions of blood vessels on endocranial surface, and part of clavicle with unhealed fracture (post-medieval St Albans, Hertfordshire, England)

formation. The normally demarcated cortex (compact bone) and medullary cavity (see Fig. 5.3) of bone are less precise. The cortex becomes thickened and spongy and the whole bone assumes a distorted and enlarged character. The sacrum, spine, femora and skull are the most commonly affected bones. Head enlargement due to skull thickening is a startling feature, and prominent meningeal vessel grooves on the endocranial skull surface, representing increased blood flow, are obvious (Fig. 8.12). The whole picture of bone deformity is complicated by frequent spontaneous bone fracture and by the occasional development of an osteosarcoma, osteoarthritis and neurological symptoms due to pressure on the body systems from enlargement of bone, although many of these sequelae are rare findings in osteoarchaeological specimens. The usual presentation is a fairly localized bone swelling and deformity, neither of which were of significance to their possessor.

Reports of the disease in palaeopathological contexts do occur, but at present the earliest example is a femur of French Neolithic date from Lozère (Pales, 1929). One of the most complete and convincing examples has been discovered in the Anglo-Saxon monastic cemetery at Jarrow, England, and dated to AD 950; in this case the disease affected almost all bones in this male body. An abnormally large skull was supported on a deformed spine. The long bones of the legs and arms were twisted, thickened and deformed. The left femur was fractured as a consequence of the underlying disorganized bone weakness of Paget's disease (Wells and Woodhouse, 1975). Other cases have recently been reported from a medieval site in Norwich, England (Stirland, 1991b) and a sixteenth-century grave at Wells Cathedral in the south-west of England (Aaron *et al.*, 1992).

Paget's disease is a condition that does not, on the basis of skeletal evidence, appear to have been as frequent in the past as today, but some of the preceding disease processes discussed in the metabolic disease classification were very common. This perhaps reflects the multifactorial nature of these 'indicators of stress' and the more precise (but yet unknown) aetiology of Paget's disease. The metabolic diseases provide a fascinating and exciting insight into past human adaptation and the factors responsible for their occurrence in human populations of earlier periods. Their potential in future palaeopathological studies is acknowledged.

CHAPTER 9

Neoplastic Disease

Corruptions peculiar unto parts.

(Thomas Browne 1605–82)

Although, today, the word tumour is, to most people, synonymous with the term new growth, this has not always been so. In strict terms of derivation, the word should be applied to all swellings, and, until the early nineteenth century, inflammatory swellings, cysts and new growths (both benign and malignant) were all considered as tumours. Neoplasms or new growths are in essence the uncontrolled growth of tissue cells. By definition, a neoplasm is an abnormal mass of tissue, the growth of which exceeds and is uncoordinated with that of the normal tissues and persists in the same excessive manner after cessation of the stimulus which evoked the change (Cotran *et al.*, 1989). They may arise in any tissue of the body, in any organ of the body and in any individual without consideration of age, sex, race, health status or social group. However, the incidence of specific neoplasms may vary within these groups for reasons ill-understood in many cases.

Individual neoplasms may consist of differentiated cells characteristic of the original tissue, or alternatively the growth may consist of totally undifferentiated cells not resembling any specific organ of the body. Neoplasms are considered as either benign or malignant. Benign neoplasms are those that remain solely at their site of origin and tend to spread only locally without a generalized bodily effect. The cells comprising benign neoplasms are generally well differentiated. They are clinically insignificant when compared to malignant neoplasms. Any symptoms from a benign neoplasm are due to the local effect of the growth on the surrounding body structures and to the sheer size of the growth itself. The malignant neoplasms are characterized by the uncontrolled local spread of the primary growth into and on to other organs of the body, and by the more sinister generalized spread of cells to distant organs of the body. This spread is achieved through the bloodstream and the lymphatic channels, and by the direct implantation of cells in such zones as the pleural and peritoneal cavities from the original growth. This autonomy of the malignant neoplasm results in the dissemination of these secondary deposits, the so-called metastases, in almost any organ of the body, with the complete disturbance and breakdown of that organ function. Without the control of the 'milieu interieur', the relentless unchecked growth of the primary malignant neoplasm and its metastases results ultimately in the death of the individual. There is clearly a resemblance of effect between the biological suicide of bacterial parasites and malignant neoplasms.

BENIGN NEOPLASMS

The multitude of soft tissue benign neoplasms, the 'warts, and everything' of Cromwell, generally leave no evidence in skeletal remains. With few exceptions, only the benign neoplasms of bone itself will be manifest in skeletal remains. These lesions, which remain discrete, albeit of varying size, are commonplace findings in skeletal remains of antiquity. As has been noted earlier, cartilage is an essential component of developing bone and neoplasms are found originating from it. For the present discussion only the more common or the more spectacular true benign neoplasms will be considered. Indeed, the full range of benign growths known today is not recognized in palaeopathological material as yet. Of course, it is quite likely that the benign neoplasms which affect humans in the twentieth century did so with equal frequency in the past.

One of the first descriptions of a bony excrescence was in the femur of *Homo erectus* of Middle Pleistocene date (Brothwell, 1967b). This bony tumour is, in fact, a post-traumatic ossification similar to that from the pelvis of seventeenth-century date illustrated in Figure 5.2. This is not a true neoplasm of bone in the strict sense, and confusion has occurred in diagnosis. An excrescence of similar outward appearance has been noted at the lower end of an Egyptian femur of the V Dynasty (Brothwell, ibid.). This lesion, an osteochondroma (Fig. 9.1), is one of the most common benign bone tumours diagnosed in modern clinical practice. Although traditionally considered neoplastic, osteo-chondromas are, strictly, developmental aberrations due to faulty ossification of the growth plate rather than true neoplasms. The onset of the lesion is during the growing period of childhood development and the tumour arises from the growing cartilaginous plate towards the end of the bone. By and large the only symptom is the inconvenience of a localized swelling on

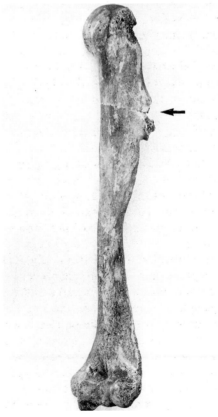

9.1 *Osteochondroma of humerus (Roman Derby, England)*

a limb. The palaeopathological literature includes a number of notable cases (Bennike, 1985; Roberts, 1985; Gregg and Gregg, 1987; Chamberlain *et al.*, 1992). Growth of the tumour ceases on completion of childhood growth. Although the osteochondroma is a single tumour, more rarely, multiple and apparently similar bony swellings may be found (Ortner, 1981; Katzenberg *et al.*, 1982). These lesions, widespread throughout the skeleton, are part of an hereditary abnormality of development called diaphyseal aclasia or exostosis multiplex. A particularly dramatic and fatal example of this latter condition has been reported from a Danish medieval cemetery (Sjøvold *et al.*, 1974). The subject was a pregnant woman. Her multiple bony excrescences were sufficiently large and ill-placed within her pelvis to prevent childbirth. The fetus contained within this poor woman's body was at full term, but both mother and unborn child perished because of the exostosis multiplex.

A particularly common finding in terms of neoplasm in skeletal remains is a small, round, smooth projection of dense bony tissue known descriptively as an ivory osteoma. These lesions are sometimes no larger than a pinhead but sometimes reach almost tennis-ball diameter, and are found most frequently on the frontal bones of the skull (Fig. 9.2). No doubt they were entirely symptomless and are today, just as

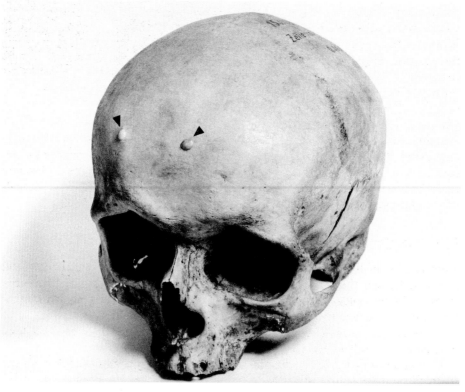

MANCHESTER MUSEUM

9.2 Osteomata of frontal bone (Zellendorf)

in antiquity, of no consequence. A less common, but equally benign, bone-forming neoplasm of bone, termed osteoid osteoma, has also been identified in skeletal remains (Gladykowska-Rzeczycka and Myśliwski, 1985). These lesions, commonly of the young, develop usually towards the ends of the tibia or femur and appear palaeopathologically as fusiform swellings which, on radiography, present a radiolucent interior (Fig. 9.3). Symptomatically, they are noted for producing considerable pain on the bone and it is easy to imagine the distressed child of antiquity with unremitting, constant and boring pain in the leg, unassuaged by the benefits of modern analgesia.

Very rarely appearing in palaeo-pathological specimens, a tumour of soft tissue may produce a bony reaction which itself resembles a neoplasm. Such is the case with a growth of the membranous covering of the brain. This neoplasm, called a meningioma, may induce, albeit rarely, a most alarming growth of the skull overlying the lesion (Rogers, 1949; Anderson, 1991). A

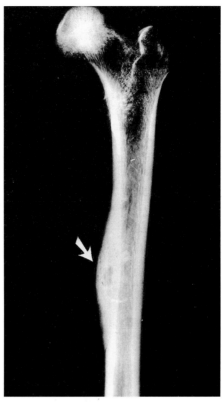

9.3 X-ray of osteoid osteoma on femur showing radiolucent interior

specimen of XX Dynasty date has such an extensive skull reaction that it is suggested that the meningioma was itself malignant. Clearly this could be confused, as will be seen, with a primary malignant neoplasm of bone. A single case of a reactive bony excrescence in a skull secondary to a neoplasm of the wall of a blood vessel has been noted, of prehistoric date (Manchester, 1980b).

MALIGNANT NEOPLASMS

However, the malignant neoplasms of bone are of the greatest palaeopathological interest, having the most terrifying clinical symptomatology and the most revealing epidemiological significance. And yet, in spite of their interest and their possible significance for modern cancer research, the malignant neoplasms of bone, both primary and secondary, are uncommon findings in palaeopathology (Ortner and Putschar, 1981; Micozzi, 1991; Strouhal, 1994).

It is a quirk of nature that the most malign and deadly tumours of humans are the malignant neoplasms affecting the young. One of the most common primary malignant neoplasms of bone, osteosarcoma, is no exception. This cancer, sometimes known as osteogenic sarcoma, arises *de novo* from the cells constituting bone tissue; it occurs principally during the growing period of life, and after the age of 30 years is comparatively rare. There is, however, a second peak of tumour development accounting for some 6–10 per cent of osteosarcomas (Cotran *et al.*, 1989). This second peak, occurring in the elderly, may be associated with Paget's disease in such people.

An osteosarcoma is so highly malignant that in the absence of treatment early death results. No doubt such was the case in antiquity before the advent of effective and radical surgery and radiotherapy, and before the introduction of cancer chemotherapy. A constant, severe boring pain, deep in the affected bone is the presenting symptom. This may be followed by spontaneous bone fracture at the site of the neoplasm, so-called pathological fracture. The early spread of neoplastic cells to other parts of the body seals the miserable fate of the victim of this most pernicious disease.

Although there are other primary sarcomas of bone known to modern practice, hitherto only the osteosarcoma is certainly recognized in palaeopathology. Perhaps the earliest example is found in a humerus of Iron-Age date from Munsingen, Switzerland. The craggy disorganized growth, with spicules of bone developing at right angles to the original bone axis, is characteristic. A burst of frenzied and uncontrolled bone growth is captured in this single humerus, which doubtless from its secondary spread was responsible for death. A possible osteosarcoma has been described from the pelvis of a mature man from Westerhus (Gejvall, 1960) but there is clearly doubt concerning this diagnosis. More certain and more dramatic is an Anglo-Saxon case from Standlake, Oxfordshire. An enormous osteosarcoma measuring about 25 cm × 27 cm was found at the right knee (Brothwell, 1967b). A pathological fracture had occurred and the individual was clearly bedridden, in excruciating pain, but was probably cared for during the terminal illness. Surely this is testimony to the fortitude of our ancestors who were denied the benefit of powerful twentieth-century pain relief. The diagnosed cases of osteosarcoma in the archaeological record are few (Suzuki, 1987). As stated, this is a tumour of the young and it is perhaps surprising, and maybe aetiologically significant, that the prevalence in antiquity was not greater, although the survival of young individuals in the archaeological record is not always good enough for observing diseases affecting this age group.

A primary bone neoplasm of similar type but differing in the cells and site of origin is Ewing's sarcoma. Whereas the osteosarcoma develops from the bone cortex, Ewing's sarcoma develops in cells in the interior of the bone. The result is a swelling, expanding tumour eventually breaking through the cortex. Although no definite diagnosis of this tumour in antiquity has been made, it seems possible to the author that a specimen exists in the pelvis of an Egyptian of the Roman period (Ruffer and Willmore, 1914). The diagnosis has yet to be substantiated.

If the young are unfortunate in their susceptibility to the osteosarcoma, the elderly are rather more unfortunate in their primary malignant bone neoplasm. The neoplasm known as myeloma is, strictly speaking, not a new growth of bone cells but is a new growth originating in the plasma cells in the blood forming tissues of the bone marrow. Myelomatosis, or multiple myeloma, so

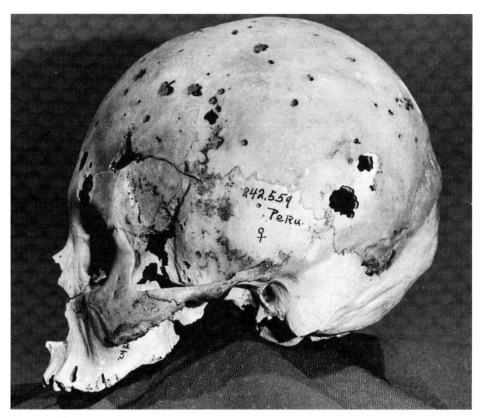

9.4 Multiple myeloma shown by multiple perforations of the skull vault: NMNH 242559, adult female, prehistoric AD 500–1530, Caudiville, Peru

called because the neoplastic lesions are widespread and multifocal in origin in many marrow cavities throughout the skeleton, is the most common of the primary malignant tumours of the skeleton. The tumour is rarely found in people below the age of 40 years and, in fact, 90 per cent of cases are found in individuals between the ages of 50 and 60 years. Males and females are equally affected. Although solitary lesions do occur, the condition usually appears as multiple lesions, which probably arise as independent developments in a systematized neoplastic bone marrow disease, rather than as secondary deposits from a single primary source. The result is a rarefaction of the bone, perforation of the cortex and possible pathological fracture. Most commonly involved sites are the vertebrae, skull, ribs and pelvis. Since the skull bones are relatively thin, perforation of the skull is perhaps an early feature (Fig. 9.4). At least in archaeological specimens, it is the feature upon which the diagnosis is usually based. The multiple and clearly destructive nature of these skull perforations distinguishes them from the perforations of chronic infections such as syphilis and from the perforations of trauma. What is more difficult in palaeopathological diagnosis is the separation of these myelomatous lesions in the skull from the skull perforations of secondary cancer (Cattaneo *et al.*, 1994). In some specimens doubt as to their specific diagnosis remains (Strouhal, 1976).

At present there are some fifteen or so cases of multiple myeloma in the palaeopathological record. In view of the expectation of longevity in antiquity discussed in an earlier chapter, it might (or might not) be thought that the neoplasm was a rarity in the past, but in prehistoric American Indian populations it was not rare at all (Morse *et al.*, 1974). In palaeopathological research the first recognition of the disease in early skeletal material was in a pre-Columbian Indian (Ritchie and Warren, 1932). The bone-destructive lesions, which were demonstrated by radiography, were widespread, being found in the skull, vertebrae, ribs, sternum, femur, pelvis and scapula. Since that time the geographic and the time spread of the disease have been extended. The earliest case so far recorded is of the fourth century BC from Kentucky (Steinbock, 1976) and the disease spread extends through the Old and the New World (Alt and Adler, 1992).

The modern practitioner familiar with the myelomatous patient who, without treatment is likely to die within 2 years from infection and kidney failure, must understand the suffering of the elderly in the past. The theme, constantly recurring in this present book, of relentless pain and increasing immobility, sharpens our awareness of the hardships of our ancestors.

In the developed countries of the world today, everyone is familiar with the problem of cancer. Indeed, in the United States, over 1 million new cases of cancer present each year, and in 1989, 500,000 deaths from cancer were recorded. As Table 9.1 shows, death from cancer has reached quite high proportions relative to other diseases. Such mortality is only exceeded by diseases of the heart and circulation. In the past, however, it was overshadowed as a cause of death by the infectious diseases. These figures do not demonstrate an increase, in absolute terms, in the number of deaths from cancer, but merely indicate a shift in the importance of cancer relative to other diseases. The prevalence of cancer suggested by the palaeopathological record does demonstrate an overall increase in malignant disease from the distant past until today. If, as seems likely, environmental changes in pollution and atmosphere, and in diet, have brought about an increase in cancer, this increase is unlikely to be of the primary bone neoplasms arising *de novo* in bone cells. It is surely in the cancers of lung, stomach, bowel, skin and breast, among others, that the increase has occurred. These are primary soft-tissue neoplasms. Their only manifestation in bone is by virtue of their secondary spread (Galasko, 1986), or more rarely their local bone invasion. Consequently the primary growths themselves are rarely in evidence in skeletal remains.

Neither must it be forgotten that death may occur before spread of the cancer to the bones. Death may ensue from intercurrent infection in the early stages of the malignant disease. In modern practice the infections occurring in the early stages of malignant disease are treated, and it is noted that today 20 per cent of fatal cancer cases possess bone metastatic deposits (Willis, 1973). Therefore, because

Table 9.1 Mortality from all cancer for males and females and by age group, United States, 1985 (data from Ca – A Cancer Journal for Clinicians *39:7, 1989)*

	Males (%)	Females (%)	Total
All ages	246,914 (53.5)	214,649 (46.5)	461,563
<15	1,042 (56.6)	798 (43.4)	1,840
15–34	4,029 (52.8)	3,608 (47.2)	7,637
35–54	25,733 (48.8)	27,001 (51.2)	52,734
55–74	136,869 (56.6)	106,299 (43.4)	243,168
75+	79,220 (50.7)	76,921 (49.3)	156,141

in antiquity the individual may have succumbed earlier in his or her cancerous illness, this figure of 20 per cent may be too high for past societies. It must also be remembered that not all cancers have the same tendency to spread to bone. Cancers of the breast, lung, stomach, thyroid gland, prostate and kidney are most likely to produce bone metastases. These metastases do not tend to be uniformly distributed throughout the whole skeleton. As was first recorded by Von Recklinghausen in 1891, the vertebrae, sternum, ribs, skull, pelvis and upper ends of femur and humerus are perhaps the most commonly affected, although the sites do vary from neoplasm to neoplasm.

A further problem in palaeopathological recognition is the fact that the secondary growths commence in the marrow cavities deep inside the bones and only later destroy and perforate the cortex to the bone exterior. Mere inspection of the dry bones of the past may fail to reveal these deep growths, which may only be demonstrated by radiography of the bone. Ideally therefore, in order to assess the true pattern of malignant disease in antiquity radiography of all skeletons from archaeological excavations should be carried out, but funding does not allow this to happen. At present the palaeopathological diagnosis rests upon finding the irregularly eroded and perforated bone surface, the skull being most commonly observed (Waldron, 1987). The lesions are usually multiple (Fig. 9.5) and, because of the similarity, confusion with multiple myeloma may occur. With the exception of cancer of the prostate, most secondary deposits cause loss of bone substance with consequent weakening. The bone at the site of the deposit is liable to fracture. Cancer of the prostate usually causes bone secondaries which themselves produce bone, albeit of a disorganized and functionless nature (Tkocz and Bierring, 1984; Anderson *et al.*, 1992b).

Occasionally in osteoarchaeological material evidence of both primary and secondary growths is found. An Egyptian skull of III–V Dynasty date exhibits invasive destruction of a primary cancer of the nasopharynx. In addition, the skull vault is perforated by a number of secondary deposits from this primary nasopharyngeal cancer (Wells, 1963). Scarcely can we imagine the suffering of this individual with a foul, fungating cancer relentlessly advancing through the roof of the mouth to protrude into the mouth itself. Death must surely have been

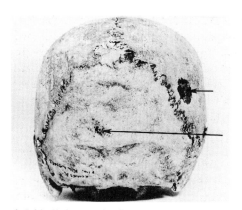

9.5 Skull showing perforations of secondary cancer

a welcome release from this bleeding, ulcerated obstruction to swallowing, talking and decent life.

Perhaps the first analytical and clinical study of metastatic cancer in a skeleton of archaeological context was that by Møller and Møller-Christensen (1952). Secondary deposits were noted in the skull of a woman from the medieval cemetery at Aebelholt, Denmark. By analogy with modern studies it was suggested that the individual may have died as a result of a primary cancer of the breast and its metastases. Other medieval cases of skull metastases have been described (Gejvall, 1960; Wells, 1964d), and indeed the span of examples, both in time and distribution, is increasing (Brothwell, 1967b; Steinbock, 1976; Allison *et al.*, 1980; Ortner and Putschar, 1981; Manchester, 1983a; Gregg and Gregg, 1987; Grupe, 1988b; Ortner *et al.*, 1991). The earliest example known at present is from the European Bronze Age. A female skull, dated to 1900–1600 BC from Mokrin, Yugoslavia, shows perforating lesions characteristic of cancer metastases, which it is suggested originated from a primary cancer of the breast (Soulié, 1980). Notwithstanding the increasing number of reports, the cases of malignancy recognized in the skeletal remains of the past are few (Micozzi, 1991). Malignant disease has, of course, been recognized in mummified remains too. An example of a malignant disease, rare today and in the past, called malignant melanoma has been noted in pre-Columbian Inca mummies from Peru (Urteaga and Pack, 1966). This pigmented growth resulted in small, dark masses within the mummy skin and in multiple pigmented lesions in the skull bones.

The clinical manifestations of malignancy have probably not changed throughout history, and only mid-twentieth-century therapy is alleviating the problem. The surgical treatment of cancer is not exclusively a modern phenomenon, however. A skull of twelfth-century date from Caen exhibits an enormous fungating malignant tumour projecting from the right side of the facial skeleton and extending into the eye-socket and the nasal cavity. An attempt, albeit unsuccessful, at surgical treatment had been made by cutting a hole in the adjacent bone (Dastugue, 1965). Perhaps the medieval patient felt that the attempted cure of his disease was more grievous than its endurance. The general ill-health, the weight loss, the anaemia, the fungating offensive and bleeding tumour, the pain and eventual death were just as much features of the medieval person as of the twentieth-century business executive. Malignant disease has no respect for creed or class.

That cancer is a disease of advancing years is well recognized today. It has been noted in an earlier chapter that the expectation of life in antiquity may not have been as great as today. Maybe the number of individuals in the past surviving to the age of 'cancer prevalence' was not as great. And yet, as is seen in Table 9.1, cancer is also a problem of younger age groups today, and therefore the presumed reduced life expectancy in antiquity cannot be the sole reason for the rarity of palaeopathological evidence. If, as seems likely, there has been an increase in malignant disease in recent times, the reasons may be related to the changing environment throughout history. That certain substances may induce cancer of the scrotum was first noted by Percival Pott in 1775 in respect of soot. Since then many agents have been found to stimulate malignant change. Most of these agents are the products of modern industrial development and would not have been encountered in the village or town life of pre-industrial societies. An entirely recent hazard, too, is the effect of radiation. The peaceful and military use of radioactive materials, which are potentially cancer inducing, is an aspect of life, welcome or otherwise, totally unknown to earlier peoples. The incidence of lung cancer in Western society has risen steeply in post-war years. The relationship between lung cancer and cigarette smoking is well attested, with a likely association also with the fumes of modern cities. But what of the cancers of the breast, prostate, stomach and so on, for which no definite environmental association or cancer-inducing agent is known? It is recognized that nasopharyngeal cancer has a higher incidence in North Africa than in other parts of the world, and similar tumour associations occur with various ethnic groups. Blood-group association with cancer has already been mentioned and is a well-recognized, but hitherto ill-explained, phenomenon. However, this does not explain the apparent increase in this dreaded disease from the sparse palaeopathological evidence of distant antiquity to the feared high incidence of today. With increasing excavation and research, perhaps the recognition of cancer in antiquity and its correlation with the environmental, geographic and ethnic conditions of the time may help to elucidate the causation of malignant disease.

CHAPTER 10

Conclusions: The Next Ten Years

Since 1983 and the first edition of this book (Manchester, 1983b) there have been many developments in the study of palaeopathology. Since the early days in the nineteenth century and the 'case study' approach there has been a major and progressive move towards population-based studies in the history of disease, and much more of a biocultural approach, i.e. integrating biological and cultural data. North America has been a leader in this respect but the rest of the world is following this lead with urgency. As Jarcho quite rightly pointed out (1966: 39) 'the investigation of single bones here and there is not a satisfactory way to undertake paleopathological studies that are supposed to illuminate history'. The biocultural approach to palaeopathology in studying large populations proves more productive.

In the final chapter of the 1983 edition a number of points were highlighted in summing up future developments in palaeopathological investigations. Sandison (1968) recommended four areas that should be considered if palaeopathology was to advance. They were: the establishment of a central registry for palaeopathological examples, a central bibliography, skeletal material with known histories and the accumulation of clear illustrations of important classic cases. One of these recommendations, the compilation of a world-wide registry for palaeopathological cases was also suggested by Manchester (ibid.) but this, of the four, is the area which has received the least attention over the past 12 years. Access to a database containing comparative data (text and images) would be an asset for everybody involved in skeletal analysis but, as yet, nothing substantial exists, unlike for forensic anthropology where cases are recorded for comparative purposes.

Many researchers work on skeletal and mummified material world-wide, either as part of a team or on an individual basis; expertise, background experience and access to training varies considerably. On the one hand, medical doctors, dentists and anatomists may study palaeopathology in their 'spare' time (if that exists in today's world!), but there are increasing numbers of people now specifically trained in the discipline of palaeopathology coming from backgrounds as diverse as archaeology, anthropology, biochemistry, genetics, biology, anatomy and ancient history. Each can contribute to the study of palaeopathology because each has his or her own special expertise; whether a person has a primarily medical or archaeological/anthropological background, both can appreciate the need for a biocultural approach in palaeopathology.

Two major health problems seen frequently today were also discussed in 1983 and their scarcity in the archaeological record noted. Those diseases were cancer (neoplastic disease) and cardiovascular-related disorders. Again, since 1983 there have been very few advances in the study of either condition. Cancer can affect both soft tissue and bone, but the majority of reports in the literature are of skeletal involvement. However, there has not yet been a collative study of the world-wide evidence for neoplastic disease to try and tackle questions of cancer, its aetiology and development in the past. Perhaps the need for extensive radiography as a diagnostic method (since many neoplastic lesions are not visible macroscopically) is daunting. The study of cardiovascular disease can only be attempted by examining mummified material and, although some studies suggest the accumulation of fatty plaques in the blood vessels of mummies, there is still no useful information about the frequency of cardiovascular disease in the past. These observations are somewhat troubling since both these diseases present major problems for mortality today. There is no reason to suspect that they were not common in the past.

Emphasis in 1983 was placed on the biocultural approach to palaeopathology; the 'date, provenance and environmental context is of paramount importance' (Manchester, ibid.: 82). No person working in this field can fail to ignore the importance of integration of biological with cultural data; assessing, for example, environmental and dietary factors operating in a population's living environment can aid in interpreting the biological data and, without it, the biological data may be biased. In addition, the need for a clinically based approach to diagnosis of disease was stressed. Diagnosis is often difficult, if not impossible, in palaeopathology, so the use of clinical data to interpret past patterns of disease is paramount in trying to diagnose disease in the past; and understanding what signs and symptoms are associated with each disease process helps to interpret the effect of health problems on an individual and populations.

However, the main point expressed in that final chapter for the future of palaeopathology was that 'it must lie in the application of scientific techniques of microscopy, radiology and biochemical analysis' (Manchester, ibid.). This is also the case today, although researchers both within and without the discipline of palaeopathology should not think that the application of methods beyond macroscopic pathological descriptive analysis will answer every question we may ask. Over the past 12 years palaeopathologically based questions have been posed and sophisticated methods of analysis have tried to answer them. However, there is still a lot of basic groundwork to do in the recording of palaeopathology in population groups. Although, in financial terms, this relatively crude methodology is a lot less expensive to perform than to analyse a skeleton for its elemental content or undertake a CT (computed tomography) scan by looking at 'slices' of a mummy, somehow the more expensive and sophisticated techniques of analysis seem to attract the attention of the media and finance of the grant-giving bodies, while fundamental problems integral to the study of palaeopathology remain unsolved.

While research councils demand grant applications on a grand scale, using the most novel and newest methods of analysis, one has to step back and remind oneself of the many very basic problems there are in the study of palaeopathology which deserve attention. For example, mortality data are essential for interpreting palaeopathology; people die because they are usually ill and therefore when people die will usually be influenced by their health status. In this respect, developments in adult ageing methods are still needed (see Chapter 2). The application of new methods of analysis are exciting, but research designs must be inherent in the use of these techniques.

Why are we entertaining these new and innovative techniques of analysis in palaeopathology? Perhaps because it might provide more information than we can obtain from examining the skeleton macroscopically. The ability of biomolecules in bone and teeth to survive long periods of burial in the ground has opened up a new opportunity in palaeopathology, that is the extraction of microbial DNA to diagnose disease. Of course, disease today can be diagnosed in modern patients using this technological advance and therefore these methods, with refinements, can then be applied to archaeological material. Paabo (1985) reported the survival of DNA in an Egyptian mummified child dated to around 2,500 years old, and Hagelberg (1989) managed to extract DNA from human bones as old as 5,450 years BP. Clearly, DNA does survive but nobody yet has done enough work to say when it survives, i.e. what burial conditions promote its survival. What may be gained from this approach? Probably the most obvious is the ability (if the DNA survives) to diagnose diseases that do not affect the skeleton, such as malaria, cholera and the plague. All these diseases were of significance at points of time in our past if the written sources are to be believed, but they cannot be detected skeletally. If we have the ability to diagnose these diseases with the isolation of DNA of micro-organisms, it may be possible to gain a better idea of their true prevalence rates (primary definitive evidence). Apart from questions of DNA survival, one more problem plagues this analytical technique; contamination of bone or soft-tissue samples is a major drawback. It is often impossible to control for extraneous DNA infiltrating the samples being used. This type of analysis is also expensive, and it is doubtful if it could ever be applied to all skeletons excavated from an archaeological cemetery site; perhaps radiography of all skeletons instead would be more productive (and cheaper). But, if this work was to be proposed, how would a research design be formulated for this analysis. For example, how does one select skeletons for sampling if the aim is to extract DNA of the plague bacillus? From plague pits? One then assumes that people buried in plague pits suffered from the plague and therefore there would be no point in the exercise. In cases such as this the curiosity factor often creeps into the research, i.e. is it possible to find preserved DNA of the plague bacillus; there is thus no research design.

The whole question of what conditions enable DNA to survive in the ground in different burial environments is one that will take years to answer (Brown and Brown, 1992), and perhaps there never will be an answer because of its potential multifactorial nature. Currently there are a few reports in the literature of attempts at microbial DNA analysis from ancient human material (Salo *et al.*, 1994) but they are certainly not prolific yet, and there have been a number of questionable published reports. Like in the nineteenth century when skulls were said to be treated like Greek vases or items of curiosity (Jarcho, 1966), DNA and disease is attracting a curious fascination, even though it is not yet answering any fundamental questions. The nineteenth-century case study approach in palaeopathology is being followed rapidly by the twentieth-century case study approach in the analysis of ancient microbial DNA. Perhaps in another 150 years there will have been some major advances in this field.

Biomolecules other than DNA are also potentially preserved and may help in the study of palaeopathology. Collagen, haemoglobin, albumin, osteocalcin and HLA antigens may also be considered if they survive burial (see Cattaneo, 1991 for a summary). For example, different HLA antigens can be associated with specific diseases, e.g. the B27 antigen and ankylosing spondylitis. This has particular potential in palaeopathology, although the field is currently wide open.

Moving backwards rather than forwards, the study of palaeopathology still needs to focus on the standardization of recording pathological lesions world-wide. Concordance between researchers about what, and how, to record abnormalities, and what can be realistically interpreted from the data will lead to more realistic reconstructions of past human behaviour. A few publications have appeared which will guide both established workers and also newcomers to the field (Rose *et al.*, 1991; Buikstra and Ubelaker, 1994). Basic descriptive recording, supplemented by illustrations and other supporting documentation, provides a basis from which to work. In addition, the assessment of differential diagnoses for abnormalities ensures a more accurate diagnosis, if diagnosis is possible. Ideally, inputting data on to a database for further analysis would be advocated, or the use of a computer-aided design (CAD) package, such as that described by Ortner (1991), to record the distribution of abnormal lesions could be invaluable. However, realistically speaking, most people do not have access to this sophisticated method of recording. Accurate basic recording is not only essential for the final interpretation and re-interpretation by other researchers, but the potential threat of reburial of skeletal remains in some countries around the world (Ubelaker and Guttenplant Grant, 1989; Goldstein and Kintigh, 1990) means, therefore, that recording the data fully and correctly is even more pressing, because, like excavation, the process cannot be repeated again if the material is reinterred.

The use of modern macerated bone specimens to understand and assess the impact of disease on the skeleton merits further development. Useful studies have already been undertaken in the joint diseases (see Chapter 6). Palaeopathology spans the divide between archaeology and medicine, and without either the study of palaeopathology would be redundant. Histological and chemical approaches to palaeopathological questions should also develop in the future as they have over the past 12 years.

Trace element analysis of ancient human bone had its origins in the 1970s (Sandford, 1992) and over the years, it seems, has generated more problems than answers to questions, particularly with respect to diagenesis; it has perhaps generated more studies on how to control for the effects on bodies of burial in the ground than any other type of analysis in this area. While trace element analysis has aimed to provide information about palaeodiet in past human groups, it still has a long way to go in terms of looking at disease processes. Perhaps the most obvious areas already considered are iron deficiency anaemia (see Chapter 8) and lead poisoning in antiquity. Despite the problems associated with the analysis of lead in bone and controlling for soil lead content, many studies have been undertaken. Stable isotope analysis, gaining in popularity over trace element analysis during the same period of development as a method of reconstructing palaeodiet, has also highlighted the obvious relationship between the dietary data generated and potential dietary deficiency or excess (Katzenberg, 1992); this area of study has great potential and will probably develop further in the future in answering specific questions about dietary related diseases. This method is not affected as much by diagenesis as the methods used for trace element analysis.

Histological changes in bone, teeth and soft tissue have also been used over the years for diagnosing disease and dietary deficiency (Weinstein *et al.*, 1981; Martin, 1991) and have potential for the future; however, it is probably with the scanning electron microscope that developments in this area may occur rapidly. Compared to other histological methods, by studying microscopic features of the surfaces of bone sections it is relatively easy to control for the effects of diagenesis. Radiography will always be a method commonly used in palaeopathological analysis as it is probably the quickest and least expensive of the analytical methods already discussed; it is also non–destructive, unlike the majority of the previous methods described. However, microradiography and computed tomography may be methods to consider in more detailed analysis of disease (see summary in Roberts, 1989b).

Despite the array of methods available to the palaeopathologist in the study of the history of disease, there are areas of study within the discipline which need attention (and answers). Three broad areas of investigation could provide useful information on past human adaptation to particular environments. The first is health and the transition to agriculture question. This area has been tackled admirably in the Americas (Cohen and Armelagos, 1984), perhaps because of the availability of the appropriate skeletal material often not seen in other parts of the world. In Europe attention should be paid to this research area as so much comparative data now exist. The second area is the consideration of the differences in health between urban and rural communities in the past. So far, in palaeopathology this has not been addressed very frequently (but see Roberts and Lewis, 1994; Brothwell, 1994). It would pay to engage some effort in assessing health and its relationship to factors operating in rural and urban environments. Today there are different stressors in these environments which prevent or predispose people to disease, and in the past a similar situation would have occurred. The third area is the gender and health issue which is becoming a focus of attention (Grauer, 1991). Multiple factors affect a person's predisposition to disease, and gender is just one of those factors. Male and female roles in society, i.e. what they do for a living, what they eat and who they come into contact with, may be factors influencing their likelihood of contracting a disease.

In terms of specific disease processes, the joint diseases warrant further attention, particularly in relation to diagnosis of particular joint diseases, and also developing a methodology that can be reliably applied to the question of whether occupation and osteoarthritis are specifically related. Indicators of stress (see Chapter 8) also pose a problem in that many have unknown specific causes; enamel defects and Harris lines are two such conditions. Both may be the result of dietary deficiency or childhood disease, and focusing on trying to determine their specific aetiologies would be useful, but 'How?' is another question. Osteoporosis has yet to be recognized as a major disorder in the past as it is today, because of the problem of diagnosis (see Chapter 8). It would pay to channel effort into establishing more accurate diagnostic methods for this condition in palaeopathology and, with the increasing attention paid to it in today's population, a wealth of literature exists.

Finally, trying to identify the 'rarities' in the palaeopathological record would add another dimension to the history of disease. For example, calcified soft tissues are common in modern populations but rarely found with burials (Steinbock, 1989). Calcifications can be found in the skull (e.g. meningioma), as joint and soft-tissue calcifications (e.g. of cartilage), as thoracic calcifications (e.g. lymph nodes), as abdominal calcifications (e.g. hydatid cysts, gall and kidney stones) and as pelvic calcifications (e.g. bladder stones). It is likely that they are either lost in the ground once covered with soil or they are probably mistaken for ordinary stones in the grave. Perhaps education of archaeologists about where these calcifications could potentially be found in relation to the body may produce more evidence. But more trained researchers in the field, able to recognize and interpret abnormalities in skeletal material with reference to the cultural derivation of the material, are especially needed. The aims of palaeopathology are to trace the history of disease over long periods of time, assess the predisposing cultural factors for disease occurrence and determine the effects of disease on past societies. As Wells (1964a) said:

> The pattern of disease or injury that affects any group of people is never a matter of chance. It is invariably the expression of stresses and strains to which they were exposed, to everything in their environment and behaviour. It reflects their genetic inheritance (which is their internal environment), the climate in which they lived, the soil that gave them sustenance and the animals or plants that shared their homeland. It is influenced by their daily occupations, their habits of diet, their choice of dwellings and clothes, their social structure, even their folklore and mythology.

These words are as appropriate today as they were in 1964. Palaeopathology has a good future backed up by a solid base of excellent research in the field. It does have limitations (as pointed out by Wood et al., 1992), but it is not alone in that respect. First, being aware of some of its potential shortcomings and, secondly, trying to control for them, have been major advances in recent years. As a discipline it is proving to be highly integrated with many other forms of evidence in reconstructing the history of disease. It provides the link between the very distant past and our present, and shows how health has changed through time and what we might expect from the future if we have a change in diet, environment, climate or living conditions. It is, by its nature, an holistic discipline which has direct relevance to future populations. The important message is not to study palaeopathology for 'its own sake'. Genuine research questions must be asked of the data; in this way a more meaningful interpretation will result.

Bibliography

Aaron, J.E., Rogers, J. and Kanis, J.A. 1992 Paleohistology of Paget's disease in 2 medieval skeletons. *Am. J. Phys. Anthrop.* 89: 325–31.

Ackerknecht, E.H. 1967 Primitive surgery, pp. 635–50 in D. Brothwell and A.T. Sandison (eds), *Diseases in antiquity.* Illinois, Charles Thomas.

Adams, F. 1849 *The genuine works of Hippocrates.* New York, W. Wood.

Aird, I. and Bentall, H.H. 1953 A relationship between cancer of the stomach and the ABO blood groups. *Br. Med. J.* 1: 799–801.

Allison, M.J., Gerszten, E., Munizaga, J. and Santoro, C. 1980 Metastatic tumor of bone in a Tiahuanaco female. *Bull. New York Acad. Med.* 56: 581–7.

Allison, M.J., Gerszten, E., Munizaga, J., Santoro, C. and Mendoza, D. 1981 Tuberculosis in Pre-Columbian Andean populations, pp. 49–61 in J.E. Buikstra (ed.), *Prehistoric tuberculosis in the Americas.* Illinois, Northwestern University Archeological Programme.

Alt, K.W. and Adler, C.P. 1992 Multiple myeloma in an early medieval skeleton. *Int. J. Osteoarchaeology* 2: 205–9.

Amundsen, D.A. and Diers, C.J. 1970 The age of menopause in Classical Greece and Rome. *Human Biology* 42: 79–86.

Andersen, J.G. 1969 *Studies in the medieval diagnosis of leprosy in Denmark.* Copenhagen, Costers Bogtrykkeri.

Andersen, J.G. and Manchester, K. 1987 Grooving of the proximal phalanx in leprosy: a palaeopathological and radiological study. *J. Archaeol. Sci.* 14: 77–82.

Andersen, J.G. and Manchester, K. 1988 Dorsal tarsal exostoses in leprosy: a palaeopathological and radiological study. *J. Archaeol. Sci.* 15: 51–6.

Andersen, J.G. and Manchester, K. 1992 The rhinomaxillary syndrome in leprosy: a clinical, radiological and palaeopathological study. *Int. J. Osteoarchaeology* 2: 121–9.

Andersen, J.G., Manchester, K. and Ali, R.S. 1992 Diaphyseal remodelling in leprosy: a radiological and palaeopathological study. *Int. J. Osteoarchaeology* 2(3): 211–21.

Andersen, J.G., Manchester, K. and Roberts, C. 1994 Septic bone changes in leprosy: a clinical, radiological and palaeopathological study. *Int. J.Osteoarchaeology* 4: 21–30.

Anderson, T. 1991 A medieval example of meningiomatous hyperostosis. *Br. J. Neurosurg.* 5: 499–504.

Anderson, T., Arcini, C., Anda, S., Tangerud, A. and Robertsen, G. 1986 Suspected endemic syphilis (Treponarid) in sixteenth century Norway. *Medical History* 30: 341–50.

Anderson, T., Wakely, J. and Carter, A. 1992b Medieval example of metastatic carcinoma: a dry bone, radiological and SEM study. *Am. J. Phys. Anthrop.* 89: 309–23.

Angel, J.L. 1974 Patterns of fractures from Neolithic to modern times. *Anthrop. Kozl.* 18: 9–18.

Antoine, S.E., Pollard, A.M., Dresser, P.Q. and Whittle, A.W.R. 1988 Bone chemistry and dietary reconstruction in prehistoric Britain: examples from Orkney, Scotland, pp. 101–6 in R.M. Farquhar, R.G.V. Hancock and L.A. Pavlish (eds), *Proceedings of the 26th International Archaeometry Symposium, Toronto, Canada, 1988*. Toronto, Archaeometry Laboratory, Department of Physics, University of Toronto.

Arcini, C. 1990 Evidence of leprosy in 10th century Lund. The earliest known cases of leprosy in the Nordic Countries. Paper presented at the 8th Paleopathology Association European Meeting, Cambridge.

Armelagos, G.J. and Chrisman, O.D. 1988 Hyperostosis frontalis interna: a Nubian case. *Am. J. Phys. Anthrop.* 76: 25–8.

Ascádi, G. and Neméskeri, J. 1970 *History of human life span and mortality*. Budapest, Akadémiai Kiadó.

Backay, L. 1985 *An early history of craniotomy. From antiquity to the Napoleonic era*. Illinois, Charles Thomas.

Bahn, P. 1989 Early teething troubles. *Nature* 337: 693.

Baker, B. and Armelagos, G.J. 1988 Origin and antiquity of syphilis: a paleopathological diagnosis and interpretation. *Current Anthropology* 29(5): 703–37.

Banks, A.L. 1959 The study of the geography of disease. *Geogr. J.* 125: 199–216.

Bass, W.M. 1987 *Human osteology. A field guide and manual*. Missouri, Archaeological Society.

Bean, J.M.W. 1962 Plague, population and economic decline in England in the later Middle Ages. *Econ. Hist. Rev.* 15: 423–37.

Becker, M.J. 1994 Etruscan dental appliances: origins and functions as indicated by an example from Orvieto, Italy in the Danish National Museum. *Dental Anthropology Newsletter* 8(3): 2–8.

Bedford, M.E., Russell, K.F., Lovejoy, C.O., Meindl, R.S., Simpson, S.W. and Stuart-Macadam, P. 1993 Test of the multifactorial aging method using skeletons with known ages-at-death from the Grant Collection. *Am. J. Phys. Anthrop.* 91: 287-97.

Bell, L. 1990 Palaeopathology and diagenesis: an SEM evaluation of structural changes using backscattered electron imaging. *J. Archaeol. Sci.* 17: 85–102.

Bennike, P. 1985 *Palaeopathology of Danish skeletons: a comparative study of demography, disease and injury*. Akademisk Forlag, Copenhagen.

Bennike, P. and Fredebo, L. 1986 Dental treatment in the Stone Age. *Bull. Hist. Dent.* 34(2): 81–7.

Berry, A.C. and Berry, R.J. 1967 Epigenetic variation in the human cranium. *J. Anat.* 101(2): 361–79.

Black, J. 1982 A stitch in time 1: the history of sutures. *Nursing Times* 78: 619–23.

Blondiaux, J. 1989 *Le cimetière Mérovingien de Neuville-sur-Escaut*. Musée Municipal de Demain.

Bloom, A. (ed.) 1975 *Toohey's medicine for nurses*, 11th edition. Edinburgh, Churchill Livingstone.

Boddington, A., Garland, A.N. and Janaway, R.C. (eds) 1987 *Death, decay and reconstruction. Approaches to archaeology and forensic science*. Manchester, Manchester University Press.

Bokonyi, S. 1977 Animal remains from the Kermanshah Valley, Iran. *British Archaeological Reports* Suppl. 34, Oxford.

Bonser, W. 1963 *Medical background to Anglo-Saxon England*. London, Wellcome Institute.

Bridges, P.S. 1989 Changes in activities with the shift to agriculture in the southeastern U.S. *Current Anthropology* 30(3): 385–94.

Bridges, P.S. 1991 Degenerative joint disease in hunter-gatherers and agriculturists from the southeastern U.S. *Am. J. Phys. Anthrop.* 85: 379–91.

Bridges, P.S. 1994 Vertebral arthritis and physical activities in the prehistoric United States. *Am. J. Phys. Anthrop.* 93: 83–93.

Brimblecombe, P. 1976 Attitudes and responses towards air pollution in medieval England. *J. Air Pollution Control Assoc.* 26(10): 941–5.

Brimblecombe, P. 1982 Early urban climate and atmosphere, pp. 10–25 in A.R. Hall and H.K. Kenward (eds), *Environmental archaeology in the urban context.* Council for British Archaeology Research Report 43. London, Council for British Archaeology.

Brooks, S.T. and Hohenthal, W.D. 1963 Archeological defective palate crania from California. *Am. J. Phys. Anthrop.* 21(1): 25–32.

Brothwell, D. 1960 A possible case of mongolism in a Saxon population. *Ann. Human Genet.* 24: 141–50.

Brothwell, D. 1967a Major congenital anomalies of the skeleton: evidence from earlier populations, pp. 423–44 in D. Brothwell and A.T. Sandison (eds), *Diseases in antiquity.* Illinois, Charles Thomas.

Brothwell, D. 1967b The evidence for neoplasms, pp. 320–45 in D.R. Brothwell and A.T. Sandison (eds), *Diseases in antiquity.* Illinois, Charles Thomas.

Brothwell, D. 1970 The real history of syphilis. *Science* 6(9): 27–33.

Brothwell, D. 1981 *Digging up bones.* London, British Museum (Natural History).

Brothwell, D. 1986 *The bog man and the archaeology of people.* London, British Museum (Natural History).

Brothwell, D. 1989 The relationship of tooth wear to aging, pp. 306–16 in M.Y. Iscan (ed.), *Age markers in the human skeleton.* Illinois, Charles Thomas.

Brothwell, D. 1991 On the zoonoses and their relevance to paleopathology, pp. 18–22 in D. Ortner and A. Aufderheide (eds), *Human paleopathology. Current syntheses and future options.* Washington DC, Smithsonian Institution Press.

Brothwell, D. 1994 On the possibility of urban–rural contrasts in human population palaeobiology, pp. 129–36 in A.R. Hall and H.K. Kenward (eds), *Urban-rural connexions: perspectives from urban-rural archaeology.* Symposia of the Association of Environmental Archaeology No. 12. Oxford, Oxbow Monograph 47.

Brothwell, D. and Møller-Christensen, V. 1963 Medico-historical aspects of an early case of mutilation. *Danish Med. Bull.* 10: 21–7.

Brothwell, D. and Powers, R. 1968 Congenital malformations of the skeleton in earlier man, pp. 173–203 in D.R. Brothwell (ed.), *Skeletal biology of earlier human populations.* Symposia of the Society for the study of Human Biology Volume 8. London, Pergamon Press.

Brown, P. 1992 The return of the big killer. *New Scientist* 10 October: 30–7.

Brown, T. and Brown, K. 1992 Ancient DNA and the archaeologist. *Antiquity* 66: 10–23.

Bruintjes, T. 1990 The auditory ossicles in human skeletal remains from a leper cemetery in Chichester, England. *J. Archaeol. Sci.* 17: 627–33.

Bryceson, A. and Pfaltzgraaf, R.E. 1990 *Leprosy.* Edinburgh, Churchill Livingstone.

Buchanan, W.W. and Laurent, R.M. 1990 Rheumatoid arthritis: an example of ecological succession. *Can. Bull. Med. Hist.* 7: 77–91.

Buhr, A.J. and Cooke, A.M. 1959 Fracture patterns. *Lancet* 1: 531–6.

Buikstra, J.E. and Cook, D.C. 1980 Paleopathology: an American account. *Ann. Rev. Anthrop.* 9: 433–70.

Buikstra, J.E. and Cook, D.C. 1981 Pre-Columbian tuberculosis in West-Central Illinois: prehistoric disease in biocultural perspective, pp. 115–39 in J.E. Buikstra (ed.), *Prehistoric tuberculosis in the Americas.* Illinois, Northwestern University Archeological Programme.

Buikstra, J. and Mielke, J.H. 1985 Demography, diet and health, pp. 359–422 in R.I. Gilbert and J.H. Mielke (eds), *Analysis of prehistoric diets*. London, Academic Press.

Buikstra, J.E. and Ubelaker, D. 1994 *Standards for data collection from human skeletal remains*. Arkansas Archeological Survey Research Series, No. 44.

Burr, D.B. and Martin, B. 1989 Errors in bone remodeling: toward a unified theory of metabolic bone disease. *Am. J. Anat.* 186: 186–216.

Burton, J.H. and Price, T.D. 1992 Rates of barium to strontium as a paleodietary indicator of consumption of marine resources. *J. Archaeol. Sci.* 17: 547–58.

Bush, H. 1991 Concepts of health and stress, pp. 11–21 in H. Bush and M. Zvelebil (eds), *Health in past societies. Biocultural interpretations of human skeletal remains in archaeological contexts*. British Archaeological Reports International Series 567. Oxford, Tempus Reparatum.

Canci, A., Minozzi, S. and Borgognini Tarli, S.M. 1994 Osteomyelitis: elements for differential diagnosis on skeletal material, pp. 88–90 in O. Dutour, G. Palfi, J. Berato and J.-P. Brun (eds), *L'origine de la syphilis en Europe avant ou après 1493?* Centre Archéologique du Var, Editions Errance.

Cardy, A. 1994 Whithorn: the late medieval cemetery. Unpublished skeletal report.

Carlson, D.S., Armelagos, G.J. and Van Gerven, D.P. 1974 Factors influencing the etiology of cribra orbitalia in prehistoric Nubia. *J. Human Evolution* 4: 405–10.

Carroll, G.A. 1972 Traditional medical cures along the Yukon. *Alaska Medicine* 14: 50–3.

Cattaneo, C. 1991 Direct genetic and immunological information in the reconstruction of health and biocultural conditions of past populations: a new prospect for archaeology, pp. 39–53 in H. Bush and M. Zvelebil (eds), *Health in past societies. Biocultural interpretations of human skeletal remains in archaeological contexts*. British Archaeological Reports International Series 567. Oxford, Tempus Reparatum.

Cattaneo, C., Gelsthorpe, K., Phillips, P., Waldron, T., Booth, J.R. and Sokol, R.J. 1994 Immunological diagnosis of multiple myeloma in a medieval bone. *Int. J. Osteoarchaeology* 4: 1–2.

Cave, A.J.E. 1939 Evidence for the incidence of tuberculosis in ancient Egypt. *Br. J. Tuberculosis* 33: 142–52.

Chakrabarty, A. and Dastidar, S. 1989 Correlation between occurrence of leprosy and fossil fuels: role of fossil fuel bacteria in the origin and global epidemiology of leprosy. *Indian J. Exper. Biol.* 27: 483–96.

Chamberlain, A.T., Rogers, S. and Romanowski, C.A. 1992 Osteochondroma in a British Neolithic skeleton. *Br. J. Hosp. Med.* 47(1): 51–3.

Cherniack, M. 1992 Diseases of unusual occupations: an historical perspective. *Occupational Med.* 7(3): 369–84.

Chundun, Z. 1991 The significance of rib lesions in individuals from a Chichester medieval Hospital. Unpublished M.Sc. thesis, University of Bradford, Department of Archaeological Sciences.

Clairet, D. and Dagorn, J. 1994 Skeletal disorders acquired in syphilis: radiographic study and differential diagnosis, pp. 32–5, in O. Dutour, G. Palfi, J.Berato and J.-P. Brun (eds), *L'origine de la syphilis en Europe avant ou après 1493?* Centre Archéologique du Var, Editions Errance.

Clark, G.A., Kelley, M.A., Grange, J.M. and Hill, M.C. 1987 The evolution of mycobacterial disease in human populations. *Current Anthropology* 28(1): 45–62.

Clark, W.A. 1937 History of fracture treatment up to the 16th century. *J. Bone Joint Surgery* 19(1): 47–63.

Clarke, N.G. and Hirsch, R.S. 1991 Physiological, pulpal and periodontal factors influencing alveolar bone, pp. 241–66 in M. Kelley and C.S. Larsen (eds), *Advances in dental anthropology*. New York, Alan Liss.

Clarke, S.K. 1982 The association of early childhood enamel hypoplasias and radiopaque transverse lines in a culturally diverse prehistoric skeletal sample. *Human Biology* 54(1): 77–84.

Clarkson, L. 1975 *Death, disease and famine in preindustrial England*. Dublin, Gill and Macmillan.

Coale, A.J. 1974 The history of the human population, in D. Flanagan (ed.), *The human population*. San Francisco, W.H. Freeman.

Cockburn, A. 1961 The origin of the treponematoses. *Bull. WHO* 24: 221–8.

Cockburn, A. 1977 Where did our infectious diseases come from? pp. 103–13 in K. Elliot and J. Whelan (eds), *Health and disease in tribal societies*. CIBA Foundation Symposium 49. Association of Scientific Publishers.

Cockburn, A., Barraco, R.A., Reyman, T.A. and Peck, W.H. 1975 Autopsy of an Egyptian mummy. *Science* 187(4182): 1155–60.

Cohen, M.N. 1989 *Health and the rise of civilisation*. New York, Yale University Press.

Cohen, M.N. and Armelagos, G. (eds) 1984 *Paleopathology at the origins of agriculture*. New York, Academic Press.

Congdon, R.T. 1931 Spondylolisthesis and vertebral anomalies in skeletons of American Aborigines. With clinical notes on spondylolisthesis. *J. Bone Joint Surgery* 14B: 511–24.

Constandse-Westermann, T.S. and Newell, R.R. 1989 Limb lateralization and social stratification in western European Mesolithic societies, pp. 405–33 in I. Hershkovitz (ed.), *People and culture change*. Proceedings of the 2nd Symposium on Upper Palaeolithic, Mesolithic and Neolithic populations of Europe and the Mediterranean Basin. British Archaeological Reports International Series 508(i), Oxford.

Corruccini, R.S., Handler, J.S. and Jacobs, K.P. 1985 Chronological distribution of enamel hypoplasias and weaning in a Caribbean slave population. *Human Biology* 57(4): 699–711.

Corruccinni, R.S., Aufderheide, A. and Handler, R.S. 1987 Patterning of skeletal lead content in Barbados slaves. *Archaeometry* 29(2): 233–9.

Cotran, R.S., Kumar, V. and Robbins, S.L. 1989 *Robbins pathologic basis of disease*, 4th edition. London, W.B. Saunders.

Courville, C.B. 1965 War wounds of the cranium in the Middle Ages: 1. As disclosed in the skeletal material from the Battle of Wisby (1361 AD). *Bull. Los Angeles Neurolog. Soc.* 30: 27–33.

Crawford-Adams, J. 1983 *Outline of fractures*, 8th edition. Edinburgh, Churchill Livingstone.

Crubézy, E. and Trinkhaus, E. 1992 Shanidar 1: a case of hyperostotic disease (DISH) in the Middle Paleolithic. *Am. J. Phys. Anthrop.* 89: 411–20.

Czarnetski, A. 1980 A possible trisomy 21 from the Late Hallstatt Period. *Proceedings of the 3rd European Paleopathology Association Meeting, Caen, France, 1980*.

Dalby, G. 1994 Middle ear disease in antiquity. Unpublished Ph.D. thesis, University of Bradford.

Daniel, H.J., Schmidt, R.T., Fulghum, R.S. and Ruckriegal, L. 1988 Otitis media: a problem for the physical anthropologist. *Yearbook of Physical Anthropology* 31: 143–67.

Danielsen, K. 1970 Odontodysplasia in Danish medieval skeletons. *Saertryk af Tandlaegebladet* 74: 603–25.

Dasen, V. 1988 Dwarfism in Egypt and Classical antiquity: iconography and medical history. *Medical History* 32: 253–76.

Dastugue, J. 1965 Tumeur maxillaire sur un crâne du moyen-âge. *Bull. du Cancer* 52(1): 69–72.

Davies, D.M., Picton, D.C.A. and Alexander, A.G. 1969 An objective method of assessing the periodontal condition in human skulls. *J. Periodontal Res.* 4: 74–7.

Dawes, J.D. and Magilton, J.R. 1980 *The cemetery of St Helen-on-the-Walls, Aldwark.* The archaeology of York. The medieval Cemeteries 12/1. London, Council for British Archaeology for York Archaeological Trust.

Day, M.H. 1977 *Guide to fossil man.* London, Cassell.

Deevey, E.S. 1960 The human population. *Scientific American* 203: 195–204.

Denny, N. and Filmer-Sankey, J. 1966 *The Bayeux Tapestry. The story of the Norman Conquest: 1066.* London, Collins.

Dequecker, J. 1977 Arthritis in Flemish paintings (1400–1700). *Br. Med. J.* 1: 1203.

Derry, D.E. 1913 A case of hydrocephalus in an Egyptian of the Roman Period. *J. Anat. (London)* 48: 436–58.

Derums, V.J. 1979 Extensive trepanation of the skull in ancient Latvia. *Bull. Hist. Med.* 53: 459–64.

Dettwyler, K. 1991 Can paleopathology provide evidence for 'compassion'? *Am. J. Phys. Anthrop.* 84: 375–84.

Dharmendra, 1947 Leprosy in ancient Indian medicine. *Int. J. Leprosy* 15: 424–30.

Dobney, K. and Brothwell, D. 1987 A method for evaluating the amount of dental calculus on teeth from archaeological sites. *J. Archaeol. Sci.* 14: 343–51.

Dobney, D. and Brothwell, D. 1988 A scanning electron microscope study of archaeological dental calculus, pp. 372–85 in S.L. Olsen (ed.), *Scanning electron microscopy in archaeology.* British Archaeological Reports International Series 452, Oxford.

Dobney, K. and Goodman, A.H. 1991 Epidemiological studies of dental enamel hypoplasias in Mexico and Bradford: their relevance to archaeological skeletal material, pp. 81–100 in H. Bush and M. Zvelebil (eds), *Health in past societies: Biocultural interpretations of human skeletal remains in archaeological contexts.* British Archaeological Reports International Series 567. Oxford, Tempus Reparatum.

Dols, M.W. 1979 Leprosy in medieval Arabic medicine. *J. Hist. Med.* 34(3): 314–33.

Dooley, J.R. and Binford, C.H. 1976 Treponematoses, pp. 110–17 in C.H. Binford and D.H. Connor (eds), *Pathology of tropical and extraordinary diseases.* Washington DC, Armed Forces Institute of Pathology.

Durand, J. 1972 The viewpoint of historical demography, pp. 370–4 in B. Spooner (ed.), *Population growth.* Boston, MA, Massachusetts Institute of Technology.

Duray, S. 1990 Deciduous enamel defects and caries susceptibility in a prehistoric Ohio population. *Am. J. Phys. Anthrop.* 81: 27–34.

Dutour, O., Pálfi, G., Berato, J. and Brun, J.-P. 1994 *L'origine de la syphilis en Europe. Avant ou après 1493.* Centre Archéologique du Var, Editions Errance.

Dyer, C. 1989 *Standards of living in the later Middle Ages.* Cambridge, Cambridge University Press.

Dzierzykray-Rogalski, T. 1980 Palaeopathology of the Ptolemaic inhabitants of Dakhleh Oasis (Egypt). *J. Human Evolution* 9: 71–4.

Eisenstein, S. 1978 Spondylolysis. *J. Bone Joint Surgery* 64B(4): 488–94.

Elliot-Smith, G. 1908 The most ancient splints. *Br. Med. J.* 1: 732–73.

Elliot-Smith, G. and Dawson, W.R. 1924 *Egyptian mummies.* New York, The Dial Press.

Elliot-Smith, G. and Wood Jones, F. *The archaeological survey of Nubia. Report on the human remains.* Report for 1907–1908, Volume II.

El-Najjar, M.Y. 1979 Human treponematosis and tuberculosis: evidence from the New World. *Am. J. Phys. Anthrop.* 51: 599–618.

El-Najjar, M.Y. and Mulinski, T.M.J. 1980 Mummies and mummification practices in the Southwestern and Southern United States, pp. 103–17 in A. Cockburn and E. Cockburn (eds), *Mummies, disease and ancient cultures*. New York, Cambridge University Press.

Enderle, A., Meyerhofer, D. and Unverfehrt, G. 1994 *Small people – great art. Restricted growth from an artistic and medical viewpoint*. Germany, Artcolor Verlag.

Epstein, S. 1937 Art, history and the crutch. *Ann. Med. Hist.* 9: 304–13.

Eversley, D.E.C., Laslett, P. and Wrigley, E.A. 1966 *An introduction to English historical demography*. London, Weidenfeld and Nicolson.

Farwell, D.E. and Molleson, T. 1993 *Poundbury Volume 2: the cemeteries*. Dorset Natural History and Archaeological Society Monograph Series 11.

Faulkner, R.A., Howson, C.S., Bailey, D.A., Drinkwater, D.T., McKay, H.A. and Wilkinson, A.A. 1993 Comparison of bone mineral content and bone mineral density between dominant and nondominant limbs in children 8–16 years of age. *Am. J. Human Biology* 5: 491–9.

Ferguson, M.W.J. 1978 Cleft palate past and present. *Paleopathology Association Newsletter* 24: 5–8.

Fife, D. and Barancik, J.I. 1985 Northeastern Ohio trauma study III. Incidence of fractures. *Ann. Emerg. Med.* 14(3): 244–8.

Fife, D., Barancik, J.I. and Chatterjee, B.F. 1984 Northeastern Ohio trauma study II: injury rates by age, sex and cause. *Am. J. Public Health* 74(5): 473–8.

Fildes, V.A. 1986 'The English Disease': infantile rickets and scurvy in pre-Industrial England, pp. 121–34 in J. Cule and T. Turner (eds), *Child care through the centuries*. British Society for the History of Medicine.

Forestier, J. and Rotès-Querol, J. 1950 Senile ankylosing hyperostosis of the spine. *Ann. Rheumat. Dis.* 9: 321–30.

Formicola, V.Q., Milanesi, C. and Scarsini, C. 1987 Evidence of spinal tuberculosis at the beginning of the fourth millennium BC from Arena Candide Cave (Liguria, Italy). *Am. J. Phys. Anthrop.* 72: 1–7.

Fornaciari, G. and Marchetti, A. 1986 Italian smallpox of the 16th century. *Lancet* 2: 1469–70.

Fornaciari, G., Mallegni, F., Bertini, D. and Nuti, V. 1981 Cribra orbitalia and elemental bone in the Punics of Carthage. *Ossa* 8: 63–77.

Fortuine, R. 1984 Traditional surgery among the Alaska natives. *Alaska Medicine* 26(1): 22–5.

Francis, J. 1947 *Bovine tuberculosis including a contrast with human tuberculosis*. London, Staples Press.

Frayer, D.W., Horton, W.A., Macchiarelli, R. and Mussi, M. 1987 Dwarfism in an adolescent from the Italian late Upper Palaeolithic. *Nature* 330: 60–1.

Froment, A. 1994 Epidemiology of African endemic treponematoses in tropical forest and savanna, pp. 41–7 in O. Dutour, G. Pálfi, J. Berato and J.-P. Brun (eds), *L'origine de la syphilis en Europe avant ou après 1493?* Centre Archéologique du Var, Editions Errance.

Galasko, C.S.B. 1986 *Skeletal metastases*. London, Butterworth.

Garraway, W.M., Stauffer, R.N., Kurland, L.T. and O'Fallon, W.M. 1979 Limb fractures in a defined population. *Mayo Clin. Proc.* 54(11): 701–7.

Gejvall, N.-G. 1960 *Westerhus, medieval population and church in light of their skeletal remains*. Lund, Hakak Ohlssons Boktryckeri.

Gelis, J. 1991 *History of childbirth*. Cambridge, Polity Press.

Gilbert, R.I. and Mielke, J.H. (eds) 1985 *Analysis of prehistoric diets*. London, Academic Press.

Gill, G.W. 1986 Craniofacial criteria in forensic race identification, pp. 143–59 in K.M. Reichs (ed.), *Forensic osteology. Advances in identification of human remains.* Illinois, Charles Thomas.

Gladykowska-Rzeczycka, J. 1980 Remains of achondroplastic dwarf from Legnica of XI–XIIth century. *Ossa* 7: 71–4.

Gladykowska-Rzeczycka, J. 1994 Syphilis in ancient and medieval Poland, pp. 116–18 in O. Dutour, G. Pálfi, J. Berato and J.-P. Brun (eds), *L'origine de la syphilis en Europe avant ou après 1493?* Centre Archéologique du Var, Editions Errance.

Gladykowska-Rzeczycka, J. and Myśliwski, A. 1985 Osteoid-osteoma from Middle Ages cemetery in Poland. *Ossa* 12: 33–9.

Glob, P.V. 1973 *The bog people.* London, Book Club Associates.

Goldstein, K. and Kintigh, K. 1990 Ethics and the reburial controversy. *American Antiquity* 55: 585–91

Goldstein, M.S. 1957 Skeletal pathology of early Indians in Texas. *Am. J. Phys. Anthrop.* 15: 299–311.

Goodman, A.H. 1991 Stress, adaptation and enamel developmental defects, pp. 280–7 in D. Ortner and A. Aufderheide (eds), *Human paleopathology: current syntheses and future options.* Washington DC, Smithsonian Institution Press.

Goodman, A.H. and Capasso, L. (eds) 1992 *Recent contributions to the study of enamel developmental defects.* Journal of Paleopathology Monographic Publications 2.

Goodman, A.H. and Clarke, G.A. 1981 Harris lines as indicators of stress in prehistoric Illinois populations, pp.35–46 in D.L. Martin and P. Bumsted (eds), *Biocultural adaptation: comprehensive approaches to skeletal analysis.* Amherst, University of Massachusetts Research Reports 20.

Goodman, A.H., Lallo, J., Armelagos, G.J. and Rose, J.C. 1984 Health changes at Dickson Mounds, Illinois (A.D. 950–1300), pp. 271–306 in M.N. Cohen and G.J. Armelagos (eds), *Paleopathology at the origins of agriculture.* London, Academic Press.

Goodman, A.H., Brooke Thomas, R. Swedlund, A.C. and Armelagos, G.J. 1988 Biocultural perspectives on stress in prehistorical, historical and contemporary population research. *Yearbook of Physical Anthropology* 31: 169–202.

Gordon, I., Shapiro, H. and Berson, S. 1988 *Forensic medicine: a guide to principles.* Edinburgh, Churchill Livingstone.

Grauer, A.L. 1991a Patterns of life and death: the palaeodemography of medieval York, pp. 67–80 in H. Bush and M. Zvelebil (eds), *Health in past societies. Biocultural interpretations of human skeletal remains in archaeological contexts.* British Archaeological Reports International Series 567, Oxford, Tempus Reparatum.

Grauer, A.L. 1991b Life patterns of women from medieval York, pp. 407–13 in D. Walde and N.D. Willows (eds), *The archaeology of gender.* Proceedings of the 22nd Chacmool Conference. The Archaeological Association of the University of Calgary, 1991.

Grauer, A. and Roberts, C.A. 1995 Paleoepidemiology, healing and possible treatment of trauma in the medieval cemetery of St Helen-on-the-Walls, York, England, in preparation.

Gray, P.H. 1969 A case of osteogenesis imperfecta associated with dentinogenesis imperfecta, dating from antiquity. *Clin. Radiol.* 21: 106–8.

Green, V.H.H. 1971 *Medieval civilisation in Western Europe.* London, Edward Arnold.

Gregg, J.B. and Gregg, P.S. 1987 *Dry bones. Dakota Territory Reflected.* Sioux Falls, Sioux Printing.

Grmek, M. 1983 *Les maladies à l'aube de la civilisation occidentale.* Paris, Payot.

Grmek, M. 1989 *Histoire du SIDA.* Paris, France Loisirs.

Grmek, M. 1992 La lèpre a-t-elle été représentée dans l'iconographie antique? *Pact* 34:147–56.

Grmek, M.D. 1994 Discussion, p. 283 in O. Dutour, G. Pálfi, J. Berato and J.-P. Brun (eds), *L'origine de la syphilis en Europe avant ou après 1493?* Centre Archéologique du Var, Editions Errance.

Gron, K. 1973 Leprosy in literature and art. *Int. J. Leprosy* 41(2): 249–83.

Grupe, G. 1988a Impact of choice of bone samples on trace element data in excavated human skeletons. *J. Archaeol. Sci.* 15: 123–9.

Grupe, G. 1988b Metastasizing carcinoma in a medieval skeleton: differential diagnosis and etiology. *Am. J. Phys. Anthrop.* 75: 369–74.

Gurdjian, E.S. 1973 Prevention and mitigation of head injury from antiquity to the present. *J. Trauma* 13(11): 931–45.

Gurdjian, E.S., Webster, J.E. and Lissner, H.R. 1950 The mechanism of skull fracture. *J. Neurosurg.* 7: 106–14.

Hackett, C. 1963 On the origin of the human treponematoses. *Bull. WHO* 29: 7–41.

Hackett, C. 1967 The human treponematoses, pp. 152–70 in D.R. Brothwell and A.T. Sandison (eds), *Diseases in antiquity.* Illinois, Charles Thomas.

Hackett, C. 1974 Possible treponemal changes in a Tasmanian skull. *Man* 9: 436–43.

Hackett, C. 1976 Microscopical focal destruction (tunnels) in exhumed human bone. *Med. Sci. and the Law* 21(4): 243–65.

Hackett, C. 1981 Development of caries sicca in a dry calvaria. *Virchows Arch. (Pathol. Anat.)* 391: 53–79.

Hagelberg, E. 1989 Ancient bone DNA amplified. *Nature* 342: 485.

Halffman, C.A., Scott, G.R. and Pedersen, P.O. 1992 Palatine torus in the Greenlandic Norse. *Am. J. Phys. Anthrop.* 88: 145–61.

Hallbäck, D.A. 1976 A medieval (?) bone with a copper plate support indicating an open surgical treatment. *Ossa* 3/4: 63–82.

Haneveld, G.T. and Perizonius, W.R.K. 1980 Trepanning practice in the Netherlands. *Proceedings of the 3rd Paleopathology Association European Meeting, Caen, France.*

Hanson, D.B. and Buikstra, J.E. 1988 Histomorphological alterations in buried bone from the Lower Illinois Valley: implications for paleodietary research. *J. Archaeol. Sci.* 14: 549–63.

Harris, H.A. 1931 Lines of arrested growth in the long bones in childhood: the correlation of histological and radiographic appearances in clinical and experimental conditions. *Br. J. Radiol.* 18: 622–40.

Hassan, F.A. 1973 On the mechanics of population growth during the Neolithic. *Current Anthropology* 14(5): 535–42.

Hassan, F.A. 1981 *Demographic archaeology.* London, Academic Press.

Hauser, P.M. 1964 The population of the world. Recent trends and perspectives, pp. 15–29 in R. Freedman (ed.), *Population: the vital revolution.* New York, Aldine.

Hawkes, S.C. and Wells, C. 1975 Crime and punishment in an Anglo-Saxon cemetery. *Antiquity* 49: 118–22.

Henneberg, M. and Henneberg, R.J. 1994 Treponematosis in an ancient Greek colony of Metaponto, Southern Italy, 580–250 BC, pp. 92–8 in O. Dutour, G. Pálfi, J. Berato and J.-P. Brun (eds), *L'origine de la syphilis en Europe avant ou après 1493?* Centre Archéologique du Var, Editions Errance.

Her Majesty's Stationery Office 1985 *Manual of nutrition.* London, HMSO.

Hershkovitz, I., Rothschild, B.M., Wish-Baratz, S. and Rothschild, C. 1994 Natural variation and differential diagnosis of skeletal changes in bejel (endemic syphilis), pp. 81–7 in O. Dutour, G. Pálfi, J. Berato and J.-P. Brun (eds), *L'origine de la syphilis en Europe avant ou après 1493?* Centre Archéologique du Var, Editions Errance.

Hess, A.F. 1929 *Rickets including osteomalacia and tetany.* Philadelphia, Lea and Febiger.

Hillson, S. 1986 *Teeth.* Cambridge, Cambridge University Press.

Hillson, S. 1992 Impression replica methods for studying hypoplasia and perikymata in human tooth crown surfaces from archaeological sites. *Int. J. Osteoarchaeology* 2: 65–78.

Hillson, S. and Jones, S. 1989 Instruments for measuring surface profiles: an application in the study of ancient human tooth crown surfaces. *J. Archaeol. Sci.* 16: 95–105.

Hinton, R.J. 1981 Form and patterning of anterior tooth wear among Aboriginal human groups. *Am. J. Phys. Anthrop.* 54: 555–64.

Hodges, D.C. 1989 *Agricultural intensification and prehistoric health in the valley of Oaxaca, Mexico. Prehistory and human ecology of the Valley of the Oaxaca,* Volume 9. Memoirs of the Museum of Anthropology, University of Michigan Number 22, K.V. Flannery (ed.). The Regents of the University of Michigan, The Museum of Anthropology.

Hodges, D.C. 1991 Temporomandibular joint osteoarthritis in a British skeletal population. *Am. J. Phys. Anthrop.* 85: 367–77.

Holcomb, R.C. 1940 The antiquity of congenital syphilis. *Bull. Hist. Med.* 10(2): 148–77.

Hollander, E. 1913 *Die medizin in der Klassischen Malerie.* Stuttgart.

Hollingsworth, T.H. 1969 *Historical demography.* Ithaca, Cornell Press.

Hopkins, D. 1980 News from the field. *Paleopathology Association Newsletter* 31: 6.

Howe, G.M. 1970 Geography looks at death. *Spectrum* 71: 5–7.

Huber, N.M. 1968 The problem of stature increase: looking from the past to the present, pp. 67–102 in D.R. Brothwell (ed.), *Skeletal biology of earlier human populations.* Symposia of the Society for the Study of Human Biology Volume 8. London, Pergamon Press.

Hudson, E.H. 1958 The treponematoses – or treponematosis. *Br. J. Venereal Dis.* 34: 22–3.

Hudson, E.H. 1963 Treponematosis and pilgrimage. *Am. J. Med. Sci.* 246: 645–56.

Hudson, E.H. 1965 Treponematosis and man's social evolution. *Am. Anthrop.* 67: 885–901.

Hudson, E.H. 1968 Christopher Columbus and the history of syphilis. *Acta Tropica* 25: 1–16.

Hulse, E.V. 1972 Leprosy and ancient Egypt. *Lancet* 2: 1024.

Hulse, E.V. 1976 The nature of biblical leprosy and the use of alternative terms in modern translations of the bible. *Medical History* 20(2): 203.

Hummert, J.R. and Van Gerven, D.P. 1985 Observations on the formation and persistence of radiopaque transverse lines. *Am. J. Phys. Anthrop.* 66: 297–306.

Hunt, E.E., Jr and Hatch, J.W. 1981 The estimation of age at death and ages of formation of transverse lines from measurements of human long bones. *Am. J. Phys. Anthrop.* 54: 461–9.

Huss-Ashmore, R., Goodman, A.H. and Armelagos, G.J. 1982 Nutritional inference from paleopathology, pp. 395–476 in M.B. Schiffer (ed.), *Advances in Archeological Method and Theory,* Volume 5. London, Academic Press.

Inhorn, M.C. and Brown, P.J. 1990 The anthropology of infectious disease. *Ann. Rev. Anthrop.* 19: 89–117.

Jackes, M.K. 1983 Osteological evidence for smallpox. A possible case from seventeenth century Ontario. *Am. J. Phys. Anthrop.* 60: 75–81.

Jackson, D.W., Wiltse, L.L. and Cirincione, R.J. 1976 Spondylolysis in the female gymnast. *Clinical Orthopaedics* 117: 68–73.

Janssens, P. 1970 *Palaeopathology.* London, John Baker.

Janssens, P. 1987 A copper plate on the upper arm in a burial at the Church in Vrasene (Belgium). *J. Paleopathology* 1(1): 15–18.

Jarcho, S. 1966 The development and present condition of human paleopathology in the United States, pp. 3–42 in S. Jarcho (ed.), *Paleopathology*. New Haven, Yale University Press.

Jenner, E. 1801 *The origin of the vaccine inoculation*. Soho, D.N. Shury.

Johnston, F.E. 1963 Some observations on the roles of achondroplastic dwarfs through history. *Clin. Pediat.* 2: 703–8.

Jones, A.K.G. 1985 Trichurid ova in archaeological deposits: their value as indicators of ancient faeces, pp. 105–19 in N.J. Feiller, D.D. Gilbertson and N.G.A. Ralph (eds), *Palaeobiological investigations. Research design, methods and data analysis*. British Archaeological Reports International Series 266, Oxford.

Jónsson, B., Gardsell, P., Johnell, O., Redlund-Johnell, I. and Sernbo, I. 1992 Differences in fracture pattern between an urban and a rural population: a comparative population-based study in southern Sweden. *Osteoporosis Int.* 2: 269–73.

Jónsson, B., Gardsell, P., Johnell, O., Sernbo, I. and Gullberg, B. 1993 Life-style and different fracture prevalence: a cross sectional comparative population-based study. *Calcified Tiss. Int.* 52: 425–33.

Jopling, W.H. 1982 Clinical aspects of leprosy. *Tubercle* 63: 295–305.

Jopling, W.H. 1991 Leprosy stigma. *Leprosy Rev.* 62: 1–12.

Jopling, W.H. and McDougall, A.C. 1988 *Handbook of leprosy*. Oxford, Heinemann Medical Books.

Judd, M. 1994 Fracture patterns from two medieval populations in Britain. Unpublished M.Sc. thesis, University of Bradford, Department of Archaeological Sciences.

Jurmain, R.D. 1980 The pattern of involvement of appendicular degenerative joint disease. *Am. J. Phys. Anthrop.* 53: 143– 50.

Jurmain, R.D. 1990 Paleoepidemiology of a Central Californian prehistoric population from CA-ALA. I Degenerative joint disease. *Am. J. Phys. Anthrop.* 83: 83–94.

Jurmain, R.D. 1991 Paleoepidemiology of trauma in a prehistoric Central Californian population, pp. 241–8 in D. Ortner and A. Aufderheide (eds), *Human paleopathology: current syntheses and future options*. Washington DC, Smithsonian Institution Press.

Kambe, T., Yonemitsu, K., Kibayashi, K. and Tsunenari, S. 1991 Application of a computer assisted image analyser to the assessment of area and number of sites of dental attrition and its use in age estimates. *Forensic Science International* 50: 97–109.

Karn, K.W., Shockett, H.D., Moffitt, W.C. and Gray, J.L. 1984 Topographic classification of deformities of the alveolar process. *J. Periodontology* 55: 336–40.

Karsh, R.S. and McCarthy, J.D. 1960 Archaeology and arthritis. *Intern. Med.* 105: 640–4.

Katzenberg, M.A. 1992 Advances in stable isotope analysis of prehistoric bones, pp. 105–15 in S.R. Saunders and M.A. Katzenberg (eds), *Skeletal biology of past peoples: research methods*. New York, Wiley-Liss.

Katzenberg, M.A., Kelley, M.A. and Pfeiffer, S. 1982 Hereditary multiple exostoses in an individual from a southern Ontario Iroquian population. *Ossa* 8: 109–14.

Keene, D. 1983 medieval urban environment in documentary records. *Archives* 16: 137–44.

Kelley, M. and Micozzi, M. 1984 Rib lesions in chronic pulmonary tuberculosis. *Am. J. Phys. Anthrop.* 65: 381–7.

Kelley, M., Murphy, S., Levesque, D. and Sledzik, P. 1994 Respiratory disease among Protohistoric and Early Historic Plains Indians, pp. 123–30 in D.W. Owsley and R.L. Jantz (eds), *Skeletal biology in the Great Plains. Migration, warfare, health, and subsistence*. Washington DC, Smithsonian Institution Press.

Kennedy, G.E. 1986 The relationship between auditory exostoses and cold water: a latitudinal analysis. *Am. J. Phys. Anthrop.* 71: 401–15.

Kennedy, K.A.R. 1989 Skeletal markers of occupational stress, pp. 129–60 in M.Y. Iscan and K.A.R. Kennedy (eds), *Reconstruction of life from the skeleton*. New York, Alan Liss.

Kent, S. 1987 The influence of sedentism and aggregation on porotic hyperostosis: a case study. *Man, New Series* 21: 605–36.

Kent, S. 1992 Anemia through the ages: changing perspectives and their implications, pp. 1–30 in P. Stuart-Macadam and S.K. Kent (eds), *Diet, demography and disease. Changing perspectives on anemia*. New York, Aldine De Gruyter.

Kilgore, L. 1989 A possible case of rheumatoid arthritis from Sudanese Nubia. *Am. J. Phys. Anthrop.* 79: 177–83.

King, S. 1994 The human skeletal remains from Glasgow Cathedral Excavations 1992–3. Unpublished skeletal report.

Klepinger, L.L., Kuhn, J.K. and Thomas, J., Jr 1977 Prehistoric dental calculus gives evidence for coca in early coastal Ecuador. *Nature* 269: 506–7.

Knight, B. 1981 History of wound treatment. *Nursing Times* 77(43): 5–8.

Knight, B. 1991 *Forensic pathology*. London, Edward Arnold.

Kolaridou, A. 1991 Harris lines as an indicator of stress in the post-Medieval population of Tours, France. Unpublished M.A. Dissertation, University of Bradford, Department of Archaeological Sciences.

Krogman, W.M. and Iscan, M.Y. (eds) 1986 *The human skeleton in forensic medicine*. Illinois, Charles Thomas.

Lai, P. and Lovell, N.C. 1992 Skeletal markers of occupational stress in the Fur Trade Period: a case study from a Hudson's Bay Company Fur Trade post. *Int. J. Osteoarchaeology* 2: 221–34.

Lallo, J., Armelagos, G.J. and Rose, J.C. 1978 Paleoepidemiology of infectious disease in Dickson Mounds population. *Med. Coll. Va. Quarterly* 14(1): 17–23.

Lambert, J.B., Xue, L. and Buikstra, J.E. 1989 Physical removal of contaminated inorganic material from buried bone. *J. Archaeol. Sci.* 16: 427–36.

Larsen, C.S. 1982 The anthropology of St. Catherine's Island 3. Prehistoric human biological adaptation. *Anthropological Papers of the American Museum of Natural History, New York* 57(3): 157–276.

Larsen, C.S. 1984 Health and disease in prehistoric Georgia: the transition to agriculture, pp. 367–92 in M.N. Cohen and G.J. Armelagos (eds), *Paleopathology at the origins of agriculture*. Academic Press, London.

Larsen, C.S. 1985 Dental modifications and tool use in the Western Great Basin. *Am. J. Phys. Anthrop.* 67: 393–402.

Laurence, K.M. 1958 The natural history of hydrocephalus. *Lancet* 29: 1152–4.

Lazenby, R. and Pfeiffer, S. 1993 Effects of a 19th century below-knee amputation and prosthesis on femoral morphology. *Int. J. Osteoarchaeology* 3: 19–28.

Learmonth, A.1988 *Disease ecology*. Oxford, Basil Blackwell.

Lee, F. and Magilton, J.R. 1989 The cemetery of the hospital of St James and St Mary Magdalene, Chichester – a case study. *World Archaeology* 21(2): 273–82.

Leestma, J.E. and Kirkpatrick, J.B. 1988 *Forensic neuropathology*. New York, Raven Press.

Leisen, J.C.C., Duncan, H. and Riddle, J.M. 1991 Rheumatoid erosive arthropathy as seen in macerated (dry) bone specimens, pp. 211–15 in D.J. Ortner and A. Aufderheide (eds), *Human paleopathology. Current syntheses and future options*. Washington DC, Smithsonian Institution Press.

Levers, R.G.H. and Darling, A.I. 1983 Continuing eruption of some adult human teeth of ancient populations. *Arch. Oral Biology* 28(5): 401–8.

Lichtor, J. and Lichtor, A. 1957 Palaeopathological evidence suggesting pre-Columbian tuberculosis of the spine. *J. Bone Joint Surgery* 39A: 1398–9.

Lilley, J.M., Stroud, G., Brothwell, D.R. and Williamson, M.H. 1994 *The Jewish burial ground at Jewbury.* The archaeology of York. The medieval cemeteries 12/3. York, Council for British Archaeology for York Archaeological Trust.

Lisowski, F.P. 1967 Prehistoric and early historic trepanation, pp. 651–72 in D. Brothwell and A.T. Sandison (eds), *Diseases in antiquity.* Illinois, Charles Thomas.

Loth, S. and Iscan, M.Y. 1989 Morphological assessment of age in the adult: the thoracic region, pp. 105–35 in M.Y. Iscan (ed.), *Age markers in the human skeleton.* Illinois, Charles Thomas.

Louis, D.S. 1990 Ramazzini and occupational diseases. *J. Hand Surg.* 15: 663–64.

Lovejoy, C.O. and Heiple, K.G. 1981 The analysis of fractures in skeletal populations with an example from the Libben site, Ottawa County, Ohio. *Am. J. Phys. Anthrop.* 55: 529–41.

Lovejoy, C.O., Meindl, R.S., Pryzbeck, T.R. and Mensforth, R.P. 1985 Chronological metamorphosis of the auricular surface of the ilium: a new method for the determination of adult skeletal age. *Am. J. Phys. Anthrop.* 68: 15–28.

Loveland, C.J., Gregg, J.B. and Bass, W.M. 1984 Osteochondritis dissecans from the Great Plains of North America. *Plains Anthrop.* 105: 239–46.

Lovell, N.C. 1990 *Patterns of injury and illness in great apes. A skeletal analysis.* Washington DC, Smithsonian Institution Press.

Lovell, N.C. 1994 Spinal arthritis and physical stress at Bronze Age Harappa. *Am. J. Phys. Anthrop.* 93: 149–64.

Lucier, C.V., VanStone, J.W. and Keats, D. 1971 Medical practices and human anatomical knowledge among the Noatak eskimos. *Ethnology* 19: 251–64.

Lukacs, J.R. 1989 Dental paleopathology: methods for reconstructing dietary patterns, pp. 261–86 in M.Y. Iscan and K.A.R. Kennedy (eds), *Reconstruction of life from the skeleton.* New York, Alan Liss.

Lukacs, J.R. 1992 Dental paleopathology and agricultural intensification in South Asia: new evidence from Bronze Age Harappa. *Am. J. Phys. Anthrop.* 87: 133–50.

Lukacs, J.R. and Pastor, R.F. 1988 Activity-induced patterns of dental abrasion in prehistoric Pakistan. *Am. J. Phys. Anthrop.* 76: 377–98.

Lurie, M.B. 1955 A pathogenetic relationship between tuberculosis and leprosy: the common denominators in the tissue response to Mycobacteria, pp. 340–3 in *CIBA Foundation Symposium on Experimental Tuberculosis.* Boston, Little Brown and Co.

Maat, G. 1982 *Scurvy in Dutch whalers buried at Spitsbergen.* Proceedings of the 4th European Meeting of the Paleopathology Association, Middelberg/Antwerpen, pp.82–93.

Maat, G. and Baig, M. 1991 Scanning electron microscopy of fossilised sickle cells. *Int. J. Anthropology* 5(3): 271–6.

Macchiarelli, R., Bondioloi, L., Censi, L., Hernaez, M.K., Salvadei, L. and Sperduti, A. 1994 Intra- and interobserver concordance in scoring Harris lines: a test on bone sections and radiographs. *Am. J. Phys. Anthrop.* 95: 77–83.

McKeown, T. and Record, R.G. 1960 Study of population for five years after birth, pp. 2–16 in *CIBA Foundation Symposium on Congenital Malformations.* Boston, Little Brown and Co.

McKinley, J. and Roberts, C. 1993 *Excavation and postexcavation treatment of cremated and inhumed remains.* Institute of Field Archaeologists Technical Paper 13, Birmingham.

MacKinney, L. 1957 Medieval surgery. *J. Int. Coll. Surgeons* 27: 393–404.

Madea, B. and Staak, M. 1988 Determination of the sequence of gunshot wounds in the skull. *J. Forensic Science Society* 28(5–6): 321–8.

Malhorta, K.C. 1990 Changing patterns of disease in India with special reference to childhood mortality, pp. 313–32 in A. Swedlund and G. Armelagos (eds), *Disease in populations in transition. Anthropological and epidemiological perspectives.* London, Bergin and Garvey.

Manchester, K. 1978a *Executions in West Yorkshire.* Scient Presentes 5. Leeds, Yorkshire Archaeological Society.

Manchester, K. 1978b Palaeopathology of a Royalist garrison. *Ossa* 5: 25–33.

Manchester, K. 1980a Hydrocephalus in an Anglo-Saxon child. *Arch. Cantiana* 96: 77–82.

Manchester, K. 1980b Jugular vein occlusion in the Bronze Age. *Yorkshire Archaeological J.* 52: 167–9.

Manchester, K. 1982 Spondylolysis and spondylolisthesis in two Anglo-Saxon skeletons. *Paleopathology Association Newsletter* 37: 9–12.

Manchester, K. 1983a Secondary cancer in an Anglo-Saxon female. *J. Archaeol. Sci.* 10: 475–82.

Manchester, K. 1983b *The archaeology of disease.* Bradford, Bradford University Press.

Manchester, K. 1991 Tuberculosis and leprosy: evidence for interaction of disease, pp. 23–35 in D. Ortner and A. Aufderheide (eds), *Human paleopathology. Current syntheses and future options.* Washington DC, Smithsonian Institution Press.

Manchester, K. 1992 The palaeopathology of urban infections, pp. 8–15 in S. Bassett (ed.), *Death in towns.* Leicester, Leicester University Press.

Manchester, K. 1994 Rhinomaxillary lesions in syphilis: differential diagnosis, pp. 79–80 in O. Dutour, G. Pálfi, J. Berato and J.-P. Brun (eds), *L'origine de la syphilis en Europe avant ou après 1493?* Centre Archéologique du Var, Editions Errance.

Manchester, K. and Elmhirst, O.E.C. 1980 Forensic aspects of an Anglo-Saxon injury. *Ossa* 7: 179–88.

Manchester, K. and Knüsel, C. 1994 A medieval sculpture of leprosy in the Cistercian Abbaye de Cadouin. *Medical History* 38(2): 204–6.

Manchester, K. and Roberts, C. 1987 Palaeopathological evidence of leprosy and tuberculosis in Britain. Unpublished SERC Report, University of Bradford.

Mann, R.W. and Owsley, D.W. 1989 Anatomy of uncorrected talipes equinovarus in a fifteenth century American Indian. *J. Am. Podiatric Medical Assoc.* 79(9): 436–40.

Mann, R.W., Roberts, C.A, Thomas, M.D. and Davy, D.T. 1991 Pressure erosion of the femoral trochlea, patella baja, and altered patellar surfaces. *Am. J. Phys. Anthrop.* 85: 321–7.

Maples, W.R. 1989 The practical application of age-estimation techniques, pp. 319–24 in M.Y. Iscan (ed.), *Age markers in the human skeleton.* Illinois, Charles Thomas.

Marcombe, D. and Manchester, K. 1990 The Melton Mowbray 'leper head': an historical and medical investigation. *Medical History* 34: 86–91.

Marlow, M. 1992 The human remains, pp. 107–18 in S.J. Sherlock and M.G.Welch (eds), *An Anglo-Saxon cemetery at Norton, Cleveland.* Council for British Archaeology Research Report 82. York, Council for British Archaeology.

Martin, D.L. 1991 Bone histology and paleopathology: methodological considerations, pp. 55–9 in D. Ortner and A. Aufderheide (eds), *Human paleopathology, current syntheses and future options.* Washington DC, Smithsonian Institution Press.

Martin, D.L., Goodman, A.H. and Armelagos, G.J. 1985 Skeletal pathologies as indicators of diet, pp. 227–79 in R.I. Gilbert and J.H. Mielke (eds), *Analysis of prehistoric diets.* New York, Academic Press.

Martin, D.L., Magennis, A.L. and Rose, J.C. 1987 Cortical bone maintenance in a Historic Afro-American cemetery sample from Cedar Grove, Arkansas. *Am. J. Phys. Anthrop.* 74: 255–64.

Masset, C. 1989 Age estimation on the basis of of cranial sutures, pp. 71–103 in M.Y. Iscan (ed.), *Age markers in the human skeleton*. Illinois, Charles Thomas.

Massler, M., Schour, J. and Poncher, H. 1941 Development pattern of the child as reflected in the calcification pattern of the teeth. *Am. J. Dis. Child.* 62: 33–67.

May, R.L., Goodman, A.H. and Meindl, R.S. 1993 Response of bone and enamel formation to nutritional supplementation and morbidity among malnourished Guatemalan children. *Am. J. Phys. Anthrop.* 92: 37–51.

Mays, S. 1993 Infanticide in Roman Britain. *Antiquity* 67: 883–8.

Meiklejohn, C., Schentag, C. and Venema, A. 1984 Socioeconomic change and patterns of pathology and variation in the Mesolithic and Neolithic of Western Europe: some suggestions, pp.75–100 in M.N. Cohen and G.J. Armelagos (eds), *Paleopathology at the origins of agriculture*. Academic Press, London.

Meindl, R.S. and Lovejoy, C.O. 1989 Age changes in the pelvis: implications for paleodemography, pp. 137–68 in M.Y. Iscan (ed.), *Age markers in the human skeleton*. Illinois, Charles Thomas.

Mensforth, R.P. and Latimer, B.M. 1989 Hamann–Todd Collection aging studies: osteoporosis fracture syndrome. *Am. J. Phys. Anthrop.* 80: 461–79.

Mensforth, R.P., Lovejoy, C.O., Lallo, H. and Armelagos, G.J. 1978 The role of constitutional factors, diet and infectious disease in the etiology of porotic hyperostosis and periosteal reactions in prehistoric infants and children. *Med. Anthropol.* 2: 1–59.

Merbs, C. 1983 *Patterns of activity induced pathology in a Canadian Inuit population*. Archaeological Survey of Canada Paper No. 119. Ottawa, National Museums of Canada.

Merbs, C. 1989a Trauma, pp. 161–89 in M.Y. Iscan and K.A.R. Kennedy (eds), *Reconstruction of life from the skeleton*. New York, Alan Liss.

Merbs, C. 1989b Spondylolysis: its nature and significance. *Int. J. Anthrop.* 4(3): 143–9.

Merbs, C. 1992 A New World of infectious disease. *Yearbook of Physical Anthropology* 35: 3–42.

Mercer, W. 1964 Then and now: history of skeletal tuberculosis. *J. R. Coll. Surg. Edin.* 9: 243–54.

Meyer, K.F. 1964 Evolution of occupational diseases acquired from animals. *Indust. Med. Surg.* 33: 286–95.

Micozzi, M.S. 1991 Taphonomy and the study of disease in antiquity: the case of cancer, pp.91–103 in M. Micozzi (ed.), *Postmortem change in human and animal remains*. Illinois, Charles Thomas.

Miles, A.E.W. 1963 The dentition in the assessment of individual age in skeletal material, pp. 191–209 in D. Brothwell (ed.), *Dental anthropology*. Oxford, Pergamon Press.

Miles, A.E.W. 1989 *An early Christian chapel and burial ground on the Isle of Ensay, Outer Hebrides, Scotland with a study of the skeletal remains*. British Archaeological Reports British Series 212, Oxford.

Miles, A.E.W. 1994 Non-union of the epiphysis of the acromion in the skeletal remains of a Scottish population of ca. 1700. *Int. J. Osteoarcheology* 4: 149–63.

Milner, G.R. and Larsen, C.S. 1991 Teeth as artifacts of human behavior: intentional mutilation and accidental modification, pp. 351–78 in M. Kelley and C.S. Larsen (eds), *Advances in dental anthropology*. New York, Alan Liss.

Mittler, D.M. and Van Gerven, D.P. 1994 Developmental, diachronic and demographic analysis of cribra orbitalia in the medieval Christian populations of Kulubnarti. *Am. J. Phys. Anthrop.* 93: 287–97.

Mittler, D.M., Van Gerven, D.P., Sheridan, S.G. and Beck, R. 1992 The epidemiology of enamel hypoplasia, cribra orbitalia and subadult mortality in an ancient Nubian population, pp. 143–50 in A.H. Goodman and L. Capasso (eds), *Recent contributions to the study of enamel developmental defects.* Journal of Paleopathology Monographic Publications 2.

Moggi-Cecchi, J., Pacciani, E. and Pinto-Cisternas, J. 1994 Enamel hypoplasia and age at weaning in 19th century Florence. *Am. J. Phys. Anthrop.* 93: 299–306.

Møller, P. and Møller-Christensen, V. 1952 A Mediaeval female skull showing evidence of metastases from a malignant growth. *Acta Path. Microbiol. Scand.* 30: 336–42.

Møller-Christensen, V. 1953 *Ten lepers from Naestved.* Copenhagen, Danish Science Press.

Møller-Christensen, V. 1958 *Bogen om Abelholt Kloster.* Copenhagen, Danish Science Press.

Møller-Christensen, V. 1961 *Bone changes in leprosy.* Copenhagen, Munksgaard.

Møller-Christensen, V. 1967 Evidence of leprosy in earlier peoples, pp. 295–307 in D.R. Brothwell and A.T. Sandison (eds), *Disease in antiquity.* Springfield, Illinois, Charles Thomas.

Møller-Christensen, V. 1969a *A rosary bead as tooth filling in a human mandibular canine tooth. A unique case from the Danish Middle Ages.* 21st International Congress on the History of Medicine, Siena, Italy.

Møller-Christensen, V. 1969b The history of syphilis and leprosy – an osteo-archaeological approach. *Abbotempo* 1: 20–25.

Møller-Christensen, V. 1978a *Leprosy changes of the skull.* Odense, University Press.

Møller-Christensen, V. 1978b *Medizinische diagnostik in Geschichte und Gegenwert.* Muchen, Werner-Fritsch.

Møller-Christensen, V. and Hughes, D.R. 1966 An early case of leprosy from Nubia. *Man, New Series* 1: 242–3.

Molleson, T. 1989 Seed preparation in the Mesolithic: the osteological evidence. *Antiquity* 63: 356–62.

Molleson, T. and Cox, M. 1993 *The Spitalfields Project.* Volume 2, *The Anthropology. The Middling Sort.* Council for British Archaeology Research Report 86. York, Council for British Archaeology.

Molnar, S. 1971 Human tooth wear, tooth function and cultural variability. *Am. J. Phys. Anthrop.* 34: 175–90.

Molnar, S. 1972 Tooth wear and culture: a survey of tooth function among some prehistoric populations. *Current Anthropology* 13(5): 511–26.

Molnar, S. and Molnar, I. 1985 Observations of dental diseases among prehistoric populations of Hungary. *Am. J. Phys. Anthrop.* 67: 51–63.

Molto, J.E. 1990 Differential diagnosis of rib lesions: a case study from Middle Woodland, Southern Ontario. *Am. J. Phys. Anthrop.* 83: 439–47.

Montgomery, P.Q., Williams, H.O.L., Reading, N. and Stringer, C.B. 1994 An assessment of the temporal bone lesions of the Broken Hill cranium. *J. Archaeol. Sci.* 21: 331–7.

Moodie, R.L. 1923 *Paleopathology.* Urbana, University of Illinois Press.

Moodie, R.L. 1927 Injuries to the head among the pre-Columbian Peruvians. *Ann. medieval History* 9(3): 277–307.

Moore, W.J. and Corbett, E. 1971 Distribution of dental caries in ancient British populations. Anglo-Saxon period. *Caries Res.* 5: 151–68.

Moore, W.J. and Corbett, E. 1973 Distribution of dental caries in British populations. Iron Age, Romano-British and medieval Periods. *Caries Res.* 7: 139–53.

Moore, W.J. and Corbett, E. 1975 Distribution of dental caries in ancient British populations III. The 17th century. *Caries Res.* 9: 163–75.

Morant, G.M. 1931 Study of the recently excavated Spitalfields crania. *Biometrika* 23: 191–248.

Morse, D. 1961 Prehistoric tuberculosis in America. *Am. Rev. Resp. Dis.* 85: 489–504.

Morse, D., Brothwell, D.R. and Ucko, P. 1964 Tuberculosis in ancient Egypt. *Am. Rev. Resp. Dis.* 90: 524–41.

Morse, D., Dailey, R.C. and Bunn, J. 1974 Prehistoric multiple myeloma. *Bull. New York Acad. Med.* 54: 447–58.

Mosekilde, L. 1990 Consequences of the remodelling process for vertebral bone structure: an SEM study (uncoupling of loaded structures). *Bone and Mineral* 10: 13–35.

Munizaga, J., Allison, M.J., Gerszten, E. and Klurfeld, D.M. 1975 Pneumoconiosis in Chilean miners of the 16th century. *Bull. New York Acad. Med.* 5(11): 1281–93.

Murphy, T. 1959 The changing pattern of dentine exposure in human tooth attrition. *Am. J. Phys. Anthrop.* 17: 167–78.

Nag, M. 1977 Anthropology and population. Problems and perspectives, pp. 41–55 in D.R. Brothwell (ed.), *Biosocial man.* Eugenic Society Publication.

Nathan, H. 1962 Osteophytes of the vertebral column. *J. Bone Joint Surgery* 44A(2): 243–68.

Nelson, D.A., Feingold, M., Bolin, F. and Parfitt, A.M. 1991 Principal components analysis of regional bone density in black and white women: relationship to body size and composition. *Am. J. Phys. Anthrop.* 86: 507–14.

Nickens, P.R. 1976 Stature reduction as an adaptive response to food production in Mesoamerica. *J. Archaeol. Sci.* 3: 31–41.

Notman, D.N.H. 1986 Ancient scannings: computed tomography of Egyptian mummies, pp. 251–320 in A.R. David (ed.), *Science and Egyptology.* Manchester, Manchester University Press.

Oakley, K.P., Brooke, W.M.A., Akester, A.R. and Brothwell, D.R. 1959 Contributions on trepanning or trephination in ancient and modern times. *Man* 59: 93–6.

Olsen, S. and Shipman, P. 1994 Cutmarks and perimortem treatment of skeletal remains on the Northern Plains, pp. 377–87 in D.W. Owsley and R.L. Jantz (eds), *Skeletal biology of the Great Plains. Migration, warfare, health and subsistence.* Washington DC, Smithsonian Institution Press.

Ortner, D.J. 1979 Disease and mortality in the early Bronze Age people of Bab edh-Dhra, Jordan. *Am. J. Phys. Anthrop.* 51: 589–98.

Ortner, D. 1981 Bone tumors in archeological human skeletons (paleopathology of human bone tumors), pp. 733–8 in H.E. Kaiser (ed.), *Neoplasms – comparative pathology of growth in animals, plants and man.* Baltimore, Williams and Wilkins.

Ortner, D.J. 1984 Bone lesions in a probable case of scurvy from Metlatavik, Alaska. *MASCA J.* 3: 79–81.

Ortner, D.J. 1991 Theoretical and methodological issues in paleopathology, pp. 5–11 in D. Ortner and A. Aufderheide (eds), *Human paleopathology.Current syntheses and future options.* Washington DC, Smithsonian Institution Press.

Ortner, D. and Putschar, W.J. 1981 *Identification of pathological conditions in human skeletal remains.* Washington DC, Smithsonian Institution Press.

Ortner, D.J. and Utermohle, C.J. 1981 Polyarticular inflammatory arthritis in a pre-Columbian skeleton from Kodiak Island, Alaska, U.S.A. *Am. J. Phys. Anthrop.* 56: 23–31.

Ortner, D., Manchester, K. and Lee, F. 1991 Metastatic carcinoma in a leper skeleton from a medieval cemetery in Chichester, England. *Int. J. Osteoarchaeology* 1: 91–8.

Owsley, D. 1994 Warfare in coalescent traditional populations of the Northern Plains, pp. 333–43 in D.W. Owsley and R.L. Jantz (eds), *Skeletal biology of the Great Plains. Migration, warfare, health and subsistence.* Washington DC, Smithsonian Institution Press.

Owsley, D.W. and Mann, R.W. 1990 An American Indian skeleton with clubfoot from the Cabin burial site (A1184), Hemphill County, Texas. *Plains Anthropologist* 35(128): 93–101.

Oyebola, D.D.O. 1980 Yoruba traditional bonesetters: the practice of orthopaedics in a primitive setting in Nigeria. *J. Trauma* 20(4): 312–22.

Paabo, S. 1985 Molecular cloning of ancient Egyptian mummy DNA. *Nature* 314: 644–5.

Pales, L. 1929 Maladie de Paget préhistorique. *Anthrop. Paris* 39: 263–70.

Pálfi, G. 1991 The first osteoarchaeological evidence of leprosy in Hungary. *Int. J. Osteoarchaeology* 1: 99–102.

Pálfi, G., Dutour, O., Borreani, M., Brun, J.-P. 1992 Pre-Columbian congenital syphilis from the Late Antiquity in France. *Int. J. Osteoarchaeology* 2: 245–61.

Panuel, M. 1994 Radiographic manifestations of congenital syphilis, pp. 36–40 in O. Dutour, G. Pálfi, J. Berato and Brun, J.-P. (eds), *L'origine de la syphilis en Europe avant ou après 1493?* Centre Archéologique du Var, Editions Errance.

Parker, S., Roberts, C. and Manchester, K. 1986 A review of British trepanations with reports on two new cases. *Ossa* 12: 141–57.

Pate, F.D. and Hutton, J.T. 1988 Use of soil chemistry data to address postmortem diagenesis in bone mineral. *J. Archaeol. Sci.* 15: 729–39.

Penrose, L.S. 1959 *Outline of human genetics.* London, William Heinemann.

Perzigian, A.J. and Widmer, L. 1979 Evidence for tuberculosis in a prehistoric population. *J. Am. Med. Assoc.* 241(24): 2643–6.

Perzigian, A.J., Tench, P.A. and Braun, D.J. 1984 Prehistoric health in the Ohio River Valley, pp. 347–92 in M.N. Cohen and G.J. Armelagos (eds), *Paleopathology at the origins of agriculture.* Academic Press, London.

Pfeiffer, S. 1991 Rib lesions and New World tuberculosis. *Int. J. Osteoarchaeology* 1: 191–8.

Pfeiffer, S. and Lazenby, R. 1994 Low bone mass in past and present populations, pp. 35–51 in *Advances in Nutritional Research* 9.

Piggott, S. 1940 A trepanned skull of the Beaker Period from Dorset and the practice of trepanning in prehistoric Europe. *Proc. Prehist. Soc.* 6: 112–33.

Pindborg, J.J. 1970 *Pathology of the dental hard tissues.* Copenhagen, Munksgaard.

Polednak, A.P. 1989 *Racial and ethnic differences in disease.* Oxford, Oxford University Press.

Polson, C.J., Gee, D.J. and Knight, B. 1985 *Essentials of forensic medicine.* Oxford, Pergamon Press.

Pounds, N.J.G. 1974 *An economic history of medieval Europe.* London, Longman Group.

Powell, M.L. 1985 The analysis of dental wear and caries for dietary reconstruction, pp. 307–38 in R.I. Gilbert and J.H. Mielke (eds), *Analysis of prehistoric diets.* London, Academic Press.

Power, C. 1992 The spread of syphilis and a possible early case in Waterford. *Archaeology (Ireland)* 6(4): 20–1.

Power, C. and O'Sullivan, V.R. 1992 Rickets in 19th century Waterford. *Archaeology (Ireland)* 6(1): 27–8.

Powlesland, D. 1980 West Heslerton – focus for a landscape project. *Rescue News* 21: 12.

Price, J.L. 1975 The radiology of excavated Saxon and medieval human remains from Winchester. *Clin. Radiol.* 26: 363–70.

Price, T.D. (ed.) 1989 *The chemistry of prehistoric human bone.* Cambridge, Cambridge University Press.

Price, T.D., Blitz, J., Burton, J. and Ezzo, J.A. 1992 Diagenesis in prehistoric bone: problems and solutions. *J. Archaeol. Sci.* 19: 513–29.

Prince, R.L., Knuiman, M.W. and Gulland, L. 1993 Fracture prevalence in an Australian population. *Aust. J. Public Health* 17(2): 124–8.

Propst, K.B., Danforth, M.E. and Jacobi, K. 1994 Replicability in scoring enamel hypoplasias: a preliminary report. *Paleopathology Association Newsletter* 87: 11–12.

Rahtz, P. 1960 Sewerby. *Medieval Archaeology* 4: 134–65.

Reader, R. 1974 New evidence for the antiquity of leprosy in early Britain. *J. Archaeol. Sci.* 1: 205–7.

Reichs, K. 1986a Forensic implications of skeletal pathology: sex, pp. 112–42 in K. Reichs (ed.), *Forensic osteology. Advances in the identification of human remains.* Illinois, Charles Thomas.

Reichs, K. 1986b Forensic implications of skeletal pathology: ancestry, pp. 196–217 in K. Reichs (ed.), *Forensic osteology. Advances in the identification of human remains.* Illinois, Charles Thomas.

Reichs, K. 1989 Treponematosis: a possible case from the late prehistoric of North Carolina. *Am. J. Phys. Anthrop.* 79: 289–303.

Reinhard, K. 1988 Cultural ecology of prehistoric parasitism on the Colorado plateau as evidenced by coprology. *Am. J. Phys. Anthrop.* 82: 145–63.

Reinhard, K. 1990 Archeoparasitology in North America. *Am. J. Phys. Anthrop.* 82: 145–63.

Reinhard, K., Geib, P.R., Callahan, M.M. and Hevly, R.H. 1992 Discovery of colon contents in a skeletonised burial: soil sampling for dietary remains. *J. Archaeol. Sci.* 19: 697–705.

Rendle-Short, J., Gray, O.P. and Dodge, J.R. 1978 *Synopsis of children's diseases.* Bristol, John Wright and Sons.

Resnick, D. and Niwayama, G. 1988 *Diagnosis of bone and joint disorders,* 2nd edition. Philadelphia, W.B. Saunders.

Richards, G.D. 1985 Analysis of a microcephalic child from the Late Period (ca. 1100–1700 A.D.) of Central California. *Am. J. Phys. Anthrop.* 68: 343–57.

Richards, G.D. and Anton, S.C. 1991 Craniofacial configuration and postcranial development of a hydrocephalic child (ca. 2500 B.C.–500 A.D.): with a review of cases and comment on diagnostic criteria. *Am. J. Phys. Anthrop.* 85: 185–200.

Richards, L.C. 1990 Tooth wear and temporomandibular joint change in Australian aboriginal populations. *Am. J. Phys. Anthrop.* 82: 377–84.

Richards, P. 1977 *The Mediaeval leper and his northern heirs.* Cambridge, D.S. Brewer.

Riddle, J.M., Duncan, H., Pitchford, W.C., Ellis, B.I., Brennan, T.A. and Fisher, L.J. 1988 Anteroposterior radiographic view of the knee: An unreliable indicator of bone damage. *Clin. Rheumatol.* 7(4): 504–13.

Ridley, D.S. and Jopling, W.H. 1966 Classification of leprosy according to immunity. A five group system. *Int. J. Leprosy* 34: 255–73.

Ripamonti, U. 1988 Paleopathology in *A. africanus*: a suggested case of a three million year old prepubertal periodontitis. *Am. J. Phys. Anthrop.* 76: 197–210.

Ritchie, W.A. and Warren, S.L. 1932 The occurrence of multiple bony lesions suggesting myeloma in the skeleton of a pre-Columbian Indian. *Am. J. Roentgenol.* 28: 622–8.

Roberts, C.A. 1985 Case report 5: osteochondroma. *Paleopathology Association Newsletter* 50: 7–8.

Roberts, C.A. 1986a Leprosy and leprosaria in medieval Britain. *MASCA J.* 4(1): 15–21.

Roberts, C.A. 1986b Leprogenic odontodysplasia, pp. 137–47 in E. Cruwys and R. Foley (eds), *Teeth and anthropology.* British Archaeological Reports International Series 291, Oxford.

Roberts, C.A. 1987 Case Report 9: Scurvy. *Paleopathology Association Newsletter* 57: 14–15.

Roberts, C. A. 1988a Trauma and treatment in British antiquity. An ostearchaeological study of macroscopic and radiological features of long bone fractures from the Historic period with a comparative study of clinical radiographs, supplemented by contemporary documentary, iconographical and archaeological evidence. Ph.D. thesis, University of Bradford, Department of Archaeological Sciences.

Roberts, C.A. 1988b A rare case of dwarfism from the Roman Period. *J. Paleopathology* 2(1): 9–21.

Roberts, C.A. 1989a Trauma and treatment in British antiquity: a radiographic study, pp. 339–59 in J. Tate and E. Slater (eds), *Proceedings of the Science and Archaeology Conference, Glasgow, September, 1987.* British Archaeological Reports British Series 196, Oxford.

Roberts, C.A. 1989b Scientific methods in palaeopathology, past, present and future, pp. 373–85 in P. Budd, B. Chapman, C. Jackson, R. Janaway and B. Ottaway (eds), *Archaeological Sciences 1989.* Proceedings of a conference on the application of scientific techniques to archaeology, Bradford. Oxford, Oxbow Monograph 9.

Roberts, C.A. 1991 Trauma and treatment in the British Historic period: a design for multidisciplinary research, pp. 225–40 in D. Ortner and A. Aufderheide (eds), *Human paleopathology. Current syntheses and future options.* Washington DC, Smithsonian Institution Press.

Roberts, C.A. 1994 Treponematosis in Gloucester, England: a theoretical and practical approach to the pre-Columbian theory, pp. 101–8 in O. Dutour, G. Palfi, J. Berato and J.-P. Brun (eds), *L'origine de la syphilis en Europe avant ou après 1493?* Centre Archéologique du Var, Editions Errance.

Roberts, C.A. and Lewis, M. 1994 A comparative study of the prevalence of maxillary sinusitis in medieval urban and rural populations in Northern England. Unpublished report to NERC, University of Bradford.

Roberts, C.A. and Rudgewick-Brown, N. 1991 CD ROM imaging in osteoarchaeology. *Int. J. Osteoarchaeology* 1: 141–5.

Roberts, C.A. and Wakely, J. 1992 Microscopical findings associated with the diagnosis of osteoporosis in palaeopathology. *Int. J. Osteoarchaeology* 2: 23–30.

Roberts, C.A., Lucy, D. and Manchester, K. 1994 Inflammatory lesions of ribs: an analysis of the Terry Collection. *Am. J. Phys. Anthrop.* 95(2): 169–82.

Roberts, R.S. 1971 The use of literary and documentary evidence in the history of medicine, pp. 36–57 in E. Clarke (ed.), *Modern methods in the history of medicine.* London, Athlone Press.

Rogers, J. and Waldron, T. 1995 *A field guide to joint disease in archaeology.* Chichester, John Wiley and Sons.

Rogers, J., Waldron, T., Dieppe, P. and Watt, I. 1987 Arthropathies in palaeopathology: the basis of classification according to most probable cause. *J. Archaeol. Sci.* 14: 179–93.

Rogers, J., Watt, I. and Dieppe, P. 1990 Comparison of visual and radiographic defects of bony changes at the knee joint. *Br. Med. J.* 300: 367–8.

Rogers, L. 1949 Meningeomas in Pharoah's people. *Br. J. Surg.* 36: 423–4.

Rose, J., Anton, S.C., Aufderheide, A.C., Eisenberg, L., Gregg, J.B., Neiburger, E.J., and Rothschild, B. 1991 *Skeletal database recommendations.* Detroit, Palaeopathology Association.

Roth, E.A. 1992 Applications of demographic models to paleodemography, pp. 175–88 in S.R. Saunders and M.A. Katzenberg (eds), *Skeletal biology of past peoples: research methods.* New York, Wiley-Liss.

Rothschild, B.M. and Heathcote, G.M. 1993 Characterisation of the skeletal manifestations of the treponemal disease yaws as a population phenomenon. *Clinical Infectious Diseases* 17: 198–203.

Rothschild, B.M. and Rothschild, C. 1994 Distinguished: syphilis, yaws and bejel on the basis of differences in their respective osseous impact, pp. 68–71 in O. Dutour, G. Pálfi, J. Berato and J.-P. Brun (eds), *L'origine de la syphilis en Europe avant ou après 1493?* Centre Archéologique du Var, Editions Errance.

Rothschild, B.M., Woods, R.J. and Ortel, W. 1990 Rheumatoid arthritis 'in the buff': erosive arthritis in defleshed bones. *Am. J. Phys. Anthrop.* 82: 441–9.

Rowling, J.T. 1961 Pathological changes in mummies. *Proc. R. Soc. Med.* 54: 409–15.

Ruffer, M.A. 1910 Remarks on the histology and pathological anatomy of Egyptian mummies. *Cairo Scientific J.* 4: 1–5.

Ruffer, M.A. and Willmore, J.G. 1914 Note on a tumour of the pelvis dating from Roman times (250 AD) and found in Egypt. *J. Path. Bact.* 18: 480–4.

Ryan, F. 1993 *Tuberculosis. The greatest story never told.* Swift Publishers, Bromsgrove.

Sager, P. 1969 *Spondylosis cervicalis. A pathological and osteoarchaeological study.* Copenhagen, Munksgaard.

Sager, P., Schalimtzek, M. and Møller-Christensen, V. 1972 A case of spondylitis tuberculosa in a Danish Neolithic age. *Danish Med. Bull.* 19(5): 176–80.

Sahlin, Y. 1990 Occurrence of fractures in a defined population: a 1 year study. *Injury* 21: 158–60.

Salo, W.L., Aufderheide, A., Buikstra, J. and Holcomb, T.A. 1994 Identification of *Mycobacterium tuberculosis* DNA in a pre-Columbian mummy. *Proc. Natl Acad. Sci. USA* 91: 2091–4.

Saluja, G., Fitzpatrick, K., Bruce, M. and Cross, J. 1986 Schmorl's Nodes (intravertebral herniations of intervertebral disc tissue) in two historic British populations. *J. Anat.* 145: 87–96.

Sandford, M.K. 1992 A reconsideration of trace element analysis in prehistoric bone, pp. 105–19 in S.R. Saunders and M.A. Katzenberg (eds), *Skeletal biology of past peoples:research methods.* New York, Wiley-Liss.

Sandford, M.K., Van Gerven, D.P. and Meglen, R.R. 1983 Elemental hair analysis: new evidence on the etiology of cribra orbitalia in Sudanese Nubia. *Human Biology* 55(4), 831–44.

Sandison, A.T. 1968 Pathological changes in the skeletons of earlier populations due to acquired disease and difficulties in their interpretation, pp. 205–43 in D.R. Brothwell (ed.), *Skeletal biology of earlier human populations.* London, Pergamon Press.

Sandison, A.T. 1980a Diseases in ancient Egypt, pp. 29–44 in A. Cockburn and E. Cockburn (eds), *Mummies, disease and ancient cultures.* New York, Cambridge University Press.

Sandison, A.T. 1980b Notes on some skeletal changes in pre-European contact Australian Aborigines. *J. Human Evolution* 9: 45–7.

Sandison, A.T. 1981 Diseases in the ancient world, pp. 1–18 in P.P. Anthony and R.N.M. Macsween (eds), *Recent advances in histopathology.* Edinburgh, Churchill Livingstone.

Santini, A., Land, M. and Raab, G.M. 1990 The accuracy of simple ordinal scoring of tooth attrition in age assessment. *Forensic Science International* 48: 175–84.

Sarnat, B.G. and Schour, J. 1941 Enamel hypoplasia (chronic enamel aplasia) in relation to systemic disease: a chronologic, morphologic and etiologic classification. *J. Am. Dental Assoc.* 28: 1989–2000.

Sattienspiel, L. 1990 Modeling the spread of infectious disease in human populations. *Yearbook of Physical Anthropology* 33: 245–76.

Saunders, S.R. 1989 Non-metric skeletal variation, pp. 95–108 in M.Y. Iscan and K.A.R. Kennedy (eds), *Reconstruction of life from the skeleton*. New York, Alan Liss.

Saunders, S. 1992 Subadult skeletons and growth related studies, pp. 1–20 in S.R. Saunders and M.A. Katzenberg (eds), *Skeletal biology of past peoples: research methods*. New York, Wiley-Liss.

Schoeninger, M.J. 1979 Diet and status at Chalcatzingo: some empirical and technical aspects of strontium. *Am. J. Phys. Anthrop.* 51: 295–310.

Schultz, B. 1985 *Art and anatomy in Renaissance Italy*. Ann Arbor, Michigan: UMI Research Press.

Schultz, M. 1979 Diseases of the ear region in early and prehistoric populations. *J. Human Evolution* 8(6): 575–80.

Schultz, M. 1994 Comparative histopathology of syphilitic lesions in prehistoric and historic human bones, pp. 63–7 in O. Dutour, G. Pálfi, J. Berato and J.-P. Brun (eds), *L'origine de la syphilis en Europe avant ou après 1493?* Centre Archéologique du Var, Editions Errance.

Schwarz, H. and Schoeninger, M. 1991 Stable isotopic analysis in human nutritional ecology. *Yearbook of Physical Anthropology* 34: 283–321.

Scott, E.C. 1979 Dental scoring technique. *Am. J. Phys. Anthrop.* 51: 213–18.

Selye, H. 1950 *Stress*. Montreal, Medical Publishers.

Sevitt, S. 1981 *Bone repair and fracture healing in man*. Edinburgh, Churchill Livingstone.

Shaw, J.L. and Sakellarides, H. 1967 Radial nerve paralysis associated with fractures of the humerus. A review of 45 cases. *J. Bone Joint Surgery* 49A(5): 899–902.

Sherratt, A. 1981 Plough and pastoralism: aspects of the secondary products revolution, pp. 261–305 in I. Hodder, G. Isaac and N. Hammond (eds), *Pattern of the past: studies in honour of David Clarke*. Cambridge, Cambridge University Press.

Short, C.L. 1974 The antiquity of rheumatoid arthritis. *Arthritis and Rheumatism* 17(3): 193–205.

Sibbison, J.B. 1990 More about fluoride. *Lancet* 336: 737.

Sigerist, H.E. 1951 *A history of medicine. Volume 1, Primitive and Archaic medicine*. New York, Oxford University Press.

Singh, A., Dass, R., Sing Heyreh, S. and Jolly, S. 1962 Skeletal changes in endemic fluorosis. *J. Bone Joint Surgery* 44b(4): 806–15.

Sjøvold, T., Swedborg, I. and Diener, I. 1974 A pregnant woman from the Middle Ages with exostosis multiplex. *Ossa* 1: 3–22.

Skinsnes, O.K. 1980 Leprosy in archaeologically recovered bamboo book in China. *Int. J. Leprosy* 48: 333.

Skinsnes, O.K. and Chang, P.H.C. 1985 Understanding of leprosy in ancient China. *Int. J. Leprosy* 53(2): 289–307.

Sledzik, P. and Bellantoni, N. 1994 Brief communication: Bioarcheological and biocultural evidence for the New England vampire folk belief. *Am. J. Phys. Anthrop.* 94: 269–74.

Smith, P. and Kahila, G. 1992 Identification of infanticide in archaeological sites: a case study from the late Roman-early Byzantine periods at Ashkelon, Israel. *J. Archaeol. Sci.* 19: 667–75.

Smith, W.D.L. 1956 Malaria and the Thames. *Lancet* 270: 433–6.

Snow, C.E. 1943 Two prehistoric Indian dwarf skeletons from Moundville. *Alabama Museum of Natural History Museum Papers* 21: 1–90.

Soulié, R. 1980 Un cas de métastases craniennes de carcimome datant du Bronze ancien; typologie des lésions. Observations paléopathologiques analogues en Europe Centrale et Occidentale, pp. 239–53 in *Proceedings of the 3rd European Paleopathology Association Meeting, Caen, France, 1980*.

Spindler, K. 1994 *The man in the ice*. London, Weidenfeld and Nicolson.

Steinbock, R.T. 1976 *Paleopathological diagnosis and interpretation*. Illinois, Charles Thomas.

Steinbock, R.T. 1989 Studies in ancient calcified soft tissues and organic concretions. I: a review of structures, diseases and conditions. *J. Paleopathology* 3(1): 35–8.

Stevens, G.C. and Wakely, J. 1993 Diagnostic criteria for identification of seashell as a trephination implement. *Int. J. Osteoarchaeology* 3: 167–76.

Stewart, T.D. 1958a Stone age skull surgery. A general review with emphasis on the New World. *Smithsonian Institution Annual Report* 1957: 461–91.

Stewart, T.D. 1958b The rate of development of vertebral osteoarthritis in American Whites and its significance in skeletal age identification. *The Leech* 28(3, 4 and 5): 144–51.

Stewart, T.D. 1976 Non-union of fractures in antiquity, with descriptions of five cases from the New World involving the forearm, pp. 396–412 in S. Jarcho (ed.), *Essays on the history of medicine*. New York, New York Academy of Medicine.

Stewart, T.D. and Spoehr, A. 1967 Evidence on the palaeopathology of yaws, pp. 307–19 in D. Brothwell and A.T. Sandison (eds), *Diseases in antiquity*. Illinois, Charles Thomas.

Stini, W. 1985 Growth rates and sexual dimorphism, pp. 191–226 in R.I. Gilbert and J.H. Mielke (eds), *Analysis of prehistoric diets*. New York, Academic Press.

Stini, W.A. 1990 'Osteoporosis': etiologies, prevention and treatment. *Yearbook of Physical Anthropology* 33: 151–94.

Stinson, S. 1985 Sex differences in environmental sensitivity during growth and development. *Yearbook of Physical Anthropology* 28: 123–47.

Stirland, A. 1986 A possible correlation between os acromiale in the burials from the *Mary Rose*, pp. 327–34 in *Proceedings of the 5th European Meeting of the Paleopathology Association, Siena, Italy, 1986*.

Stirland, A. 1991a Pre-Columbian treponematosis in medieval Britain. *Int. J. Osteoarchaeology* 1(1): 39–49.

Stirland, A. 1991b Paget's disease (osteitis deformans): a classic case? *Int. J. Osteoarchaeology* 1: 173–7.

Stirland, A. 1994 Evidence for pre-Columbian treponematosis in medieval Europe, pp. 109–15 in O. Dutour, G. Pálfi, J. Berato and J.-P. Brun (eds), *L'origine de la syphilis en Europe avant ou après 1493?* Centre Archéologique du Var, Editions Errance.

Stirland, A. and Waldron, T. 1990 The earliest cases of tuberculosis in Britain. *J. Archaeol. Sci.* 17: 221–30.

Stone, J.L. and Miles, M.L. 1990 Skull trepanation among the early Indians of Canada and the United States. *Neurosurgery* 26(6): 1015–20.

Stout, S. 1992 Methods of determining age of death using bone microstructure, pp. 21–35 in S.R. Saunders and M.A. Katzenberg (eds), *Skeletal biology of past peoples: research methods*. New York, Wiley-Liss.

Stroud, G. and Kemp, R. 1993 *Cemeteries of St Andrew, Fishergate*. The archaeology of York. The medieval cemeteries 12/2. York, Council for British Archaeology for York Archaeological Trust.

Strouhal, E. 1976 Tumors in the remains of ancient Egyptians. *Am. J. Phys. Anthrop.* 45: 613–20.

Strouhal, E. 1994 Malignant tumors in the Old World. *Paleopathology Association Newsletter* 85: 1–5.

Stuart-Macadam, P. 1985 Porotic hyperostosis: representative of a childhood condition. *Am. J. Phys. Anthrop.* 66: 391–8.

Stuart-Macadam, P. 1987 A radiographic study of porotic hyperostosis. *Am. J. Phys. Anthrop.* 74: 511–20.

Stuart-Macadam, P. 1989a Porotic hyperostosis: relationship between orbital and vault lesions. *Am. J. Phys. Anthrop.* 80: 187–93.

Stuart-Macadam, P. 1989b Nutritional deficiency disease: a survey of scurvy, rickets and iron deficiency anaemia, pp. 201–22 in M.Y. Iscan and K.A.R. Kennedy (eds), *Reconstruction of life from the skeleton.* New York, Alan Liss.

Stuart-Macadam, P. 1991 Anemia in Roman Britain: Poundbury Camp, pp. 101–13 in H. Bush and M. Zvelebil (eds), *Health in past societies. Biocultural interpretations of human skeletal remains in archaeological contexts.* British Archaeological Reports International Series 567. Oxford, Tempus Reparatum.

Stuart-Macadam, P. 1992 Anemia in past human populations, pp. 151–70 in P. Stuart-Macadam and S.K. Kent (eds), *Diet, demography and disease. Changing perspectives on anemia.* New York, Aldine De Gruyter.

Stuart-Macadam, P. and Dettwyler, K.A. (eds) 1995 *Breastfeeding: biocultural perspectives.* New York, Aldine De Gruyter, in press.

Sumner, D.R., Morbeck, M. and Lobick, J.T. 1989 Apparent age-related bone loss among adult female Gombe chimpanzees. *Am. J. Phys. Anthrop.* 79: 225–34.

Sussman, R.W. 1973 Child transport, family size, and increase in human population during the Neolithic. *Current Anthropology* 14(5): 285–9.

Suzuki, T. 1985 Paleopathological diagnosis of bone tuberculosis in the lumbosacral region. *J. Anthrop. Soc. of Nippon* 93: 381–90.

Suzuki, T. 1987 Paleopathological study on a case of osteosarcoma. *Am. J. Phys. Anthrop.* 74: 309–18.

Tanner, J.M. 1968 Earlier maturation in man. *Scientific American* 218(1): 21–7.

Teaford, M.F. 1991 Dental microwear: what can it tell us about diet and dental function? pp. 341–56 in M. Kelley and C.S. Larsen (eds), *Advances in dental anthropology.* New York, Alan Liss.

Tkocz, I. and Bierring, F. 1984 A medieval case of metastasizing carcinoma with multiple osteosclerotic bone lesions. *Am. J. Phys. Anthrop.* 65: 373–80.

Trevor, J.C. 1950 Notes on the human remains of Romano-British date from Norton, Yorkshire, pp. 39-40 in *Roman Pottery at Norton, East Yorkshire.* Roman Malton and District Report 7.

Trinkhaus, E. 1983 *Shanidar Neanderthals.* London, Academic Press.

Trinkhaus, E. 1985 Pathology and posture of the La Chapelle-Aux-Saints Neandertal. *Am. J. Phys. Anthrop.* 67: 19–41.

Trotter, M. 1970 Estimation of stature from intact long limb bones, pp. 71–83 in T.D. Stewart (ed.), *Personal identification in mass disasters.* Washington DC, National Museum of Natural History, Smithsonian Institution.

Turkel, S.J. 1989 Congenital abnormalities in skeletal populations, pp. 109–27 in M.Y. Iscan and K.A.R. Kennedy (eds), *Reconstruction of life from the skeleton.* New York, Alan Liss.

Turner, C. 1993 Cannibalism in Chaco Canyon: the charnel pit excavated in 1926 at Small House Ruin by Frank H.H. Roberts jr. *Am. J. Phys. Anthrop.* 91: 421–39.

Ubelaker, D. 1979 Skeletal evidence for kneeling in prehistoric Ecuador. *Am. J. Phys. Anthrop.* 51: 679–85.

Ubelaker, D. 1987 Estimating age at death from immature skeletons: an overview. *J. Forensic Sciences* 32(5): 1254–63.

Ubelaker, D. 1989 *Human skeletal remains. Excavation, analysis and interpretation.* Washington, Taraxacum Press.

Ubelaker, D. 1992 Hyoid fracture and strangulation. *J. Forensic Sciences* 37(5): 1216–22.

Ubelaker, D. and Guttenplant Grant, L. 1989 Human skeletal remains: preservation or reburial? *Yearbook of Physical Anthropology* 32: 249–87.

Urteaga, O. and Pack, G.T. 1966 On the antiquity of melanoma. *Cancer* 19: 607–10.

Van Beek, G.C. 1983 *Dental morphology. An illustrated guide*. Bristol, P.S.G. Wright.

Vaughan, V.C. and MacKay, R.J. 1975 *Textbook of paediatrics*. Philadelphia, W.B. Saunders.

Vernon-Roberts, B. and Pirie, C.J. 1973 Healing trabecular microfractures in the bodies of lumbar vertebrae. *Ann. Rheum. Dis.* 32: 406–12.

Vrebos, J. 1986 Cleft lip surgery in Anglo-Saxon Britain: The Leech Book (circa A.D. 920). *Plast. Reconstr. Surg.* 77: 850–3.

Vreeland, J.M. and Cockburn, A. 1980 Mummies of Peru, pp. 135–74 in A. Cockburn and E. Cockburn (eds), *Mummies, disease and ancient cultures*. Cambridge, Cambridge University Press.

Wakely, J. 1993 Bilateral congenital dislocation of the hip, spina bifida occulta and spondylolysis in a female skeleton from the medieval cemetery at Abingdon, England. *J. Paleopathology* 5(1): 37–45.

Wakely, J., Manchester, K. and Roberts, C. 1991 Scanning electron microscopy of rib lesions. *Int. J. Osteoarchaeology*, 1: 185–9.

Waldron, T. 1985 DISH at Merton Priory: evidence for a 'new' occupational disease. *Br. Med. J.* 291: 1762–3.

Waldron, T. 1987 Lytic lesions in a skull: a problem in diagnosis. *J. Paleopathology* 1(1): 5–14.

Waldron, T. 1989 The effects of urbanisation on human health, pp. 55–73 in D. Serjeantson and T. Waldron (eds), *Diet and crafts in towns. The evidence of animal remains from the Roman to the post-Medieval periods*. British Archaeological Reports British Series 199, Oxford.

Waldron, T. 1993a The distribution of osteoarthritis of the hands in a skeletal population. *Int. J. Osteoarchaeology* 3: 213–18.

Waldron, T. 1993b The health of the adults, pp. 67–89 in T. Molleson and M. Cox (eds), *The Spitalfields Project*. Volume 2, *The Anthropology. The Middling Sort*. Council for British Archaeology Research Report 86. York, Council for British Archaeology.

Waldron, T. 1994 *Counting the dead. The epidemiology of skeletal populations*. New York, Wiley.

Waldron, T. and Cox, M. 1989 Occupational arthropathy: evidence from the past. *Br. J. Industrial Med.* 46: 420–2.

Waldron, T. and Rogers, J. 1991 Inter-observer variation in coding osteoarthritis in human skeletal remains. *Int. J. Osteoarchaeology* 1: 49–56.

Waldron, T. and Rogers, J. 1994 Rheumatoid arthritis in an English post-Medieval skeleton. *Int. J. Osteoarchaeology* 4: 165–7.

Walker, E.G. 1983 Evidence for prehistoric cardiovascular disease of syphilitic origin on the Northern Plains. *Am. J. Phys. Anthrop.* 60: 499–503.

Walker, P.L. 1986 Porotic hyperostosis in a marine-dependent Californian Indian population. *Am. J. Phys. Anthrop.* 69: 345–54.

Walker, P.L. 1989 Cranial injuries as evidence of violence in prehistoric Southern California. *Am. J. Phys. Anthrop.* 80: 313–23.

Walker, P.L. 1994a Biases in preservation and sexism in sexing: some lessons from historical collections for the paleodemographers. Unpublished manuscript.

Walker, P.L. 1994b Skeletal evidence for child abuse in earlier populations. Abstract,

Paleopathology Association 10th European Meeting, Gottingen, Germany. *Homo* 45: 139.

Walker, P.L. and Hollimon, S.E. 1989 Changes in osteoarthritis with the development of a maritime economy among southern Californian Indians. *Int. J. Anthropology* 4(3): 171–83.

Walker, P.L., Dean, G. and Shapiro, P. 1991 Estimating age from tooth wear in archaeological populations, pp. 169–78 in M. Kelley and C.S. Larsen (eds), *Advances in dental anthropology*. New York, Wiley Liss.

Walker, R., Parsche, F., Bierbrier, M. and McKerrow, J.H. 1987 Tissue identification and histologic study of six lung specimens from Egyptian mummies. *Am. J. Phys. Anthrop.* 72: 43–8.

Warren, H.V., Delavault, R.E. and Cross, O.H. 1967 Possible correlations between geology and some disease patterns. *Ann. New York Acad. Sci.* 136(22): 657–710.

Webb, S. 1988 Two possible cases of trephination from Australia. *Am. J. Phys. Anthrop.* 75: 541–8.

Weiner, A.S. 1970 Blood groups and disease. *Am. J. Human Genetics* 22: 476–83.

Weinstein, R.S., Simmons, D.J. and Lovejoy, C.O. 1981 Ancient bone disease in a Peruvian mummy revealed by quantitative skeletal histomorphometry. *Am. J. Phys. Anthrop.* 54: 321–6.

Weiss, D.L. and Møller-Christensen, V. 1971a An unusual case of tuberculosis in a mediaeval leper. *Danish Med. Bull.* 18: 11–14.

Weiss, D.L. and Møller-Christensen, V. 1971b Leprosy, echinococcosis and amulets: a study of a Mediaeval Danish inhumation. *Medical History* 15(3): 260–7.

Weiss, K.M. 1972 On the systematic bias in skeletal sexing. *Am. J. Phys. Anthrop.* 37: 239–50.

Wells, C. 1962 Three cases of aural pathology of Anglo–Saxon date. *J. Laryng. Otol.* 76: 931–3.

Wells, C. 1963 Ancient Egyptian pathology. *J. Larygngol. Otol.* 77(3): 261–5.

Wells, C. 1964a *Bones, bodies and disease.* London, Thames and Hudson.

Wells, C. 1964b The study of ancient disease. *Surgo* 32(1): 3–7.

Wells, C. 1964c Chronic sinusitis with alveolar fistulae of Mediaeval date. *J. Laryng. Otol.* 78(3): 320–2.

Wells, C. 1964d Two medieval cases of malignant disease. *Br. Med. J.* 1064: 1611–12.

Wells, C. 1965 Osteogenesis imperfecta from an Anglo-Saxon burial ground at Burgh Castle, Suffolk. *Medical History* 9: 88–9.

Wells, C. 1967 Pseudopathology, pp. 5–19 in D. Brothwell and A.T. Sandison (eds), *Diseases in antiquity*. Illinois, Charles Thomas.

Wells, C. 1973 A palaeopathological rarity in a skeleton of Roman date. *Medical History* 17(4): 399–400.

Wells, C. 1974a Osteochondritis dissecans in ancient British skeletal material. *Medical History* 18(4): 365–9.

Wells, C. 1974b The results of 'bone setting' in Anglo-Saxon times. *Medical and Biological Illustration* 24: 215–20.

Wells, C. 1976 Romano-British pathology. *Antiquity* 50: 53–5.

Wells, C. 1977 Disease of the maxillary sinus in antiquity. *Medical and Biological Illustration* 27: 173–8.

Wells, C. 1978 A medieval burial of a pregnant woman. *The Practitioner* 221: 442–4.

Wells, C. 1980 The human bones, pp. 247–374 in P. Wade-Martins (ed.), *Excavations at North Elmham Park 1967–1972*. East Anglian Archaeology 9.

Wells, C. 1981 Discussion of the skeletal material, pp. 85–111 in R. Reece (ed.),

Excavations on Iona 1964–1974. London, Institute of Archaeology Occasional Paper 5.

Wells, C. 1982 The human remains, pp. 135–202 in A. McWhirr, L. Viner and C. Wells, *Romano-British cemeteries at Cirencester.* Cirencester, Excavations Committee.

Wells, C. and Woodhouse, N. 1975 Paget's disease in an Anglo-Saxon. *Medical History* 19(4): 396–400.

Wenham, S. 1987 Anatomical interpretations of Anglo-Saxon weapon injuries, pp. 123–39 in *Weapons and warfare in Anglo-Saxon England.* Oxford University Committee for Archaeology Monograph 21.

White, W. 1988 *The cemetery of St Nicholas Shambles.* London, Museum of London and the London and Middlesex Archaeological Society.

Whittaker, D.K. 1993 Oral health, pp. 49–65 in T. Molleson and M. Cox (eds), *The Spitalfields Project.* Volume 2, *The Anthropology. The Middling Sort.* Council for British Archaeology Research Report 86. York, Council for British Archaeology.

Whittaker, D.K., Molleson, T., Daniel, A.T., Williams, J.T., Rose, P. and Resteghini, R. 1985 Quantitative assessment of tooth wear, alveolar crest height and continuing eruption in a Romano-British population. *Arch. Oral Biology* 30(6): 493–501.

Widmer, W. and Perzigian, A.J. 1981 The ecology and etiology of skeletal lesions in late Prehistoric populations from Eastern North America, pp. 99–113 in J.E. Buikstra (ed.), *Prehistoric tuberculosis in the Americas.* Illinois, Northwestern University Archeological Programme.

Wienker, C.W. and Wood, J.F. 1987 Osteological individuality indicative of migrant citrus laboring. *J. Forensic Sciences* 33(2): 562–7.

Wiggins, R., Boylston, A. and Roberts, C.A. 1993 Report on the human skeletal remains from Blackfriars, Gloucester (19/91).

Willis, R.A. 1973 *The spread of tumors in the human body.* London, Butterworth.

Wintrobe, M. 1974 *Clinical hematology.* Philadelphia, Lea and Febiger.

Wiseman, R. 1696 *Eight Chirurgical Treatises.* London, Tooke and Meredith.

Wood, J.W., Milner, G.R., Harpending, H.C. and Weiss, K.M. 1992 The osteological paradox. Problems of inferring prehistoric health from skeletal samples. *Current Anthropology* 33(4): 343–70.

Woods, R. and Woodward, J. 1984 Mortality, poverty and the environment, pp. 19–36 in R. Woods and J. Woodward (eds), *Urban disease and mortality in 19th century England.* London, Batsford.

Woodward, M. and Walker, A.R.P. 1994 Sugar consumption and dental caries: evidence from 90 countries. *Br. Dental J.* 176(8): 297–302.

Woolf, A.D. and St John Dixon, A. 1988 *Osteoporosis: a clinical guide.* London, Martin Dunitz.

Zias, J. 1985 Leprosy in the Byzantine Monasteries of the Judean desert. *Koroth* 9(1–2): 242–8.

Zias, J. and Mumcuoglu, K. 1991 Pre-pottery Neolithic B headlice from Nahal Hemar Cave. *Atiquot (Jerusalem)* 20: 167–8.

Zias, J. and Numeroff, K. 1987 Operative dentistry in the 2nd century BCE. *J. Am. Dental Assoc.* 114: 665–6.

Zias, J. and Pomeranz, S. 1992 Serial craniectomies for intracranial infection 5.5 millenia ago. *Int. J. Osteoarchaeology* 2: 183–6.

Zias, J. and Sekeles, E. 1985 The crucified man from Giv'at Ha-Mivtar. *Israel Exploration Society* 35: 22–7.

Zimmerman, M.R., Yeatman, G.W. and Sprinz, H. 1971 Examination of an Aleutian mummy. *Bull. New York Acad. Med.* 47(1): 80–103.

Index

Page numbers in *italics* denote an illustration. Page numbers in **bold** denote a main reference to the subject.